Y0-AWG-693

BRIGHT SILENCE

RAISING HEARING IMPAIRED CHILDREN

By Margaret H. Ferris

Classroom Experiences — Contributors

Parents of Hearing Impaired Children

Hearing Impaired Students as Young Adults

Professionals in Education, Testing, and
Services for Hearing Impaired Children

Reviews from Professional Journals

Grant from SIGMA STATE, DELTA KAPPA GAMMA — 1988

Copyright© 1994
Margaret H. Ferris
Bright Silence Press

All rights reserved
Reproduction in whole or in part
of any portion in any form
without permission is prohibited.

First Edition

Library of Congress Catalog Number: 94-71173
ISBN: 0-9641044-0-7

Printed in USA by
Palmer Publication, Inc.
Amherst, WI 54406

BRIGHT SILENCE

Dedicated to the Memory of

Mrs. Ruth Beck
Preschool Aide
1959 to 1970 ⇨
Years of Service

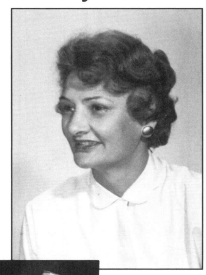

Cynthia Streblow
1955 to 1968
⇩

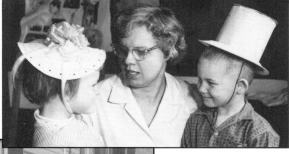

*Mark Mathison exchanged this hat for a baseball cap and motorcycle helmet. He is now the father of a teenage son.

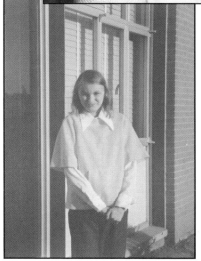

Debra Lyn Wesenberg
1959 to 1987
⇦ *Oshkosh West*
High School

Debra made her yellow over-blouse.

Her Perfect Baby

He plays quietly in his play pen.
He always smiles his dimpled grin.
With upstretched arms he asks
For mother's hug and kiss.

He crawls and tries to stand.
She steadies him with her hand.
He waits for her warm embrace.
She laughs and holds him close.

She calls to him as he awakes.
He does not turn his face.
Her heart stops in fear.
Her baby does not hear.

Margaret H. Ferris

Bright Silence
Preface

A hearing loss is the most devastating educational handicap a child can endure. But hearing impaired children do become contributing adults and live satisfying lives in the mainstream of society.

For this to happen there must be early identification of a hearing loss, immediate fitting of hearing assistive devices, and intervention services for the children and their families.

The parents initial reaction is most traumatic and they need counseling so that they can get on with helping the child to develop socially as well as educationally.

A hearing impaired child born to deaf parents does not cause the trauma that a hearing impaired child does for hearing parents. Deaf parents, whether oral or those who sign, immediately begin communicating with their child. But the vast majority of young parents have no background or experience with either deaf adults or children.

It is for these parents, the hearing parents, who need to cope with their own feelings, to help their child, and to get on with their lives, that this book was written.

The level of education of the parents is of little consequence in this task of recognizing a hearing loss. I recall an incident in 1957 of parents, both professionals, who were concerned that their four-year-old son did not talk. While waiting in a train depot Tom, age four, was playing nearby. A gentleman sitting near them remarked, "I see your child is deaf." That was the first time they even considered their son's problem was a hearing loss.

Not only were these parents educated people, but the mother was a diabetic. Today there is a High-Risk Registry that is a part of every hospital's nursery program. Any infant born with low birth weight, Rh factor, hearing loss in the family, and premature birth, anatomical malformations, bacterial meningitis or influenza, and any congenital or perinatal infections or health problem of the mother, will be referred by a pediatrician for an audiological test. Now 18 states require all newborns to be routinely tested.

At least 150 Audiologists throughout Wisconsin have attended workshops in techniques for testing infants. And so it is throughout the United States. Hopefully testing will be done before the child is six months old.

Part H of Public Law 99-457 strives for early intervention programs designed to meet educational, intellectual, social needs, and also a variety of therapeutic and medical needs of children from birth to age three. The project was to be in place in 1992, working toward a comprehensive, county-based, family-focused services for young hearing impaired children and their families.

Why is childhood hearing loss, even a mild loss, such a handicap? And why are parents so in need of help to meet the needs of their child?

Instead of telling parents what they should do, I hope to take them into the classroom and the homes as we begin the communication program. All social interaction depends upon communication—parent with child, child with parent and peers, and all of education is predicated upon communication. The infant, any and all infants, live in the immediate present; learn that things, people, events and activities have names. They need to learn to express their feelings in accepted ways.

Read what the parents of hearing impaired children have learned. They share their concerns, their efforts, and the every day problems of raising a deaf or hard of hearing child.

One of the first questions the parents asked was, "What will my child do when he grows up?" I have asked these now young adults to tell their stories—each so different. There are many ways to a fulfilling life and career.

Among the professionals who have contributed are Dr. Jack E. Kile, Audiologist, and Leslie K. Halvorsen, Speech Therapist and Interpreter. They give the technical information so necessary to understand the importance of early auditory assistance and communication methods for the educational and social development of the hearing impaired child. Dr. Kile and Mrs. Halvorsen are hearing people.

The other contributors are deaf. Their poignant stories clearly challenge parents and teachers to attend to the emotional and social needs as well as the best methods of educating our hearing impaired children.

Today many options exist—partial or complete mainstreaming, self contained classes, residential schools, resource teachers; and assistive listening devices or interpreters in regular classes. Parents must understand and evaluate these possibilities. They must become partners in setting goals and cooperating with the schools.

And school personnel need to understand the needs of the hearing impaired child—both deaf and hard of hearing.

Today, as never before, there is a bright future for our hearing impaired children.

Margaret H. Ferris
Neenah, Wisconsin

Introduction

This book covers fifty years of Deaf Education in Wisconsin, so check the date of the story or article to place it in the time frame. Several other stories by students raised in other locations have been included as they give a wider understanding of deaf education during this same time. A short history shows how we arrived at the education available today.

Terms used in the articles and stories reflect the time the events took place. The story about the first teacher of *deaf-mutes* reflects the 16th century. The term *retarded* was used in past times, while today we usually say *Adaptive Education*. Today the *Deaf* do not like the term *impaired*. They prefer the one word *deaf*.

Then it became necessary for those with lesser degrees of hearing loss to use the term *hard of hearing*. However, I have often used *hearing impaired* as an inclusive term.

Parents and former students tell their stories of their experiences. Each family and each hearing impaired young person has a different story.

No one method is the perfect path to satisfying adulthood. There have been many changes in the educational approaches, yet there remains the basic problem of learning to communicate.

Beware of the swing of the pendulum. There must be a middle ground where the best of each approach is chosen to fit the needs of the child in his particular family and setting.

All little children learn to talk with such ease that we assume it is easy. Yes, it is easy if done at the biological time when the brain is so programmed.But encase the child in silence and the tremendous task becomes apparent.

The highest praise goes to the students, their parents and the teachers. They did it! They worked together and all did their best.

There will be a brighter future.

. . . . .

Acknowledgements

To Professor Emeritus, Alice H. Streng, instructor in Deaf Education at Milwaukee State Teachers College (now the University of Wisconsin—Milwaukee) goes my gratitude, lasting appreciation and affection.

To my daughters, Margaret and Sue, who taught me early childhood development and on through the teenage years, goes my love. Now my five grandchildren amaze and delight me.

How do I thank the parents of my students? We worked together. They made toys and refreshments, they helped in the scholarship activities. They were advocates for their children and the school.

The esprit de corps that exists among the teachers of hearing impaired students is special and lasting.

My students have grown into fine men and women. Many honored me with their stories. To the many others, you too are remembered with fondness.

An added thanks to the young adults from other backgrounds who extended the scope of educational programs.

My membership in Self Help for Hard of Hearing People allowed me hands-on experience with today's remarkable technology.

Having a Governor's appointment to the Wisconsin Council for the Deaf and Hard of Hearing has broadened my knowledge of the concerns of this population.

Members of the Epsilon Chapter, Delta Kappa Gamma—a Women Educators Society, encouraged me to apply for the Sigma State Award. This grant has allowed me to do the research to prepare this book.

My gratitude goes to the many librarians, artists, and photographers who added their expertise. And the professionals who read and made suggestions for this book. Finally the layout rested in the capable hands of Kelly Meronk at Palmer Publications.

* * * * *

Table of Contents

Chapter VII — Audiology

Chapter VIII — Special Education Hearing Children, 1970

Chapter IX — Multiple Handicapped Deaf Children, 1971

Chapter X — Home At Last, 1978

Chapter XI — Don't Skate On The Wrestling Mat

Chapter XII — Sign Language

Chapter XIII — Young Adults

I

DAVID'S STORY

1959-1993

David

David was a holder of things; objects that he could clutch in his fist, put in his mouth, stuff in a box, or squeeze into a discarded lozenge box. His concern for his treasure-trove was all consuming. He could not share it, nor could he put it down.

Meningitis had left David with a profound hearing loss at age two when he was beginning to learn to talk. Several months later when he entered nursery school for deaf children all memory of using speech had faded. He was mute. Cut off from the continuous flow of speech that surrounds the hearing child he appeared stunned and lost in his silent world.

Perhaps that is why David was engrossed with his belongings.

The manipulation, the very contact, held his only link to the real world. He no longer had his mother's reassuring voice. Even though babies do not understand the words spoken to them, they respond to the emotion and meaning carried by the tone of the voice itself. Now encased in silence and surrounded by loneliness David reached out for bright, small objects. It was as if he were compelled to have, to hoard, to clasp as his very own, every small thing. It was an obsession.

With tiny deaf children one watches for what interests the child to open the door to meaning. A stick with a bit of broken balloon still tied to the end held warm remembered happiness. But what of a thimble, a button, a bottle of fingernail polish, or the fastener from a broken zipper? And what of the day he had his pockets stuffed with stockings? David's possessions were so bizarre that the first thought was to have him put these "distractions" down—in full view, but beyond easy reach. But in trying to persuade him to let go the whole teaching situation collapsed. We would have to function with his possessions, or not function at all.

David had chosen for his toys oddments which do not appear on the Dolch Word List. But never mind, I too had a choice of toys. My choice was a small car with a boat trailer and a boat. We worked alone in a small enclosed area sitting before a large mirror. Below the mirror extended a shelf nine inches wide upon which we put the toys. Ideally, both the child and the teacher sit so as to face the mirror. We can manipulate the toys and from time to time easily watch both our faces. There is a large auditory trainer on a shelf to one side and a set of ear phones for the child. The teacher wears the microphone.

David was willing to put his toys into the boat, move the car back and forth along the shelf, park the car, disconnect the trailer and boat, play at sailing it, have the toys fall out and reload. Meanwhile I talked about what we were doing. I used simple complete sentences. The purpose was that David would see the words "boat" and "car" on my lips time and time again and would gradually associate the lip movements with the toys. There was only one flaw in this assumption. David never looked at me either directly or in the mirror.

2

But I persisted day after day, varying the toys and the game. I used pictures and cut-outs and games as well as the miniature toys. The days passed and I began to feel as though I were talking to myself. If I were to succeed in getting David to watch me, I thought, I have to be all there is in our enclosure. We have to establish rapport before we begin to associate words with objects. I cleared the work area and managed to force David's hoard into his shirt pocket and then grasped his hands firmly to prevent his attempts to retrieve his toys. I sat him astraddle my lap, placed his hands on my cheeks and made a variety of sounds—mooing, barking, buzzing, humming and nonsence waggling my tongue. David objected, butting my face and pinching my cheeks. Suddenly he reared backwards and if it were not for my determined grip on his strong, fat hands, he would have fallen off my lap onto the floor.

So we played this new game, "Down you go. Up you come." Then I began to leave him down longer and longer, and said over and over, "Up, up, up." We repeated this until my shoulders were exhausted. But David never looked at me.

Our periods together continued during the fall and winter, but with no progress. David could not learn to lip read if he did not look at my face. Besides this exacting drill, there was the casual approach. It, however, still necessitated David's watching me. My only hope was that he was looking at me out of the corners of his eyes so to speak. Except for our few minutes together, David was part of the general activity in the busy room of ten little deaf children. While I did precise drill and speech development, an aide was watching and directing the play. Most of our activities were done together, for the children had to learn to share and understand other's rights and needs.

I watched David at play. The nursery room was filled with toys and play equipment. A walk-in play house had a stove, sink, and cupboard (made by David's father). There were tables and chairs, dishes and pans, and empty food containers to pretend to fix meals. There was a real phone given to us by a telephone repair man we met on one of our walks. The children always saw that the loose wire was attached to a chair leg or pipe. Large blocks and small, a climber, bikes, and a wagon. Cars, boats, and trains were best loved. There was an abundance of quiet work, not only for fun, but to develop observation of detail.

This included puzzles, games of matching, and creative materials. And many books and pictures. David did not really play with the other children, but he did behave normally for a two year old. He rode the bike. He worked puzzles and built towers. He put his possessions in purses, boxes, and carried these larger encumbrances about. Meticulous and determined, he insisted that my purse always be put away on the same shelf, that his shirt sleeves be turned up exactly even before washing, and that the straws in the milk cartons for mid-morning snacks be patted into equal degrees.

My aide and I talked to the children about whatever the activity was at the moment. We talked as you would to hearing children in simple, but complete sentences, and in a normal voice. A problem situation was even more ripe for learning language than a calm one. And like all tiny, jostling, vitamin filled children, ours were in constant motion. David could not be part of these activities without some impressions being imprinted in his nervous system that would eventually accumulate and grow into meaning. Maturation was on my side. This intense, self-centered phase would pass and his world enlarge. There appeared to be nothing in the disease of meningitis that had effected more than his hearing, or for a few months, his balance.

He was steadier now. So the first year passed. The only noticeable difference was that David had grown taller.

Fall came. David's two hours a day were now extended to the full morning session. The children, mere babies, bewildered and frightened that first morning of the last year, now strode into the room, found their favorite toys and we were off. Not a tear, not a problem. All actually sat in a row to have a "lesson". David joined the group, but he did not sit for long—possibly 73 seconds. But he now looked at me, obliquely, from time to time, as if to question what I had done with his toys. He was now interested in animals. So I gathered any number of small plastic, but realistic looking, toy dogs, monkeys, ponies, cows, ducks, and chickens. We loaded them in trucks, put them in coops and boxes, in pens and pools.

Through all this David had remained mute. Sound has to be recognized as sound and vibrations before words can be developed. The mike was scarred and scratched where the other children had hit and bumped it in their eagerness and joy of making noise, often meaningless to the hearing adult, but the beginning of speech for them. We rang bells, blew horns, hummed against a balloon to magnify the vibrations, made noises like animals, clapped blocks together, pounded on drums—fast, slow, soft and loud. Eventually the children would be willing to close their eyes and identify the sounds. Discrimination had to be developed. They had to learn to listen. We drilled vowels and consonants and built them into words. They had pictures of the words and simple phrases. We wrote the sounds and then words on the board and on the papers the children took home.

David, however, would have nothing to do with the ear phones which might have brought him, even if faintly, some sound. There is no child who can not learn to feel vibrations with his hands, on the teacher's face, on his own face. And then become aware of vibrations in his ears. But David would not tolerate the ear phones for more than a few seconds; apparently he received no sound or was distracted by the pressure and weight of the head set.

David's play had become more meaningful, but he still resisted me. In my eagerness to reach him, I had become like David. My purse and pockets were filled with small objects. A small sponge baby duck was in a package with a new tooth brush—perhaps that was why I bought it. Its bill could be made to move, its wings to flap, it could be made to waddle and quack.

I showed it to David and all the wonderful things it could do. "Quack,

4

quack, quack," I said, manipulating its bill. David turned to me and formed silent quacks with his lips. I placed his hand on my cheek to feel the vibration of my voice. I let him hold the toy duck, pressed his face to mine and quacked and paused, and quacked again so he could feel the difference. But David was no longer interested in my kind of fun. The duck was his. The rest of the morning it was never more than a few inches from his hand.

At Christmas time we had a huge paper Santa with a toy bag. David pointed to each toy and made an appropriate gesture to identify it. He pretended to blow the horn, bounce the ball, and march to the beating of the drum. He was symbolizing, developing inner language. My task was to substitute the lip reading and speech for the objects and the motion. He was ready to begin lip reading lessons. Perhaps, I thought, if David saw how the other children responded, he would mimic them.

I devised a lesson for Kevin and David. Kevin was several months younger than David, but had some residual hearing and was a good lip reader. He could also say the approximations of many of the words we drilled. I selected three toys very dissimilar in lip reading; a ball, a truck, and an airplane.

We did not work in our speech area, because I wanted to create a new behavior pattern. We worked in the corner of the room, David and Kevin facing me so that there was no opportunity for the activity in the room to move into their vision.

My intention was that a little competition would goad David into watching and doing as Kevin did. There was competition all right. Enough to run blood on the floor, and it nearly did. Instead of my teaching, I was merely the referee. Each item, part of our regular, every day play equipment, patched, old, and missing parts, was writ large with MINE. Each wanted to clutch as his very own all three of the toys.

I had lost another round. I withdrew to review the situation and regroup. I reasoned that an older child would not be at David's level of self-centered extreme possessiveness, and would be a more reliable partner. Curtis was the natural choice.

He was five, but new this year, nor was he so advanced but that he would benefit from the drill.

The objects for the lesson had to be interesting, but not overpowering so. The words had to show a contrast on the lips. I decided to use smaller toys, but not fist size, and to put them in a deep cylinder box. This would require fishing, and when one child had his arm in the box, it would not be possible for the other child to snatch the toy. I had built this lesson carefully; chosen the participants, the toys, the location, the modus operandi. I had hedged against every contingency, there remained for me only the task of making this activity the most interesting game in all Christendom.

The three toys were in my lap. I held up the airplane near my face and said, "See the airplane." I gave it a few swoops and returned it to a position again

5

near my face and repeated, "This is an airplane. The airplane flies. The airplane goes up high." And then I dropped it in the box.

And so with the toy cow and the ball. I talked about each, repeating the names of the toys several times. Then I shook up the contents of the cylinder with the expectancy of a conjuror.

"Curtis, find the airplane." I gave him the box. He fished up to his arm pits and came up with the airplane. I clapped with delight and praised him. "You found the airplane. What a good boy." His eyes sparkled with pleasure.

"Now, David, find the cow that says moo, moo, moo. Find the cow." He came up with the ball.

"No," and I shook the ball back into the cylinder. "Find the cow." I repeated it several times. This time he was right. Curtis was as delighted as I was. We shook up the toys again and gave David the first turn. We played the game over and over. David guessed more times than he knew. But he was cooperating.

He was learning to lip read.

Our journey had finally begun. David and I had scaled the first mountain. Around us lay the shining world of meaning. And David had accepted me as his guide. Before us stood two more formidable peaks, that of speech and language. With David's new skill and his desire to learn, our perilous trip would be more sure and rewarding.

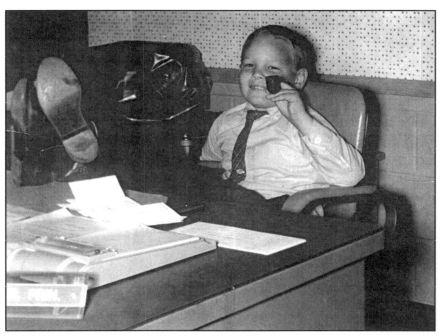

David now has everything under control.
Photo by *Oshkosh Daily Northwestern*

David's Mother Writes

Recently Mrs. Rawson wrote about David's school days after leaving Wisconsin which had an oral program.

When David went into the junior high program in California, the program was Total Communication only. He did well—sign language was easy for him, but not for us. Then the school system went into SEE signs which, as you know, is Signing Exact English. Mr. Rawson, our daughter Cheryl, and I went to classes. The kids soared, Mom and Dad did fairly well! But when David got out of school everything went back to American Sign Language (ASL). We were lost because they go too fast and we go too slow!

Luckily David can talk—if he wants to. We communicate quite well when he is here or we are there. Hearing aids were tried three different times in David's school life. None worked for him at all.

Tenth Coin

David traveled with a gospel group known as the Tenth Coin.[1] The group gave programs in sign language, not only in the United States, but in Korea, Japan, Philippines, England, Scotland, Barbados, Jamaica, Puerto Rico, and Havana.

He has also traveled to World Deaf Games in other countries.

He attended North Central Bible College earning a Bachelor of Arts Degree. He is now the Pastor of the Pleasant View Church for the Deaf in Spring Lake Park in Minnesota.

Rev. David Rawson—Prayer

Dear Heavenly Father, we thank You for today, for where we live, wherever that may be, throughout life, from birth to death, upon this world.

Help us all to understand each other as a parent would help his children. That this may include Deaf and Hearing. That they may understand one another in areas like culture and communication. For I know for a fact about Deaf. And Lord, I pray for hearing parents to accept their children who are deaf, and help them to understand how to communicate, not only this, but also be willing to get along with them and to accept Deaf people as a whole, even with their different background and culture.

Lord, I pray that You give wisdom to hearing parents of deaf children. Show them the way to get along with one another, and show their love and let it reach out and touch their children, as You do with your inner heart, and accept and care for them.

I thank God that my parents accepted who I am as I grew up.

Lord, I pray that all of you parents will feel the same way.

In Jesus' name, Amen.

1. Luke 15:8-10

A Recent Visit To Russia
Fall of 1993

Rev. David Rawson

In a TT phone call from David a few weeks ago he reported that he had been to Estonia and Russia.

Rawson: I have been traveling a lot lately as guest speaker. I have been to Estonia, former Russia, two times. Last two weeks I have been in Russia near Moscow to meet deaf people there. I know big different way they live. They are about 40 years behind us.

Ferris: Can you tell me about the schools? Are they oral or do they use signs?

Rawson: Both ways. They use sign more, but they do oral in school. But I met kids. They sign to me. I understand. I learn fast. Funny, older people try to tell me to learn oral in Russia. I could not read lip good. I feel lost. I told them better for me to see sign. Ha Ha. They try to help me oral. I get lost.

Ferris: There must be some similar signs that make it easy for you to learn those while speaking Russian would be difficult to learn even if you could hear.

Rawson: True. One man traveled with me. He is hearing. He told me try learn speak in Russia. He (would) like learn sign better. I have been to deaf school in Estonia. They have two different schools. One deaf school and one hard of hearing school.

I was surprised. I think go back to Russia this summer. I am not sure yet—have to wait to decide.

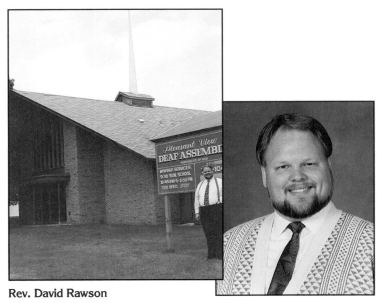

Rev. David Rawson

8

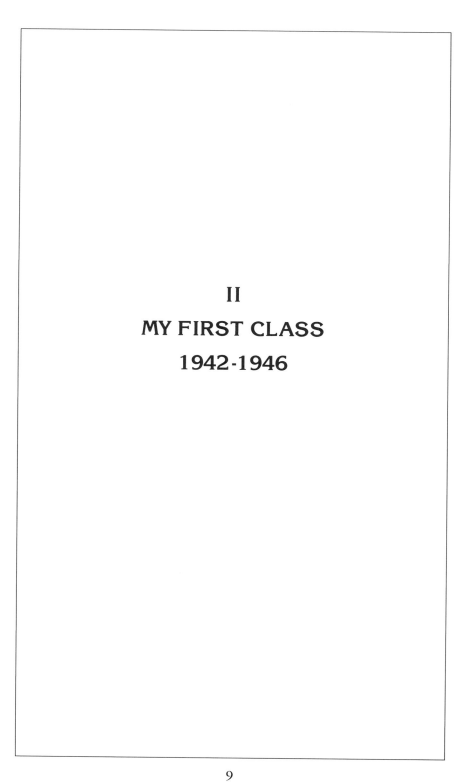

II

MY FIRST CLASS

1942-1946

A Straight Course

My mother was a teacher before she married and my father an accountant. He began to lose his hearing when I was four years old. His mother and sister had also became deaf in early adulthood.

It was otosclerosis, one of the inherited causes of deafness. It develops in early adulthood. Otosclerosis is the growth of spongy bone in the middle ear and around the parts connecting it with the inner ear resulting in progressively increasing deafness. My interest in becoming a teacher was natural. What would I teach? Deaf children. The fact that I had never seen a deaf child did not deter me. I had helped my father with his lipreading lessons, so I thought I knew something about the problem. Four years of study and many years of teaching revealed the differences between childhood hearing loss and adult acquired hearing loss.

Milwaukee State Teachers College, now the University of Wisconsin-Milwaukee, had a renowned course in Deaf Education. I enrolled. I studied. I graduated and was hired to teach the primary deaf class in Appleton, Wisconsin.

I had to have normal hearing and dentition to be accepted in the program which was oral.

I taught four years and was married during that last year. My young man came from Maine, so it seemed doubtful that we would settle in Wisconsin. The superintendent called me into his office—Morgan School housed special classes and the administration offices—and he suggested I ask my young man to look for work in Appleton. Garwood did return and found work in the Valley, however, I did not continue teaching the next year. I did keep an interest in school affairs and was elected to the Appleton Board of Education on my 30th birthday.

During the Korean Conflict my husband was recalled and we moved to Eglin Air Force Base in Florida. When I was gone over two months I had to resign from the Board of Education.

When we returned to the Valley, we did not live in Appleton. Several years later I tutored a trainable child in my home for a year. My work with Bobby, even though he was a hearing child, led to my eventual interest in working with the multiple handicapped deaf children. That experience and the many problems I met in the preschool classes of deaf and hard of hearing infants led to my search for answers.

In our literature one reads of the early history of deaf education. One statement, only one sentence, mentions a Spanish Benedictine monk, Pedro Ponce de Leon, the first oral teacher of the deaf. When I did not have the answers for teaching when I had professional training, worked with other teachers of the deaf, and had 150 years of professional journals—how did the monk do it? Research made me appreciate his devotion and success. And I hope you will enjoy his story. Ponce de Leon was born in 1520.

My course was set in 1938 when I entered college, graduating in 1942. Our three day 50-year reunion in 1992 was a delightful trip down memory lane. Five of us spent one afternoon with our instructor, Professor Emeritus, Alice Streng. May we all be as interesting as she is in her eighties. She touched our lives and we went out to conquer the world.

* * * * *

*"Those who cannot remember
the past are condemned to
repeat it."*
George Santayana

My First School
1942-1946
Morgan School, Appleton, Wisconsin

In March of my senior year, in 1942, at Milwaukee State Teachers College I was hired to teach the Primary Deaf Class in Appleton, Wisconsin to start in September. The teacher of the class had married at Christmas and was forthwith discharged. Married women could not teach in the Appleton schools. This was the school policy as it was in many schools and places of business. In the Depression Days it was thought that married women would take the jobs of family men. The fact that there was no teacher available was of no concern to the Appleton School Board. Finally a Speech Correctionist took over the class, but by May she was anxious to test grade school children in preparation for her students for the next year. So the superintendent returned to the college and sought permission from my instructor, Alice Streng, and Dr. Samuel Kirk, Director of Special Education, for me to start teaching immediately. It was agreed that I would finish my college program that summer.

On May 10, 1942 I began my four years of teaching. The final assignment in Deaf Education was to write a curriculum for a typical class of deaf students. This was to include students of different ages, age of onset of the hearing loss, the I.Q. and academic achievement. It was to include lessons in speech, the academic program, and activities to carry out this plan. Miss Streng, my supervisor, spent a day with me in Appleton to evaluate my students. I was to write the curriculum for my actual class.

The first morning in the classroom the students came in and stared at me. To them this was still another change. But we got off to a good start as the routine and lessons were on-going.

The auditory trainer in the classroom was the size of a large cabinet. This equipment had been donated to the school by a service club in 1934. The microphone stood alone, but had suffered so much abuse as we moved about doing our activities, that the janitor mounted it on a cement pedestal such as you would mount a stop sign at the corner. The children had to sit in a row and wear heavy head sets which were on short cords. None of the children had individual hearing aids.

The Public Works Administration (PWA) had built a large doll house, taller than the children, furnished with every conceivable piece of furniture. And the large dolls in the play area had clothes made by the PWA. The material was washable and had firm snaps and buttons.

The Encyclopedia Britannica made excellent movies of animals, fire fighters, policemen, trips to the city and on the farm.

Our classroom was a corner room on the second floor. One afternoon while the children were out for recess, I put the new vocabulary and drew pictures on the board for the next lesson. I had just finished when fire trucks arrived to put out the fire in a house across the street. The superintendent, whose office was down the hall, came into my room to see what was happening. When he turned from the window and looked at the board, a quizzical expression showed his surprise. The lesson I had prepared was about fire fighters, their trucks, their hats and slickers, the hoses, and a house aflame. I had used colored chalk, so it looked real.

We always had projects. Easter time we went a few blocks to town to Sears to buy baby chicks. The teacher across the hall came from the country and would take the chicks to her parents' farm. At speech time Lois complained of a queer noise. I put on the head set and I could hear the chicks peeping.

During the winter or bad weather all the students went down into the basement, where the shop and home economics classes were, to make projects. Morgan School had been a senior high school for many years. We played games in the gym. This took an adaptive approach as the orthopedic students were not able to run, the retarded students took longer to learn the rules, and our deaf ones could not hear the directions. But we had fun.

I was often invited to take my class to meetings of civic organizations and service clubs to show how the children learned to lipread and speak. Lois, a seven-year-old, had good speech, so at the close of the demonstration she would give the Pledge of Allegiance. There wasn't a dry eye in the audience.

In December of the fourth year I was married. The school system had relaxed the policy preventing married women from teaching. During World War II many teachers were married as their young men came home on leave. The system could not stand the loss of half the teaching staff. However, I resigned in June. I left my valuable collection of pictures as I was not going to return to teaching. I was expecting a baby and knew my life would change. Once a married woman started a family, she stayed home to care for the children. That is how it was in the 40s.

The class at Morgan School continued for a few years, then the students

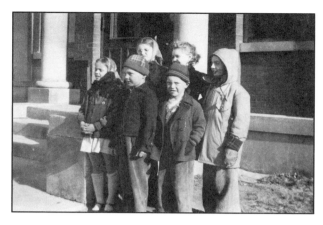

My First Class

went on to the Wisconsin School for the Deaf at Delavan, a residential school, or to Day Classes in either Oshkosh or Green Bay.

I did some tutoring with children from parochial schools which did not have speech correctionists. And later, after the polio epidemic, I worked with several recovered, but speech handicapped children.

I still often spoke to groups about my teaching. One such talk many years later to a church circle resulted in my being called to return to teaching. In fact it was David Rawson's mother who several years later, after David had meningitis, recalled my talk, and gave my name to Peter Owsley, the Principal of the School for the Deaf and Hard of Hearing in Oshkosh.

* * * * *

Little Lamb

Sue was my first new pupil even though it was my second year of teaching. Sue was four, she had been born deaf.

I frantically searched my memory of lecture notes as to what to do with a new child. All practice teaching takes place in well established rooms with experienced teachers, the class already flowing and into routine.

Sue's mother was talking, "Sue can't say anything, but she is smart. She colors, can set the table, and tie bows. She likes to play with her dolls. She swings and can ride her tricycle."

Fortunately my professionalism returned and I assured the mother, as all kindergarten teachers do that first morning, "Sue will be fine. Leave quickly. It will be better that way."

I turned a bright smile on the tiny child who was still pressed against the

13

wall. "Come, Sue, let's look at the dollies." I took her plump little hand and drew her to the play corner.

"This dolly should be dressed. She can't go to school in her pajamas," I said in a normal voice as you would speak to any child.

I held out a bright dress, and Sue deftly slipped off the doll's pajamas. She spied the box of doll clothes and found panties and a slip. With ease Sue buttoned the dress and tied the sash. I noted with pleasure her good coordination.

The first day went happily along. The older children vied with one another to show what they remembered. Only Sue regarded me as mere equipment, necessary like a chair. She watched the other children as one would watch a passing crowd on the street, without interest or involvement.

Each morning I lined the children in a row for voice building exercises. They stood on their little oak chairs so their faces were nearly even with mine. I held a child's hand, the open palm, against my cheek, and the child's other hand against his own cheek so he could compare the vibration.

"Ba ba ba ba, la la la la, mmm mmm mmm, ho ho ho, fe fe fe fe. You say it Ted." We practiced taking deep breaths, did the exercises fast and slow, soft and loud. Sue's fat hand rested on my cheek, but her bright blue eyes regarded me without interest. She made no attempt to mimic. I smiled encouragingly, but my heart sank a bit each day. Every lesson throughout the days left Sue untouched.

She was full of her made up signs and gestures to express her desires to the other children. At that time Morgan School in Appleton housed classes for physically handicapped children, and the retarded. In the halls, in the lunch room, and on the playground Sue leapt to the assistance of the other children. In no time she was the official jacket buttoner, and shoelace tier.

Lipreading lessons fared no better than the voice drill. Her attitude plainly said that moving my lips did not have any meaning. With no knowledge of speech or language, how was Sue thinking? Yet her actions said she was an intelligent child and aware of what went on around her. It was my fault that she did not make the connection between actions and words.

Days passed into weeks. I watched her play and chose her favorite toys to put on the table for lipreading: the doll, her own hair bow, a bowl and spoon. "You hold the baby doll. Oh, she is crying," and I looked sad and held the doll and patted it, and looked again at it. "Maybe she is hungry." I gave the spoon to Sue and indicated she should feed the doll. She did.

Then I repeated each word, indicating the object, pointing to each. Again I repeated a word and waited for Sue to respond. She only looked at me.

Six weeks had almost passed and I had reports to write. The other children had learned new vocabulary and simple sentences. They were beginning to add. Their printing was good. But here was Sue, bright, attentive, a good child, friendly and helpful, but not making progress in the very things she was in school to learn.

Sue was my first new pupil. No beginning. No promise.

I had to put more meaning into the lessons. I had to find a way. We were still at that first hour, Sue pressed against the wall.

The October morning was bright. The children all had news. The brothers Ted and Gilbert each clutched a bedraggled bunch of bittersweet. Patty had a small pumpkin with a face cut in it. Sue had a stuffed animal, a lamb. Not a black sheep, but decidedly not white, a beloved toy. At lipreading time for Sue I got the pumpkin and the doll. When Sue put her lamb on the table, my heart skipped a beat.

Smiling reassuringly, I talked about each toy. "Here is the Jack-o-lantern. Look, it has a nose, mouth, and eyes" pointing to each several times. And then indicated the doll. And we went through the same exercise. Then I looked surprised that the lamb too had eyes, nose and mouth.

Then I said, "This is your lamb." Then I asked, without pointing, "Where is your lamb?"

Sue's fat hand reached out and tentatively rested over her lamb. Stars danced in her eyes.

I gathered up Sue and the lamb and hugged them so vigorously that I broke my rimless glasses!

Across that barrier of silence, I had finally reached this little child. Sue had waited, not understanding what was expected, not seeing the connection of my speaking to her world. Dear old lamb, her comfort in the quiet dark night, soft and warm, led her to the world of meaning.

Buried in my lecture notes was: "Infants are nine months to a year and a half before they say their first words, but they have been listening and making associations since birth."

Sue had been seeing the word "lamb" on her parents' lips for several years, but only that morning in October did she finally make the association. Sue rapidly acquired a lipreading vocabulary and the beginning speech. The next year when Sue was five she could read, write, and say simple sentences.

· · · · ·

Lipreading

Lipreading, or speech reading as it is also called, is an art. It can be taught and it does improve with practice, yet the skill is difficult to describe.

It is assumed that your child is wearing his hearing aid at all times. He will need to wear it at home, at play, as well as at school. This will give him the added help in learning to lipread.

Hearing people can lipread better than deaf people — even those who have had training, because people with normal hearing are familiar with the language and vocabulary of every day conversation and the technical jargon.

So why is it so difficult for the deaf or hard of hearing child?

We are back to the difficulty of learning language. The young deaf child has to grasp the idea that things and actions have names. He learns slowly that the fleeting movements of the lips convey a message, have meaning. And to have meaning, talking must follow the "code" or the word order of the language.

Lipreading is of two types:

Casual: You are talking as events unfold, not pre-planned. This will, however, occur over and over in similar situations. Every night at a given time you will say, "It is time for bed." This repetition of situations and expressions will eventually hold meaning. If, however, you said it in the middle of the morning, your child would not lipread this as it would not be "cued" into the situation.

Specific: This is a planned lesson in which one takes a related group of words, sentences, questions or phrases about activities and drills them. This the teacher must do to teach math, geography, for a reading lesson, and the rules for a game.

In the beginning we are constantly "putting in". The child is "taking it in" just as a baby listens for the first year and a half before he says his first words. We have to give our hearing impaired children even longer to "soak up" meaning.

Now the hard facts: Only 40 percent of what is spoken can be read on the lips. *Yet we must use complete sentences, ask complete questions, give idioms—of which our language is rich.*

The little words, called function words, "is, on, of, with, and," cannot be seen on the lips or are so fleeting as not to be recognized. Function words do not have meanings of themselves. You cannot picture an "of". Word endings are often lost. We group many words together such as prepositional phrases. The list goes on. Not only are many words not seen, but many sounds are made in the back of the mouth such as /g/ /k/ /ng/ /s/ /r/. Don't cry just yet. There are many sounds that look alike. "d-t, m-b-p, s-z". You would not put "red and green" in the same sentence—they look the same as does "baby, mama, and papa".

Single words are more difficult to read than phrases or sentences. Avoid telegraphic language which leaves out the function words. Constantly caution members of the family to talk in complete, age appropriate sentences. The grandmother who told her grandson "boots car" had to be reminded that she must say, "Put your boots in the car."

16

Give the child "live language" at his interest level. In the beginning don't ask the child, "What do you want?" He does not know the name or word for what he wants. You ask, "Do you want a cookie? Do you want your red car? Do you want your Teddy Bear?" You may put emphasis on the key word and it is good if it comes at the end of the question.

If the child has just pointed and is not looking at you when you asked if he wanted a cookie—hold it in a stop motion and he will give you a glance to see why the delay, and then you can repeat it. He will soon be conditioned to look at your face.

Your child will never be through learning to lipread. His vocabulary should be constantly expanding with new words and ever more new ideas.

Some people are easier to lipread than others. People who bob around, have mannerisms, have a mustache, do not move their lips will always be more difficult to lipread.

The light should be on your face. If your back is to the window, your child has difficulty seeing your face. A well lighted room is a must.

He will get many cues from your facial expressions and posture—it has to substitute for the tone of your voice for the hearing listener.

Look directly at your child to begin the conversation, so he knows you are speaking to him. Then if you change your position as you help him, he can read your profile. If you are looking at the newspaper, at some one else, or watching your own activity, he will not make the personal contact, the "chemistry" of communication. You and the child have to be "tuned in".

In the classroom during a lesson I speak directly to each child—just to say it to the class in general accomplishes nothing. There has to be the I-Thou relationship.

To review:
> Talk in full sentences.
> Have the light on your face.
> Give the child the words and sentences in the situation.
> Know that he must watch for a long time before meanings and relationships are mastered.
> Your child will always be learning to lipread.
> He must have a clue about what you are talking about.
> Always use a normal voice and a normal talking pace. Mouthing words distorts the form of the words and sentences.
> If after repeating an idea and your child is still puzzled, re-word the sentence. Choose a more visible word.

All this seems a tremendous task, but soon it will become routine and you will do it naturally and without any great effort.

* * * * *

In The Beginning Was The . . . Thought

All children are brothers. Hearing children in whatever country or savage tribe have mastered language by the age of four. Man is driven by psychological and social needs to communicate. He appears to do so effortlessly as all language seems simple to its own speakers. But it is an illusion to think that a child learns to talk with ease or that it gives him the freedom to think and to be a rational human being. Indeed, we are blissfully unaware that our very culture is structured according to our language.[1] And language is locked in a mold with rigid rules which ordain how we communicate. How we categorize and channel our reasoning and how we build our house of reality.[2]

English is one of the most complex and baffling languages on earth. How do our children master this language? Normally the infant is in a sea of sound and talking from his first days, yet he listens for at least a year before he grasps simple concepts and controls his speech mechanism sufficently to mimic perhaps a dozen words. He has been babbling—exercising the muscles of his lips, tongue, and larynx, been reinforced by fond parents and simply enjoys listening to own voice. Gradually the experience is distilled so he understands that certain verbal patterns accomplish his wish. He is nearly two years old when "language" —more than one word sentences—appears. Then rapidly his mind unlocks the code and his muscles learn to glide through intricate motor patterns. Never again will he be so receptive to learning to talk. He has become an articulate human being. He is age four.

How then does our deaf child learn to talk? And how does it differ from this normal pattern? Early childhood deafness is a two fold handicap. First it is physical. Nerves may be dead or the hearing mechanism has malfunctions. But the greater handicap is educational. For all education is predicated on the idea of communicating knowledge by speaking, signing, or in written form. And deafness in a young child cuts across this very humanizing force— the need and the power to communicate. It is thus that deafness is the most devastating handicap the child with a normal mind can endure. In the absence of sound in his environment and without normal channels for communicating, the deaf child's perception of reality is reduced and his experiences are structured differently. One could add a third handicap—the psychological. He is limited and frustrated in his attempt to learn.

Therefore, immediate intervention is of the utmost importance. When an otherwise normal infant does not seem to react to environmental sounds, does not show the startle reflex to a sudden noise, or does not turn his head

---

1. American Sign Language (ASL) is considered the basis for the Deaf Culture.

2. These ideas about the acquisition of language by all children are from *Language, Thought & Reality from Selected Writings of Benjamin Lee Whorf,* 1956, Massachusetts Institute of Technology.

when spoken to, parents must seek immediate medical advice. And request a thorough examination. Doctors must take parents' apprehension seriously and schedule an audiological examination.

High-risk babies should be examined at birth. High-risk infants are those whose prenatal or delivery presented problems: those whose mothers had medical conditions, and family histories that might indicate a hearing loss. Certainly all children who indicate the possibility of having a hearing loss can and should be tested before the age of six months.

Infants can be fit with hearing aids. Parent counseling must start immediately and continue on a regular basis. Audiologists can guide the parents through the trauma of accepting the child's loss, and learning how to care for the hearing aid. At the same time the professionals in the area of early childhood hearing loss must guide parents in ways to stimulate listening and the beginnings of language development.

Parents must understand that the day a child is fit with a hearing aid is his "hearing birthday". A hearing impaired child needs time to "listen to voices and environmental sounds". Like the hearing child, he must be given this time. If you, a hearing individual, found yourself stranded in China—you would hear everything, but the language would have no meaning. If a hearing infant has been listening and learning for over a year and a half—you have to give your hearing impaired child time to "interpret" meaning and even longer to understand language and speech.

A professional will see the family perhaps once or twice a week. The parents must be shown how to engage in play that leads to learning. Parents without early encouragement and guidance or who delay getting hearing aids for their infant tend to stop talking to their toddler as he does not respond. But parents and siblings must continue talking with the infant. Even in families where Signed English is incorporated, speech must continuously be used.

For the time table for learning to talk is ticking for the hearing impaired child just as it does for all children.

Parents who can and do use sign language—whatever system—intuitively know that the stimulation and communication starts immediately. And they too must encourage the development of listening skills.

Without this early stimulation the hearing impaired child would forever dwell in his restricted world, without depth of thinking or complete understanding. He would be immature and uneducated. And this would be so for all hearing impaired children regardless of the educational achievements of his family. A lawyer's child would be as impoverished as an orphan roaming the paths of a war torn country.

The statement that 85 percent of all knowledge is acquired through vision—according to manufacturers of visual aids—is not even true for the hearing child. Pictures and films are never presented without labels, captions, or sound track, or the teacher's or parent's explanation. So here is our normal child relying upon this most valuable tool known to man—language. Certainly, then, the mere passing of life before the deaf child will not be enough for him to comprehend what is happening.

Our hearing impaired children gain a feeling for the flow of language through hearing aids, assistive listening devices, lipreading, and signs. All add to his understanding.

Regardless of how much or little he hears, there will always be help in learning to listen and to develop speech. Speech must be preceded by an understanding of language. Just to learn a list of words would be no more help than memorizing a spelling book. True, words are like bricks of a building, but a pile of bricks is not a house. Nor is speech a static position, but a flow of sounds and movement. *And always it has to be a result of meaning—either the child wants to tell us something or to get his wants fulfilled.*

To return again to language. Language is the code, the structure of thinking. It must come first for the child with a hearing loss just as it does for the hearing child. *All children have this innate ability to understand and formulate ideas in the acceptable language "code" of their mother tongue.*

. . . . .

Margaret Brown
July 16, 1945

Summer School, Columbia University,
Lexington School for the Deaf
New York City

Daily Report on a Speech Demonstration

Today's demonstration caused within me a strange reaction. I think it has to do with "patience". Years ago when I helped my father with his lip reading lessons based on the "foo, foo, foo" method, I suffered a mental or emotional feeling so strong as to almost make me ill. Often during my observation periods in college, I felt this again. But once I got into the field actively—I have never felt it.

It is the necessity of going over and over and over and over a drill; the necessity to be vital and encouraging; to be able to not over-do the child's patience; to make the drill meaningful and satisfying that calls for patience.

I've been studying Spanish at vocational school so I can appreciate what it is to form words and handle a new language pattern. How keenly I feel the child's struggle.

Not only is successful teaching based upon sympathetic participation in an activity, but the whole mental outlook of the teacher is important. It is not what we teach, it is what we "are" that counts. The teacher must be able to reach out beyond the day's horizon, she must be normal and human. She must be what she wants her children to be—normal and human.

. . . . .

Sue and Jim Perhai

We live in Bloomington, Illinois for over 30 years. We bought a house when we had our son. Later we bought 30 acre land with shed and well. Only 20 miles north of our house, so we can go for our pleasure and hobby like gardening, riding our ATV four wheelers, etc. We have dogs since we got married. We have fifth-wheel trailer there. My husband Jim always says, "It is my summer home."

I met my husband at the institution (residential school, Wisconsin School for the Deaf) as I know his two deaf older sisters.

My husband and I love to travel all over the U.S. and other countries like Mexico, Fiji Islands, Australia, and New Zealand while World Games of the Deaf was presented. We love to watch all people from other countries using their own sign language than ours.

I work for Country Companies for 24 years (Jan. 27, 1969). At present I am office specialist clerk for Country Life Insurance Co. My responsible job is to receive all life applications from the agents all over in Illinois and ten out of states and check for the amount of cash, signatures of Insurers or Applicants and dates before depositing all checks. The applications are processed before delivering to the underwriting department. Also I take care of all collection cards (first premium) with money from agents for their commissions.

I think the hearing impaired infants would be beneficial to see and learn quickly by using sign language. Even the hearing infants, like my son, learn and sign before one-year-old and speaking. Using fore finger point to the head fore for "da da" or point to the palm of hand for "cookie" or point on the lips for "water" and close hand squeeze and loose back and forth for "milk". My son used to sign when he was seven or eight months old.

For deaf babies after one-year-old or to pick up several words in sign language, then they try to speak. Nowadays with better hearing devices, if success they could go to the regular or mainstream schools. My opinion— For half of childhood go to the mainstream school and the other go to the

21

deaf institute, both of which I am glad that I did.

I really enjoyed at the institution where I involved in all kinds of deaf activities like sports and clubs. I met and made many friends. Before I went to the institution, I had more time with my family till I got older (11 years old that separated from my family).

How did I raise my son? I had experience with one of three brothers who was the youngest when I was almost 17 years old. I watched and helped my mother with my brother while infant became a toddler. I continued tending with him till I got married when he was only three years old.

Then I had my baby son three years later.

* * * * *

Jim and Sue Perhai are now grandparents. Little Hannah who is 17 months can sign over 50 words. (She is a hearing child.)

Recently Sue wrote that they bought a larger home next door to their home. And are busy decorating it.

Jim, she writes, has worked for Pantagraph for 30 years. He got a clock.

We attended the first annual reunion at Wisconsin School for the Deaf Alumni Association and had fun seeing old friends. Then we drove on to Denver to the NAD (National Association of the Deaf) where over 3000 people attended.

* * * * *

Jim and Sue were both at the Morgan School reunion several years ago. The five girls I taught in Appleton at Morgan School were there. Some are grandmothers. All are capable women who have raised families and many worked outside of the home. Like them, I enjoy reunions.

* * * * *

Unspoken Tale
Deaf Storyteller Lets Fingers Do His Talking

By Dorene Lomanto
Reprinted courtesy of *The Indianapolis News*

All eyes will be on Ted Myhre this weekend as he tells his tale of the discovery of electricity. But most ears will be listening to his interpreter.

Myhre, who is deaf, is one of 25 storytellers participating in the Second Annual Hoosier Storytelling Festival.

"He has what every storyteller needs: a good choice of stories and a good way of telling them. You get caught up in the way Ted signs, and he really know how to do that," said Robert Sander, executive director of Stories Inc. a festival sponsor. "It knocks down the bridges and misconceptions people have about deaf people telling stories."

Myhre's storytelling tale begins in Wisconsin during his middle school years when he was introduced to the art.

"I grew up in a deaf school and the dorm had no TV," Myhre said through his interpreter, Mary Glenn Cullison. "The deaf supervisors would tell stories, and the girls and boys stayed in the dorms on the weekends just to hear the stories.

"I would sit back and listen. And sometimes the boys and girls would tell stories. I never told stories myself," he said, crossing his arms and shaking his head, "until I came here."

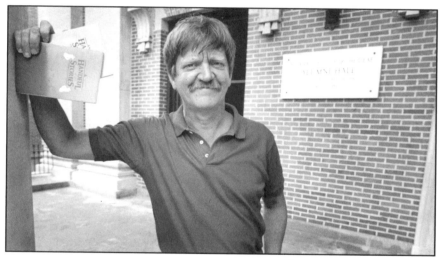

Ted Myhre as the story teller
Photo by Mike Fender, *The Indianapolis News*

Here is the Indiana School for the Deaf, 1200 E. 42nd Street where Myhre has been a teacher since 1975. Some students behaved so poorly, Myhre said, that the only way to calm them down was to tell them stories. Soon the students' requests were joined by those of teachers who also wanted to be swept up into Myhre's fables.

"For a signing storyteller, there's a lot of eye and body language. You get a picture of the story," he said. "If a hearing person and I tell the same story, you'll see American Sign Language is much more expressive."

Even in simple conversation, Myhre makes his language a rich art form. His hands become a blur as he weaves them in and out. His eyes gaze at his "listener." His face reddens as he contorts it to show frustration, sorrow and happiness.

It was during a ghostly Halloween story session at the school last year that Sander was captivated by Myhre's visual presentations.

"He was so lively, animated and humorous," said Sander, he then invited Myhre to a Stories Inc. meeting to perform. "He was a hit. It seemed like the next logical step was to invite him to the festival."

Myhre likes to tell animal stories to children. "I remember when I was small, a hearing principal came to my classroom and told us the story of Blaze. It is about a boy who always wanted a horse and his parents get him one. I loved that story," he said, embracing himself to sign the word "love". "I use that story occasionally."

But perhaps Myhre's favorite yarns to spin into fine threads of theater are deaf folklore. He chose Roslyn Rosen's story "1776: Deaf People's Contribution" to tell at the festival.

"Ben Franklin happened to have a deaf person work for him at his print shop. One night Franklin heard that Congress supported war against England to free the colonies. He wanted to get this in the paper. He ran to his print shop late at night." Myhre said, slapping his hands together and throwing one forward, "but he didn't have a key to get in the shop.

"He remembered his deaf assistant had a key, so he went to his home . . . and banged on the door," he signed by pounding his fist against an imaginary wall. "But he got no response. Ben saw a light on on the second floor and got a wonderful idea.

"He got a real big kite and started flying it back and forth in front of the window." Myhre said by forming an outline of a kite and then by swaying his arms back and forth as though holding on to its string.

The story goes on to a happy, but unexpected ending of electricity being discovered. "I have many funny stories," Myhre said.

Myhre was born in Neenah, Wisconsin. For three years, his parents who could hear, weren't sure their son was deaf. "They thought maybe I was OK, or just a little quiet," Myhre said. "They never learned ASL. They knew the signs for "water" and "eat" and "mow the lawn". Most things related to work. I lived in a hearing world. I never really enjoyed it. I missed so much."

At nine, Myhre entered a new world when his uncle told him about a deaf school in Wisconsin. His father resisted sending Myhre there until he met school officials. "I loved it there. I didn't want to go home at the end of the semester in December. But I had to . . . I cried and cried," he signed by dragging his finger down his cheek.

Party Boys — Several years after the Appleton class was discontinued. Ted, Larry and Gilbert

"People's consciousness about the deaf community has changed since those days," Myhre said. "More and more parents are learning to sign. Through the media it has improved. Communication is getting better."

Countries hardly serve as barriers to communication. Myhre found out during travels in Europe and Asia. Although the deaf communities there rely on oralism and fewer signs, that didn't stop Myhre from meeting deaf people.

"In Moscow I saw two deaf people in the market. I saw them moving their hands and I ran over to talk to them." Myhre said. "They asked me where I was from. I made a picture of USA with Florida down here," he said forming the outline of the Southern states. "Next day I had a lot of deaf Russians come to my hotel room to chat."

Myhre isn't exactly sure what is next for him. "Maybe I'll get involved in community affairs through storytelling. I don't want to tell my stories just to deaf people. I'd like to see the public library have deaf storytelling with skilled signers so you can go and hear and listen. You need to inform the public."

Author's Comment

Ted Myhre and his brother Gilbert, a couple years older, were in my first class.

After I left the Appleton system, the program continued for a year or two and then the students moved either to Oshkosh or Green Bay day classes or on to Delavan, The Wisconsin School for the Deaf. That was where Ted found himself. And he went on to Gallaudet and became a teacher. As this article points out, Ted Myhre traveled widely.

* * * *

III

SPECIAL EDUCATION
A Hearing Child

1954

Multiple Handicapped

Conditions which cause childhood hearing loss are many. And, unfortunately, often other handicaps appear. An infection such as meningitis effects the central nervous system. High fevers of undetermined origin have often been blamed. An Rh condition, measles, mumps, in early childhood can also damage more than the hearing mechanism.

Some conditions are inherited. Generally inherited conditions are singular in just the cause of hearing loss.

Birth injury, prenatal conditions can cause added problems.

The following story was my introduction to the handicapped child who had hearing. This year with a Trainable Retarded child allowed me to study what this handicap meant. I was then able to understand the multiple handicapped deaf child.

My experience with Bobby points the direction my teaching eventually took. It was 1954-55:

Give Every Child The Chance To Learn
1954-1955

After a summer of unrelenting heat, August 30 dawned chilly and gray. The appointment for Bobby Fennor's test was for 1:30. The Standford-Binet Test was important to Bobby's mother for Bobby was a brain-injured, retarded child of seven.

Through the years Mrs. Fennor had made the heart-breaking trek from doctors to psychologists. They said Bobby's slow physical development, his slightly spastic movements, and his mental retardation were probably caused at birth. What would today's test show?

The test was important to me, his teacher this past year, in still another way. Would Bobby finally respond to the testing situation?

I arrived at the Fennor home before the young man who was to administer the test. Mrs. Fennor greeted me warmly. When Bobby heard me, he came down the stairs one step by one step. He wore a beautiful blue shirt, his eyes the same clear blue. He grinned, "How are you?" To Bobby this was just another pleasant day, as all his days were.

We went into the living room to wait for Mr. Blessing from the Wisconsin Bureau for Handicapped Children. The large living room was chilly, so Mrs. Fennor lit a fire in the fireplace. Soon the flickering light brought warmth to the comfortably furnished room. Bobby touched my arms and my earrings. He chattered, "How are you? Pretty. Build a fire. Turn it off. Bobby sweep."

Mrs. Fennor and I talked quietly, but encouragingly, about Bobby's progress over the year.

The year before when Bobby was six, his attention span was so short and he was so vacillating that the Standford-Binet Test had been impossible to administer. After two attempts the tester had given an "educated guess" that Bob was very mentally retarded. She had said that he was below the level acceptable in the Special Education Room in the public school system.

Mrs. Fennor refused this verdict. She said to the Elementary Grade Supervisor who received the test results, "You can't condemn my child for all time because of this one test! He has to have the chance to try to learn. You are segregating him from children, and denying him a happy school experience. I am sure Bobby could learn with special help."

The supervisor then patiently explained, "There are no facilities for the very retarded child in the public school system. The slow learning children in the Special Education rooms will eventually be capable of beginning reading. Bobby will never be able to read. To place him in a school situation where he cannot cope with the problems would certainly not be a happy experience. It would cause frustration and most likely lead to emotional disturbances and behavior problems."

"But how do you know he can't learn?" pleaded Mrs. Fennor. "If only his attention span can be increased, he will learn many things."

And it was in this desperate hour that a friend had said, "I know a woman who can teach handicapped children."

When Mrs. Fennor called me, I had to tell her, as kindly as I could, that I had taught deaf children who had normal, average intelligence. I was not qualified to teach the mentally retarded. However, at her insistence, I agreed to see Bobby.

The next morning she brought Bobby to my home. I knew I could not promise this mother anything. Still, being a mother of two lively girls much the same age as Bobby, I could not refuse to help. Perhaps I was fortified with the belief that any handicapped child needs everything a normal child does, only more so.

Bobby was to come to my home every school day morning from 9:00 to 11:00 a.m. My Sue, who was five years old and going into afternoon kindergarten, would be a companion for Bobby.

Sue was self contained and loving. Each morning began with hugs and kisses, but did not go like hearts and flowers to the end of the period. For Bobby was indeed restless, as is typical of many brain-injured children. He moved from toy to toy, pulling at each, but without curiosity to play. Books were pulled to the floor and left; doll dishes put on the play table and forgotten; a few blocks stacked and kicked over.

A room full of toys was too distracting. This was never more evident than at story time. I had to clear the area completely and then clutch Bobby to my side. And all to no real avail in the beginning, for he continued to punctuate every sentence that I read with, "Read it! Read it!" And he constantly wriggled to get free or to pull at Sue.

He had to be coaxed to touch the tricycle! And then I had to work his legs up and down to get him to pedal. Guiding the bike was too complicated. The moment I removed my hold, he got off, throwing his leg awkwardly over the handle bars.

But each nice day Sue and the many little neighbor children rode their bikes up and down the walks. Soon Bobby began to peddle along with the rest.

Inside, in the basement, we played tag, marched, walked like elephants, crept like Indians, and learned to jump. In the fall Bobby could not jump. Obviously he couldn't learn to jump over any object. Working from the sound psychological law of learning that meaningful activity is the more quickly learned, I drew chalk pictures on the sidewalk or basement floor. I drew a candle and said:

"Jack be nimble,   Jack be quick,   Jack jump over   The candle stick."

I held his hands and helped him jump. And so Bobby learned.

To train his concentration I began with keys on a ring. All children love to jingle keys. The first day I gave Bobby the open ring and put four keys on the otherwise clear table. I said, "Bobby, put the keys on the ring." He pushed at the keys as though they were repulsive. The next lesson period, I put the open ring in his hand, a key in the other hand and then guided his hands. Time after time I helped him put the keys on, snap the ring closed or open it and remove the keys.

A period of intense concentration such as working with keys, learning to snap or unbutton clothing, screw large nuts and bolts, or working simple five piece wooden puzzles was never attempted for longer than two or three minutes at a time. As soon as Bobby showed signs of tension, we stopped and had marching, running, or free activity.

At ten each morning was snack time with crackers and milk. Sue and I looked forward to this time as did Bobby.

Washing doll dishes was a favorite activity, and Bobby did it expertly. But music was his forte! He would select the record he wanted from the thirty we had and tell which side to play. He listened enraptured; sang many of the songs; and gradually learned to dance to "Looby-Loo, and "Did you ever see a Lassie."

Sue played happily along. The most frustrating thing for her was that she wanted to continue an activity long after Bobby lost interest. We solved the puzzle dilemma to everyone's satisfaction. Sue worked more complicated puzzles. They had races where Bobby could win fair and square and have a real feeling of accomplishment. What a supreme experience for a slow child who is usually left behind and left out of life's little competitions!

By March Bob could unbutton his coat. He was fighting for a turn on the bike. Spring took us outdoors again, and with the many neighbor children, ages three and four, Bobby learned to play. The children rode bikes, ran on the grass in happy games, rolled and tumbled, swung, played in the sand and mud. While Bobby really never turned a somersault, still he had the happy, joyous feeling of being one with the children. A real moment of achievement came when Bob joined the children sitting on the steps or in a circle on the lawn while I read stories with all eyes attentive and only the normal wiggling. These little children accepted Bobby completely, never saying an unkind word. They shared running, laughing, companionship—togetherness.

This was Bobby's neighborhood. Unfortunately, his home neighborhood had no other young children.

Retarded children retain so little they learn unless it is constantly repeated that it was not without trepidation that Mrs. Fennor and I wondered, that August afternoon, what three months of vacation had done to Bobby's small gains.

Mr. Blessing arrived. He was warm-natured, a quiet young man, a father himself. He asked for a card table and quickly arranged his testing materials. Bobby sat opposite him in a large comfortable chair. Mrs. Fennor and I were in the sun room to the back of Bobby so he could not see us and be distracted.

Mr. Blessing began the Standford-Binet Test. He worked effortlessly, drawing Bobby's attention, holding it kindly, firmly. Mr. Blessing put three small objects on the table, possibly a toy doll, a tiny engine, a spoon. He had Bobby point to each and name it. Then he put a cardboard shield between Bobby and the objects. He covered one object with a small box. He removed the shield and asked Bobby, "What is under the box?"

Bobby missed the first trial, but succeeded in the next two. The test was going well. Bobby was responding his very best.

Mrs. Fennor and I watched silently.

Mr. Blessing continued through the many exercises of the test which is so constructed that it tests the component parts of a child's intelligence and reveals his mental age. Since an individual's I.Q. does not usually vary greatly from year to year, it affords a basis for predicting his probable future achievement. The value for school placement is apparent.

Bobby began to grow restless and when he could no longer give correct answers, Mr. Blessing stopped. Bobby moved away. I took a seat at the table. Mrs Fennor stood behind me. As Mr. Blessing scored the test, I knew it would be an accurate measure of Bob's intelligence. I sensed that Mrs. Fennor girded her courage.

Mr. Blessing looked up kindly, and in his quiet way said, "I wish my news were better . . ."

Up to this very utterance, I knew Mrs. Fennor had hoped Bobby would be "only a little slow". The implication of his words must have washed over her hopes like iced water. Her stillness behind me was tense.

Mr. Blessing continued in a tone such as a doctor would use in diagnosing an incurable condition—as indeed Bobby's was. "Bobby falls below 50 I.Q., into a group we call 'trainable'. It means he probably will never learn to read. He has learned remarkably this year because of the 'rich' environment. He will be able to learn to care for himself and do many simple tasks under direct supervision.

Mrs. Fennor spoke for the first time to ask, "Is there no school for Bobby?"

Mr. Blessing hesitated. "There are institutions."

"No!" Mrs. Fennor was firm.

Mr. Blessing offered, "There are several day classes in the state for this trainable level. But the nearest one has its quota." He continued, "If there are other children in this area at Bobby's level, such a class could be organized here."

Hope returned to the room. Mrs. Fennor accepted the challenge. "If other handicapped children like my Bobby live in this city, I will find them."

Mr. Blessing directed, "Then you parents must petition your local school board for the class. The board will then request our department to make a survey to determine if these children require this special help."

"How many children will be needed for a class?" Mrs. Fennor wanted to know.

"The law says six children between the ages of seven to 16, with an I.Q. of 35 to 50," he stated. "Also there are other factors to be considered. The child has to be able to adjust to a social group. So each child is enrolled on a trial basis."

"Why haven't we heard about these classes?" I asked.

"The concept of day classes at this level is very new," he said. "The first one in the state was in Milwaukee in 1950, and that was privately sponsored by the National Association of Parents and Friends of Retarded Children."

"The cost. Will that be a stumbling block?" I thought out loud.

"No. Because the state pays nearly 100 pecent of the cost of this special class."

Eagerly Mrs. Fennor asked, "How many Trainable classes are there in Wisconsin?"

"There are 19 with approximately 190 children enrolled."

Then I asked, "How does that compare with the number in our state institutions for the mentally retarded?"

"There are 3,060 children in the state's institutions. And it costs twice as much to maintain them there as it does to pay for training in a day class." He added, "So you see our department is very willing to help a community where the need exists."

"Is Wisconsin unique in establishing these classes?" I inquired.

"Yes, we are among the five states in our nation with tax-supported classes under the administration of the Department of Public Instruction."

"I feel I will find real help for my Bobby," Mrs. Fennor concluded.

Because one mother would not accept defeat, our community will soon have a Trainable Class. One mother felt that home life with love and care was her son's birthright. Every child must have the chance to learn and develop to the fullest of his ability.

. . . . .

Serving The Trainable Child Today

Bobby's mother did find other children so that a class could be established in our community. A church offered the use of the church school rooms and a teacher and an aide were hired.

In a few years the program moved to an elementary building. This elementary program continues. Then when the students became teenagers, several communities combined their efforts and located a small school to the edge of the city. There were two classrooms and a well equipped kitchen including a washer and dryer. Eventually a gym was added. Here 27 students learned self help skills and developed work projects. They learned to shop for food and prepare their lunches. They learned to maintain the building and grounds.

Then in the 80s came the integration requests. Each community became responsible for the education of the severely handicapped students in regular school settings. Neenah, now with only a few students, returned to the junior and the senior high school. Here they continue much the same program. The students attend school pep rallies, auditorium programs and many regular students help them with their projects. Parents feel that peer relationships, limited as they are, prove beneficial for their children. And looking to the future, hopefully the general population will show compassion and understanding, and most importantly, see that these programs continue.

At age 21 the severely handicapped adults move into Group Homes. They work in sheltered workshops and have responsibilities in the homes. Bobby, whose parents have died, now has a legal guardian. He lives in a private residential setting.

. . . . .

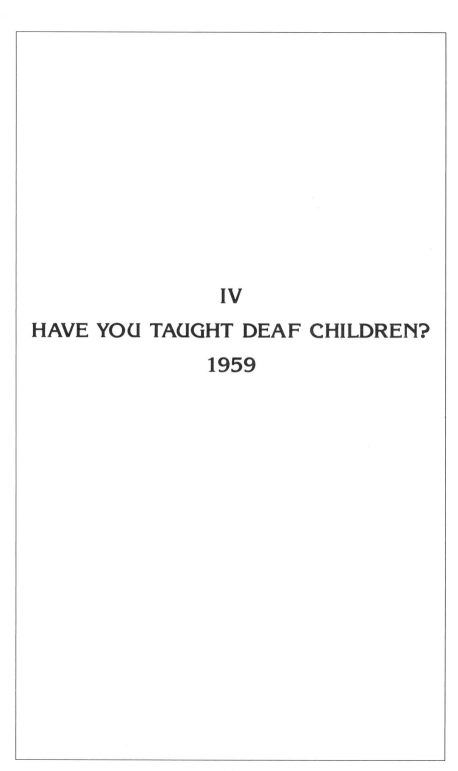

IV
HAVE YOU TAUGHT DEAF CHILDREN?
1959

Have You Taught Deaf Children?

It was a morning in mid-August in 1959 when I received a phone call from the Principal of the School for the Deaf and Hard of Hearing, a department within the Oshkosh Area Public School System in Wisconsin.

Peter Owsley asked, "Have you taught deaf children?"

"Yes, over ten years ago in Appleton, Wisconsin."

"We need a preschool teacher. Would you be interested?"

The following morning I drove the twelve miles from my home in Menasha to Oshkosh. As we talked I was concerned that driving through Wisconsin's winter weather might be a problem.

"Don't worry. If the weather is that bad we cancel school."

"I have developed a mild hearing loss in one ear."

"We'll hang a hearing aid on you."

"But to teach speech?"

"You do not appear to have a significant problem. You were trained by Alice Streng in Milwaukee State Teachers College and you say you attended a summer session at the Lexington School for the Deaf in New York City. You won't have any problem."

Next to his office was a small sound proof room for testing hearing. Mr. Owsley was a certified audiologist as well as a trained teacher of the deaf. With this reassurance, I accepted his offer to teach.

He put through a call to the superintendent who immediately came over with the contract.

I looked forward to teaching in this new building when he said, "Now let's go over to the building where you will have your class."

Longfellow School was a typical older elementary school. My room to be was a large, empty room on the second floor up a steep flight of stairs—not my idea of a location for a preschool. It did have big windows and was flooded with sunshine.

The next few days some little oak tables and chairs were moved in. There were only a few toys. And an auditory trainer was positioned in one corner.

If ever the expression, "Fools rush in where angels fear to tread." It applied to me.

That first morning the parents or drivers brought ten tiny toddlers, the oldest barely four. Fortunately they wore identification tags so after class the drivers knew which children to take.

Some parents cried. In regular kindergarten the children cry. But here I

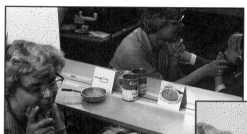

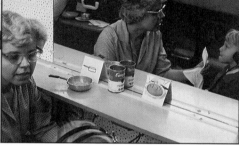

These two pictures seem similar, but they illustrate two methods of teaching speech.

In one, the teacher holds the child's hand against her cheek and the child's hand on the child's face.

The other illustrates the visual help by seeing the puff of air on the tissue. This illustrates the initial /p/ for pan and the final /p/ in soup.

Photos by James Auer

had parents crying. I did not know that many of the children were to live in boarding homes and the parents would not see them until Friday noon.

Peter Owsley had given a six weeks summer session for the parents of these toddlers. He covered the problems of raising hearing impaired children. Without this background my first year would have been traumatic.

The first morning I took my ten-year-old daughter Sue, now a seasoned baby-sitter and knowledgeable about handicapped children. Also each day I had volunteer aides. Each had been assigned a morning.

One mother later said she didn't expect me to last the year. Twenty-three years later she was at my retirement dinner and was still mystified that I had remained.

You will now meet some of these "toddlers" who today are successful young adults.

* * * * *

Parents' Summer Sessions
Heidi Evans, Parent
1960

The Tidings
The 1960 Yearbook
Oshkosh School for the Deaf and Hard of Hearing

Last June a group of mothers went back to school for a six week period. We had an average of 10 to 12 "students" a day. I think we could all agree

35

that it was one of the nicest schools that we ever attended; we had coffee breaks, with doughnuts, strawberry shortcake, pies and cakes. There was no homework, and no tests to cram for. Also every once in a while we were honored by the presence of a father or two.

Some of the topics discussed were: What can I talk about, How can I make him aware that I'm talking, Why is language so difficult for my child, The ear and how it works, Things to know about hearing aids, and many others. We also discussed the problems we had with our children. We now know all about decibels and frequencies, and how to read an audiogram. We even took turns giving one another hearing tests, and found we all had quite good hearing.

About once a week we had a guest speaker, as Mr. Owsley was afraid we would get tired of listening to him all of the time. Mr. Tipler, Superintendent of the Oshkosh Schools, told us how the school operates, and something about its budget and future plans. Mrs. Wood visited us and told us about beginning auditory training, and how to make use of the calendar at home. Mr. Evans told about art experiences for children and how we could encourage them. Mr. Samuel Milesky, from the State Bureau for Handicapped Children, told of his work throughout the state. One of the school nurses of Oshkosh visited us one day. She told of some of the communicable diseases, and of the immunization clinics held each year. Dr. Emrich also spoke to us. He told about the ear and how it works. One nice thing about all our speakers was that they were all glad to answer our many questions.

A supervised playground was held during the two hours we met every day. Jan Cowan and Judy Britton did a very nice job of supervising the many children left in their charge.

In July we had a family picnic at Winnebago County Park, with everyone bringing something for dinner. The children had a chance to swim in the afternoon. A good time was had by all.

All in all it was a profitable summer and we all gained much (about five pounds each) knowledge about our children and what we could do to help them.

Author's Comment

After I signed the contract, Mr. Owsley took me to the Evans' home where I met Pam, their three-year-old daughter, who would be in my class.

* * * * *

Reliable Roy, Dependable Roy

Philosophers and saints spend a lifetime in meditation in order to obtain equanimity of spirit. Roy was born with inner calm and acceptance of life.

Whatever the etiology of his hearing loss, the removal of enlarged tonsils and abnormal adenoids at age three resulted in a marked improvement in his hearing in the speech frequencies. Roy was the fourth child with an older brother who had a long history of chronic running ears with a slight hearing loss.

Roy was fitted with a hearing aid with dual receivers and he tolerated amplification well. He vocalized and had a good quality of voice. There was some nasality, perhaps a hold over from the adenoid growth. However, his speech was minimal.

Roy had been very immature, clinging to his mother, so much so that the recommendation during the summer was that he not be entered in school until the following February, and then only on a trial basis. But after the operation and acquiring the hearing aid, he developed rapidly. He entered school that fall, and aside from not being toilet trained, he was outgoing and self-possessed. He was friendly and cooperative. He came willingly for lessons. He used gestures and pantomime because he had good inner language. (Means a child can visualize objects and actions.)

This nursery class was composed of 10 children all very close in age. Even though Roy was the youngest, he willingly sat with the group and took an active part. He was remarkable in accepting the necessity of taking turns. For exacting lipreading and speech development, Roy could work with any other

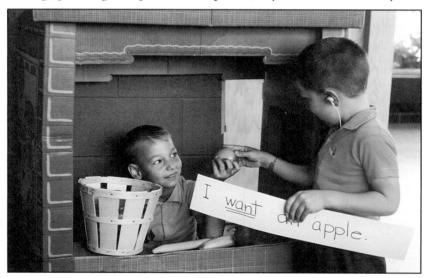

Role playing helps establish speech and language. Roy is buying an apple from Mark.

Photo by James Auer

child, and had a calming effect upon the more restless ones.

There were usually two periods each morning of group activity after which the children made a picture or object to take home so the parents could give extra lipreading drill.

In the beginning Roy could not color or paste, but he was helped to do these things and, if necessary, given the sample to take home. By the time he was four he could cut on the line, draw his own boat or car. His mother reported that at home if his coloring went over the line, Roy would attempt to brush it back with his hand—enough to indicate it should stay within the outline.

To illustrate the progression of these activities: The theme would be a simple, one word, concrete object such as "boat". We started with toys and pictures of different kinds of boats. The first day we had construction paper boats in two parts—the boat and the sail. The next day a ship and smoke stacks. Then a row boat or canoe. The paper already had the water crayoned in. Perhaps another day, not necessarily in day to day development, ship and a row boat were in the same picture to illustrate "a big boat, a small boat". Then came the day we added people. Our picture file contained all kinds of children and people cut out of catalogues. The children could choose their own "family" to put in the row boat. Of course, the boys wanted a motor. And we drew in the fishing pole and the fish. And we talked about catching the fish—a little fish, a big fish, and how many fish. Meanwhile the speech and lipreading of these settings had progressed, also the phonetic reading and printing by the four and five year olds. By the time the children were able to draw their own boat scenes, they were able to print and say, "Daddy caught a fish. I caught two fish." And they brought pictures from home showing their fishing experiences.

All the children had blackboards at home and the ease with which they printed showed they had been practicing.

Consonants were given their phonetic names, and vowels were at first presented in Alcorn Symbols.[1] These symbols are the mouth positions of the vowels, some 16, drawn on the faces of children on the cards in a chart. Eventually the regular spelling was used.

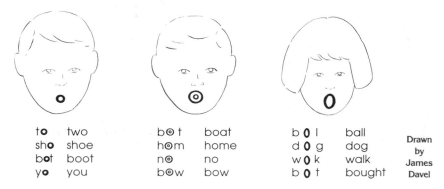

t**o**	two	b**⊙**t	boat	b **0** l	ball
sh**o**	shoe	h**⊙**m	home	d **0** g	dog
b**o**t	boot	n**⊙**	no	w **0** k	walk
y**o**	you	b**⊙**w	bow	b **0** t	bought

Drawn by James Davel

Roy could soon read several consonants and six Alcorn symbols (vowels). He could read most of the names of the children in the class and was never mistaken on his own name.

Besides this exacting drill, the day was filled with natural language rising from our living and working together. Roy understood this readily and used many expressions. By the end of the year he did not have all the sounds, but had plasticity in speech movements and the prognosis was excellent.

Roy had great concern for the other children and though he was boy-rough, he was never intentionally mean. Roy was an all around good guy.

1. Sophia Alcorn developed 16 symbols representing the mouth configurations. Reference: *Hearing Therapy for Children.* Streng, et al. New York, Grune & Stratton, 1958.

* * * * *

Meet Mr. Roy Kessler

Roy, profoundly deaf now, is a Computer Program Analyst for an insurance company in the Valley. He is one of three who is on duty all the time. He has a terminal at home and is apt to be called anytime during the night. The trouble is called in and he brings up the program and works out the problem.

He wrote briefly about his work and his activities:
"Special services were offered at the Fox Valley Technical College, but I did not need them. I used lipreading, notes my friends would share, and I studied from my books very hard. The teachers often helped me after class.

My lipreading helps me most at work. And my project manager reviews with me what is talked about at the meetings.

I did carpool, but now I trade driving with a co-worker.

Yes, I bowl, golf, jog, play racquet ball, and a little soft ball. Most of my friends are deaf, but I have hearing friends at work. My family does not sign. I have a TDD.

My opinion: All deaf children should learn speech as a first language and sign language second so they can communicate with people outside the deaf world. I am always thankful that I learned speech and lipreading. I would not have my job without it.

* * * * *

The Wild, Wild World of Peter

The mental image of Peter's guardian angel is of a creature with tattered feathers from constantly darting and soaring, halo askew, bent and chipped, eyes bleary from sleeplessness.

Plainly the task was beyond the capabilities of a mere guardian angel and lesser beings were called upon to help. It began the first hours after Peter's birth. An Rh baby, Peter required three complete blood interchanges the first week. The jaundice level, considered critical at 20, went up to 27. His birth weight was five pounds and slipped to two pounds. Peter was the fifth child in the family.

Within the first year it was obvious that Peter had a substantial hearing loss. Examinations at Madison University Hospitals verified a sensory-neural hearing loss in the speech frequencies and accompanied by general hypertension.

Peter attended half-morning sessions at the Oshkosh School for the Deaf and Hard of Hearing at age two years four months.

There were ten children in this class, two others with volatile personalities and possible brain damage. The ages ranged from Peter's two years four months, to five years two months. This was the first year for all the children with an exception of some class experience the spring before. Nearly all the mothers had attended a six-week summer session concerning school and home problems of the hearing handicapped child which Peter Owsley (later Peter Owsley, Ph. Ed.) the principal, taught.

This was my first experience with preschool, and it was not until this group of children moved on that I realized the importance of parent education.

The first half of the morning was spent in individual speech and lipreading development. There were volunteers to assist and direct the play. These were local women, some ten of them who were scheduled so that one came each morning.

Peter responded immediately to speech development. He hungered for the music and rhythm through the group biaural hearing aid. Because of Peter's joy of listening, Peter Owsley, our principal and also a certified audiologist, soon fit him with a body type hearing aid. But Peter would have nothing to do with it except to dismantle it.

Peter's three years in the nursery-kindergarten can best be characterized by "tremendous hyperactivity". He was not entirely motivated by curiosity, but by the inability to pay attention for more than a few seconds at a time.

It is said that listening is recognized to be part of the complex mechanism of consciousness, awareness, and attention. And therefore it is readily apparent that the ability to pay attention is acquired gradually and demands a certain organic and functional integrity of a large part of the central nervous system.

This being the case, the deaf child has had no experience watching and being attentive above and beyond his basic natural curiosity. Learning to talk for the deaf child is the most difficult task known, so it is little wonder he shows no native desire to merely watch the lips and to try to mimic. The hard of hearing child who at least gets the vibrations and hears phrasing, if not actual speech, will have more attention training. Peter got no sound without the aid which he refused to wear.

He had no constructive play habits. While one was picking up the pieces of one destructive episode, he had wrought havoc in several wide spread areas. He was constantly escaping the room, or playground which was not fenced. He manipulated everything and left it in shambles. The controls on the hearing aids, both group and individual, held much fascination for him. Aside from the cost involved, the minute adjustments were constantly disturbed. Finally our only recourse was to have the auditory repair man, who lived in by necessity, set the controls and then remove the knobs.

For every episode I experienced, Peter's mother could report a more spectacular one. In Peter's defense, his mother and I agreed to require both of our signatures on referral papers to the residential school hoping we would not both have a "bad time of it" on the same day.

While Peter was not wild by intent, still a certain mischievousness entered the picture. While I was working with Peter individually, he responded well. But all the children had to have individual lessons. Group work with Peter was impossible except in gross motor development exercises and learning to lipread commands. My assistants were not trained teachers, much less familiar with children with special problems. So I was constantly having to take Peter.

The second year he stayed the whole morning. He wanted to learn to cut. He braced his left hand with the scissors against his leg and fed the paper into it. He cut every which way, but we guided his hands, and he learned. His mother reported how well he cut. He cut everything—drapes, tableclothes, and clothing.

By his third year he could draw his own pictures. On one occasion he drew a truck with considerable detail and then proceeded to scribble over it with his crayon. I did the same to my drawing on the easel and said it was a mess. He turned over his paper and immediately redrew and neatly colored his truck.

His thoughtless, over-exuberant actions nearly resulted in an accident. He pushed a child down a long flight of steps. Fortunately an up-coming line of older children blocked the child's fall. When I expained how he might have hurt his friend, he put his arms around him and kissed him. And for days after that when we went up or down the stairs Peter would tell me, "Do not push".

The area in which I taught the individual lessons was blocked off from the activities of the rest of the class. The mike picked up much of the room noise, but at least the child could not see what the others were doing. Deaf children are so easily distracted by movement. They use their eyes to assess each new situation. In this little area with Peter he was able to be attentive. We used toys, and he had the opportunity to manipulate them. He learned the names of the toys and animals, and sounds they made. Both lipreading and beginning speech developed rapidly. Then in small groups of two, and then three children, we worked on commands— "Stand up. Walk. Skip. March. Give the airplane to Greg. Put the milk on the table. Feed the fish." We had flash cards with the commands printed on them. The children took turns being the teacher. Each child had his picture on a card, so it was easy to put a name card in the chart and choose a command. So reading developed right along with lipreading and the first attempts of speech.

And stories were started at a very early stage. It is more fun to drill "bed, chair, and bowls" in the story of *The Three Bears*, or the animals and the parts of the animal's body in *The Gingerbread Boy*.

Peter learned to love books. He would sit in the book corner and "read and read".

He learned to print, large letters on the board, and large letters on his paper. We used the phonetic approach. And number concept developed easily. This particular class learned to count pockets! How many pockets a child had was important, a status symbol. One day Peter's mother was visiting and we showed her how he counted. And that day he had four pockets. She was so delighted that at home she got out a strip of shelf paper and Peter showed his brothers and sister how he counted and wrote 4. Then someone noticed he had a shirt pocket too. They tried to help him write 5. But this number was new. He could count to 10, but not print all of them. He could not get it, so he brushed them aside and wrote 4 and 1, and spread his five fingers over both numbers. He had the concept of addition.

Peter moved on to the primary room, but not until he tried to enter a regular first grade in our building. I was near by so I could give him speech and additional help. After a couple days the first grade teacher said he was not ready. On a test from a workbook she asked the children to underline the pictures of the vegetables and draw a circle around the pictures of fruit. Peter could see what the children were doing and he immediately drew circles around all the items. He knew the names of most of the fruits and vegetables, but it was my fault for I had not taught the language of directions: draw a line under, or draw a circle around. Nor had I taught categories: the class words; vegetables, fruit, dessert. I had taught carrots, potatoes, oranges, apples, ice cream, cake.

Peter then moved on to the primary room for the deaf. He was the youngest in that room. He had excellent natural language, he wore the head phones all day. He could read and write and made an "A" in conduct. Only under stress did he show signs of having difficulty coping. On the Ontario

Performance Test he scored above average. Prognosis excellent.

Peter was integrated at the fourth grade level.

* * * *

Peter Today

Peter attended Gallaudent University graduating with majors in psychology and physical education. Physical education was a natural choice as Peter grew tall and well coordinated. He was a basketball star in high school. Our class of preschoolers played in the gym across from our classroom and Peter could make baskets even then.

Jobs were not easy to find when he graduated. He did work in the Post Office in Oshkosh and transferred to one in Illinois.

He is married and has two beautiful children. A son, now in third grade, teaches his classmates sign language. Even though Peter has residual hearing and did manage to mainstream from 4th grade through high school, depending upon his hearing aids and lipreading, his wife is deaf so the family uses sign language.

He does say that mainstreaming was stressful. With high intelligence, a good education, and warm family support, there are still problems. A hearing loss puts additional stress on every day living.

Peter's guardian angel must still be on duty.

* * * *

Letters To Parents

Following are excerpts from letters to parents. They tell the little things that make up our days. We talk about these activities just as you can at home.

September 1965

We do only one little paper a day, but we work and play at many things each day. The children all play so constructively. The boys thoroughly enjoy playing house. Mark and Terry wash the doll dishes with soap and water and a big dish towel—and do a good job! They all hang up the doll clothes with many clothes pins. For two days Dean has done a mountain of ironing. He puts the laundry basket up on a chair so he can reach the clothes easily. He wants the end of the iron cord taped (connected) to something. They all take turns pushing the doll stroller up and down the sidewalk. Boys do not have

43

much opportunity to play house and seem to enjoy doing so. Terry is so gentle when he puts the the doll to bed. Tod and Jenny were working a puzzle and a piece fell on the floor on Tod's side. He indicated that she should get it. She hopped off her chair and went around and got it for him.

They all enjoy the Master Viewer of the many wild animals and our little plastic ones. They like the farm animals, and the new big barn that Jenny's grandfather built. And of course, the small and large cars, trucks and airplanes. They move the large blocks about. They certainly are busy every minute!

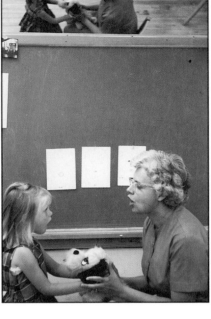

Note the mirror above the board. When the children sit in a row for a lesson, they can monitor their speech.
"Dog" is easy to say and lipread. The cards on the board are the Alcorn Symbols.

Photo by James Auer

We run, jump, march, and salute to records with different rhythms. However, we try to walk in the hall, but that is most difficult for little folk.

We are learning to listen. It is important to recognize environmental sounds. We have an old alarm clock that each can hold and turn on and off. Bells, pounding the drum, and horns—one for the bike too. This for fun as well as learning to recognize sounds in and around the house and play areas.

It is saying the simple little expressions and sentences over and over in similar circumstances that gradually brings meaning. We get the most spontaneous speech at milk and cracker time, and when we are outdoors playing.

One day I will draw attention to someone's cap or raincoat, another time to shirts, or pockets or shoes. If someone gets a hair cut, that is news and we put up a picture of a child in the barber's chair. Last week Dean's mother mailed us a box of cookies. We got out her picture and put it next to Dean's name card and a picture of cookies.

Mrs. Tucker gave us a fat hamster in a cage. So far we have not taken it out, but we will learn how to hold it gently. Her own little children had it as a pet all summer, so it is used to children.

Yesterday a big spider crawled across the floor. We put it in a bottle so we could study it. While we were talking about it, Mrs. Beck got out the many pictures of spiders and then we drew the body on brown construction paper. The children cut out the body and we cut strips. Each child had to count eight strips for legs. That explains the large spiders each took home. When all the children left, I discovered the sample one had been placed in the doll bed!

Whatever happens to little children, whatever catches their interest, whatever they do or like to do, or should do, or are naughty or good, these things we talk about. Just living together, with the bumps and the fun—those are the things our days are made of. In the beginning they are merely soaking up the experiences, and then one day they will begin to talk—because we are learning to say the sounds, the words and the phrases and simple sentences. *Speech has to be meaningful and fun and natural.* Accept and encourage every attempt to talk. Expand what they say into phrases and simple sentences just as you do for your hearing children who are learning to talk. The important thing is that there is *meaning and necessity for all*

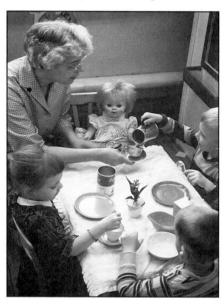

talking. It will be a long time before whole sentences, correctly spoken come out. Because our children are used to being helped and encouraged to repeat, they will become more exact. Accept your child's motions. Give him the words and sentences that he is trying to tell you. It is acceptable to motion back to be sure he has the meaning, but immediately give him the simple sentence or phrase.

Parents and teachers and care givers must participate in all activities to introduce vocabulary and language.
Left to right:
Quinn, doll, Mark and Tom

Photo by James Auer

All should have blackboards. Stick figures will do. When I drew the picture of the hamster on the board and a carrot for it, Tod immediately drew several more. Guess he thought the hamster looked hungry.

I hope we get some good weather—dry and warmer. We will walk over to the park to see and feed the deer and ducks. And to see the bear cubs, the fox and the wolf.

I see that our room is to arrange for the first PTA meeting on October 15. Doughnuts or pumpkin pie squares should be seasonal. The school has a large coffee maker. The PTA pays the cost and we usually put out a dish for coffee money. Parents may wish to bring friends and relatives. The Ben Casey movie about a deaf child has been ordered. The PTA officers will send out flyers to get an estimate of how many will attend. It will be in the library at Webster Stanley Junior High. See you there.

July 1967

The Institute for Parents of Pre-school Deaf Children at Delavan will start August 6 through August 9. There will be a limited number of baby sitters. Mr. Huff wrote: "We just can not take care of youngsters under three years old."

Last year I taped all the meetings at the three day Institute, so as the year progresses, we can review them. It will not be the same as being there in person to see the school, yet we will cover the same topics in our evening meetings.

We will plan eight evening meetings for this coming year: four in the fall, and four in the spring.

There have been seven new children asking for admittance into our school so far this summer, ages 5 through 13. Our school is looking for an additional teacher. All this has bearing on the Infant Program.

Two hour sessions are all the little ones can profit from.

Because of the dangers in transporting such small children and there will be no older children in the return home, we must consider this carefully.

Most cities complain about the mid-day extra trip and cannot always arrange it. (Appleton picked up the five-year-olds at 11:10 and often did not get the children home until after 1:00 p.m. We cannot tolerate this with three-year-olds.)

Drivers must be 21, pass a driving test by the state patrol, carry heavy insurance, and be under contract to the school district—therefore, parents cannot just form a car pool. Your insurance companies will not hear of it—that is, will not allow it.

The recent rubella epidemic has increased our Infant enrollment. In the past only one to three little ones have entered in September. So far this July we have 13. So this calls for changes and innovations.

We hope to continue the parent oriented program and this is the proposed schedule.

1. Monday, Wednesday and Friday—Mothers bring the children and stay in the classroom 9:00 to 11:00 a.m.
2. Tuesday and Thursday—Mothers stay with the children 9:00 to 11:00 a.m.
3. One afternoon a week, Mothers and children, 1:00 to 3:00 p.m.

We suggest that the children who will be three by November take advantage of the three mornings a week.

Four children on my list have not yet had approval for school and must do so before September from the Supervisor of the Bureau for Handicapped Children.

I will continue to make home calls during the year, October through April. The hope is that you will learn to instinctively take advantage of everyday, on-going experiences in the home to encourage your child to lipread and to talk. It is the all day, constant awareness of talking about what is going on that will give your child the head start he needs.

Let me know which schedule you feel you can follow. And what problems this may mean for you and your family.

Last year three mothers drove. There are usually about six mothers driving in all grades. I think there is a total of 16 drivers, one Fond du Lac, two Neenah-Menasha, and four Appleton and Oshkosh two. Transportation is our biggest problem, next to finding teachers and classroom space.

Definite schedules will not be made until the last week in August when the teachers return and the enrollments are put into final line.

Enclosed is the order form for the identification bracelets. On line two put the parent's name, on the last line put your phone number and the word deaf. Don't bother about age.

Send in the possible plan you think will be best for you. This will help in our planning. Do send any other suggestions you may have.

1968 to 1969

Comment: By this school year all the post-rubella children had been enrolled and the program included 26 preschoolers. Four periods were necessary to accommodate classes of no more than nine students. The total school enrollment was 90 with ten teachers.

This was before the high school program was initiated. The older students continued to have classes at the junior high school. The older students had typing, shop and home economics and physical education, and art class.

The large enrollment meant that the elementary classes had moved to three grade schools—wherever there was room. It was another year or so until the program developed so that all the elementary students were together in one building. The final plan put the students in an elementary building that fed into one junior high school and then on to one senior high so that friendships continued. And most important, the regular staff and the teachers of the deaf worked together.

· · · · ·

Shirley

1961-64

After removing items from Shirley's mouth such as an open safety pin, a bit of chewed construction paper, a bent tack, someone else's gum, a rubber band, a puzzle piece or chewed crayon—and lastly, her thumb, the lesson could begin. Well, not quite yet. She would no doubt fall between the chairs, have her shoe off, want to love you, knock over the equipment, and have to get a drink of water. Through all this Shirley stayed remarkably good natured, was thrilled when it was her turn for a lesson, and wanted to please in every way. At the end of her second year in school she had made great strides in all her endeavors.

Shirley, the eighth child, came into the world prematurely as her mother hemorrhaged and Shirley was delivered Caesarean section. Her mother died two days later of internal bleeding. At five months Shirley had meningitis. She was left profoundly deaf.

Shirley had a great deal of motor involvement. Fortunately the speech muscles were not as severely included in this injury. However, her eyes were, in that she had difficulty focusing—but mostly it was a matter of perception. The first year in school, at age three, she was constantly moving and into everything. We had to come to harsh terms about touching things on my desk and the belongings of the other children. She had to be helped down the seven steps to our room, and was rigid when doing so. She fell constantly, but got gayly up. She could not ride the bike nor sit in the swing. She was toilet trained.

Shirley's first year was, fortunately, Peter's third. Other than for individual lessons, Shirley did not have the attention span or the ability as yet to be part of group work. She could not, simply could not sit for any activity. The women who helped in the nursery dearly loved Shirley. She had to be continually watched. Eventually she was almost the only child who went up and down the steps in an adult fashion—rather than one step at a time. She had to be put on the bike and her legs made to pedal. She could not guide the bike that first year.

Now in the third year she still had to be right in front of the example on the easel to be able to make a copy. She was so easily distracted by the other children and could not focus more than two arm lengths away.

The day we made construction paper tulips, most were able to cut out the parts. For Shirley I pasted the stem and leaves in place. Shirley put the flower more or less in place, but the pot was at a haphazard angle right in the middle of it all.

She did not care much for puzzles. And after three trials with Casuist Form Board she continued to make the same mistakes and could not solve it without suggestions. The Kohs Block Designs were impossible. All the other

48

profoundly deaf children could construct several patterns—many without help.

Shirley's speech was progressing. She was a natural mimic. But on her own she said only a few words. Lipreading was poor as her visual memory was limited. However, she had learned to handle a scissors and could color neatly. She could draw a few things on her own. She could button her coat, and sit for a story or movie.

Her limitations were great, but she was a happy child and anxious to please.

Shirley would enjoy whatever life had to offer.

Author's Comment
Shirley was employed at the Oshkosh Work Adjustment Services, Inc. I found her in charge of a project.

· · · · ·

Wautoma, WI
January 23, 1965

Dear Mrs. Ferris:
Thank you so much for your prompt encouraging letter. If at all possible, Dean and I shall try to be there for the time you can set aside for us. If not, I will let you know; but I do so want to bring him. I will try my hardest to get someone to take care of my other 21 month old son and the one yet to be born this February.

Dean is now working on the 7th and 8th lesson in the John Tracy Course. We started with the course a year ago and probably would have been done by now, but we slipped up somewhat during the summer months due to the fact that most of our time was spent outside. Even now, I find Dean is happier if he can be out in the barn helping daddy, pulling milk cans at times to the barn on his sled, or grading snow off the front walk with his grader.

Dean understands quite a few commands in lipreading, and we are quite sure he understands the following words- "hot, baby, bye-bye, shoe, potty, milk, bed, mama, daddy, car, ball, tractor, bottle, and boots." We are working on "apple, airplaine, snow, bread, butter". We always try to use these words in sentences. He has moved his lips to the word "hot" and does a fairly good job of saying "bye-bye". We are also working on animal names and colors.

Dean is a very active little three-year-old. He sleeps well at night, but isn't too fond of afternoon naps lately. There are times when he shows a great interest in learning, and will even go to the cupboard for his lesson material. Then again there are times when he'd rather go ahead with his own interests rather than be bothered by lessons. It is usually best at these times to let him play, as nothing much gets accomplished without both of us getting upset, so we try our best to take advantage of these times when he is willing to cooperate.

Like most boys his age, Dean enjoys playing with trucks and tools (screw drivers, wrenches, hammers, etc.). Just recently he has shown more of an interest in watching television than ever before. Lots of the programs, I find, have good lipreading. Also, he likes to cut paper to pass the time or play with clay.

He likes to be helpful in the house as well as in the barn. He will help clean, wash and wipe dishes, bake, dress his brother Brian. Brian doesn't especially care for this, but Dean enjoys trying. I have been encouraging Dean to dress and undress himself and he is coming along quite well.

I hope this covers most of the things requested, and will be of some help. If you should think of anything else, do let me know. (Oh, Dean weighs 30 pounds and has a good appetite most of the time if he doesn't lunch too much between meals.)

On the boarding home policy, I believe the child must be four years of age when he starts or will be that old the same year.

Sincerely yours,
Mrs. James Blader.

* * * * *

Dean and Katie Blader

Dean's Mother Continues

Dean and Katie Blader were married April 1986 and live in a new mobile home on Dean's grandfather's farm. He learned a lot about farming from his father. Dean and Katie hope to eventually buy the farm.

Dean attended the day classes in Oshkosh until age nine when he transferred to the Wisconsin School for the Deaf in 1970. He graduated with a scholarship in 1980 enabling him to attend technical school. All of the other students were hearing, but with the aid of an interpreter he took classes in agriculture mechanics and learned about machinery repair.

He also worked for Katie's father on their farm in Columbus where he learned about the milking parlor, harvester silos and the computer feeding systems. He also worked for a tobacco farmer.

Dean met Katie through their mutual friends and all the young people have remained close. They are all married and were attendants in each other's weddings.

A year after his marriage, he had a serious illness, but has completely recovered. He now has a job at the Square D Company in Oshkosh that makes electrical and medical supplies. He helps his parents on their farm when needed especially when Brian is traveling.

Katie attended school in Madison and had speech therapy. She has excellent speech even though her mother and father and four sisters are all deaf or hard of hearing. Katie feels Dean lost the speech he had by depending on sign language.

Katie worked for Electric Data Systems before moving on the farm. She now has a job with an insurance company. She likes to cook and can. They both like to garden and they are raising a few beef.

Dean and Katie will eventually own the farm as farming is in their blood.

Author's Comment
Mrs. Barbara (James) Blader furnished the details of her large, energetic family. She wrote an article for the John Tracy Clinic and one for the United Methodist Women. She has much to say to parents who have hearing impaired children. Her stories give hope and encouragement.

· · · · ·

Robyn, A Sister's Story

Siblings are as important as the parents in the life of hearing impaired children. Robyn's story about her feelings for her brother, Dean Blader, emphasis this importance.

Dean, My Brother
The first and for most significant event that put my thoughts into perspective was a brother handicapped by illness. Because of my brother's deafness, I have learned to respect and admire handicapped people. I probably would have shunned or shied away from people with handicaps. I now look up to them. I have learned a whole new language. I find sign language to be interesting as it is beautiful. If you've never seen a song signed, you've really missed something. It's the most beautiful, fascinating thing you could ever witness. Two of my favorite songs were signed at my brother's wedding.

My brother Dean had spinal meningitis when he was 14 months old leaving him profoundly deaf. My parents were devastated. They knew so little about deafness, yet they were determined to make their little boy's life as normal as possible. Mom enrolled in the John Tracy Correspondence Course. Through this course we learned how to communicate with Dean. It

51

was fun and exciting and Dean was eager to learn.

Before Dean was four years old he began classes at Oshkosh School for the Deaf and Hard of Hearing. He had to stay in a boarding home during the week. This was a sacrifice we all had to make. We knew the adjustment would not be easy even for a hearing child. He was able to come home every weekend. The going back was always the hardest thing for everyone, especially Dean.

Before his ninth birthday, he began classes at Wisconsin School for the Deaf in Delavan, Wisconsin. Oshkosh at that time did not have vocational training for the deaf. Also Dean could learn sign language which he really needed because of his profound hearing loss. The adjustment was even harder for us because we could not get him home every weekend. He had to stay for a longer period of time. During this time we could write Dean.

In 1980 Dean graduated with a scholarship enabling him to attend technical school. We were all so proud of him. We felt our efforts had been richly rewarded.

Last year, April 19, 1986, was Dean's wedding day. The wedding was beautiful, and the interpreters signed the songs so gracefully. Friends and relatives talked of the beauty and joy of that day for quite sometime. We all thought Dean had found true happiness. He married a beautiful girl who, too, is deaf. After a ten day trip to Hawaii, they returned home to stay with us until their new trailer home was ready.

After some searching, Katie, Dean's wife, found the job she wanted with an insurance company, and Dean started working for dad on the farm.

All seemed to be going well until Dean started having health problems. After much testing, the doctors confirmed he had cancer. We were all devastated. The doctor gave us encouragement by saying this type of cancer responded well to treatment and many people had been completely cured. Dean showed us all a lot of courage and will-power going through this ordeal. He got very sick and lost a lot of weight from the treatments.

Dean was cured.

From watching Dean over come such extreme misfortunes, I've learned a lot about courage and determination. I have also learned there is no obstacle so great that it can't be overcome.

· · · · ·

Jenny

1987

I really enjoyed our conversation over the phone (TDD) the other night. I have found some time to write about my school and work.

52

Starting at age three (1965), I got my initial start at receiving excellent education from Mrs. Ferris and other teachers. I remember very well learning to speak and read lips, reading and writing, as well. I had remained in the program for the Deaf at the Oshkosh schools until the end of my eighth grade. At the suggestion of both my mother and Mrs. Ferris, I was asked if I wanted to attend my local high school. I always wanted to, so my mother went in to fight the teachers, school board officers, and those who were opposed to the idea. We won the battle, therefore I had later more than fulfilled my mother's wishs. I made the honor roll and was inducted into National Honor Society. Boy, did I ever prove that even I, with the aid of an interpreter, could do it in a public high school! Upon graduation from high school, I attended Fox Valley Technical Institute (now College) for two years, studying Pulp and Paper Chemical Technology. I received my Associate Degree in that field.

Presently, I am employed by Nicolet Paper Company, DePere, WI, as a lab technician. I get along with the people at Nicolet very well and they are very well aware of my "invisible" handicap and limitations. Some of these people are curious about the way I cope with my problems. I tell them about myself, so they can understand better about where I stand. They have been very helpful to me. They know I am very uncomfortable in group discussions and that I understand best on one-on-one. If all else fails, I do it by paper and pencil. It can be very frustrating for me, but I try to ask questions and learn.

My favorite saying is, "Every time I speak, I practice. With practice, I improve." My previous experience with lipreading and speaking during my high school and post high school years play a big part in coping with the problems I encounter at work every day.

I married a wonderful man not too long ago. He has been very helpful and patient with me. I guess you could say we both are in the same boat, for he is hard-of-hearing. He understands my problems only too well because he has the same problems. He is able to speak on the phone and tries his best to interpret some things like the news on television (which are not closed-captioned for the hearing impaired). We both wear hearing aids in both ears. We have two phones with volume control. We have a TDD and I am always calling my mother, sister, and my sister-in-law, all of whom have TDDs. We also have Tele-Caption device so we could enjoy the closed-captioned programs even more. My husband did some wiring in our house; now I know when the phone is ringing when I am in the living room or in the bedroom (with the use of Fone Flasher, which can be purchased at Radio Shack). I have a flashing alarm clock. It is also very nice to have the Relay Service so I can call my friends who don't have a TDD or even order a pizza!

Author's Comment

Recently I attended the baptism of Jenny and Mark Dillard's third daughter—all hearing children.

Mark worked in Appleton as an airplane mechanic until the Midwest

Express transferred to Milwaukee.

His father was a pilot in the Air Force in Guam when Mark was born. To find good schooling for Mark, he retired and became a commercial pilot. Mark learned to fly as a teenager. He has a pilot's license and can fly in and out of small fields using sight as he does not hear well enough to contact the control tower.

Jenny's mother, Mrs. Van Straten, drove Jenny to school the thirty five miles every day when Jenny was three until she finished eighth grade. Mrs. Van Straten started a business in Oshkosh rather than make two round trips.

Their stories point up the tremendous effort their families exerted to obtain a good education for their children.

· · · · ·

Are You The Fellow
Who Is Taking Us Guys Home?

Gregg was a perfectly normal almost four-year-old lad. One morning he turned on the TV cartoons, as he always did, but he got no sound. He was furious.

He had lost his hearing over night.

The family doctor was puzzled and made immediate arrangements for Gregg to be seen at the Mayo Clinic. In taking his medical history the nurse asked his mother what childhood diseases he had or had been exposed to. His mother reported that his sister had mumps several weeks earlier, but Gregg did not catch it—he had no fever, no swollen glands, was not irritable. He did not have mumps his mother stated.

Ah, but he did. The virus did not show the usual symptoms, but the infection attacked the eighth nerve and his hearing loss was severe. It is rare that mumps attacks both ears, but it had in Gregg's case.

Gregg entered my class in December immediately upon the return from the Mayo Clinic. The family doctor was married to a former teacher of deaf children and he knew how important it was to get Gregg immediately enrolled in the nursery class.

He still had perfectly normal speech. One day a different driver called for the children and Gregg asked him, "Are you the fellow who is taking us guys home?" A deaf child, deaf from birth or before developing language and speech, would not be capable of such a complicated question for many years.

However, as time went on, Gregg spoke less and less. I could not encourage him to continue the normal four-year-old chatter. He was interested in the cars and trucks in the classroom and enjoyed playing with the other children. But getting him to talk about the play activities was not often successful. Lipreading is not learned immediately. Paying attention to facial expressions or lip movements were not able to interest Gregg, even though he had a wonderful background in language—nearly all the language forms he would ever need. That changeover was not easy. He received no feedback when he talked to the children or adults, so he used his speech less and less. Research revealed that is a normal experience when a young child suffers a sudden severe hearing loss.

The following years he learned to read easily because he had the rich language background. However, his speech lost much of its naturalness. This is true for adults who suffer severe hearing loss—they too lose natural intonations. We monitor our speech by that used in our community. Our hold on the quality of our speech is that tenuous.

Gregg continued in the Oshkosh program for the hearing impaired and was helped somewhat by wearing hearing aids. Signed English was introduced while Gregg was in the elementary grades. His mother acted as a teachers' aide in his school, so the whole family learned how to communicate with Gregg.

Gregg reports that in junior high it was so noisy that he discontinued wearing the aids. Interpreters accompanied the students to regular math and science classes as well as other classes.

In junior high he participated in track and basketball and continued basketball in high school. Regular school transportation was not offered for after school activities. He writes he was, "Thankful to my Mom and Dad for their encouraging me to play in these sports and for their time to drive from Appleton to Oshkosh for the years I played in these sports."

Gregg's wife Jackie is also deaf and had attended Delavan, so sign language is the choice at home.

Trapper, their faithful Hearing Ear Dog, has helped them for eleven years. He alerts them to environmental sounds. And he can accompany them whenever they go on a bus, airplane, in a restaurant or store. He has a license and a special leash.

Gregg works in the Oshkosh Post Office as do several other hearing impaired people, both men and women.

Gregg teaches CPR through the Red Cross to hearing impaired people and to interpreters and teachers of deaf and hard of hearing people. He says, "I will not work with hearing individuals who are not familiar with sign language as there might be confusion due to the interpreters."

In a phone (TT) conversation with Gregg he says, "Hearing parents can learn sign language to communicate such as my family does. It is important that there is love and patience. My family had these and we continue to have our love bond as we all have patience with one another. That is the key to success—to develop communication between two different worlds—Hearing and Deaf."

Love and patience. Can anyone ask for more.

· · · · ·

Patrick Laux—Civil Engineer

Margaret asked me to write a short story about my education while growing up as a deaf child. She can be very persistent and has a way of making you feel guilty.

My deafness was caused by a bout of spinal meningitis at 3½ years old. Actually it was some drugs that did the damage to my ear nerves. The hospital stay was about 13-14 days, mostly in isolation from other patients. Meningitis is a very contagious disease. There is this one vivid memory from the hospital stay. The nurse asked me if I wanted a glass of water. I just knew what she said, but I did not hear her. Another memory is when my dad was putting on my clothes and getting ready to go home.

Soon afterwards my parents noticed something was wrong with me. They thought it was a balance problem—something with my bones. And my voice trailed off at each word. There was failure to respond correctly to questions and to respond to noise.[1] After several medical diagnoses, a hearing examination showed complete loss in the right ear and 90 dB loss in the left ear.

Schooling began early at 4½ years of age at the Oshkosh oral program. Mrs. Ferris was my first teacher. My first recollection was always wondering what was going on behind the wall divider. Mrs. Ferris would come over and take someone behind the wall divider. Mrs. Ferris always smiled. Finally my turn came. There in that room the word "ball" was connected to the subject matter—a red ball.

Mom said that I was looking forward to going to school every day, waiting for the driver to take me there.

My next three teachers in the deaf program were Mrs. Kiser, Mrs. Sitte, and Mrs. Mitcheler. In Mrs. Kiser's class there was always this thing with the

---

1. Patrick Laux's parents recall the many doctors they visited to get an answer to Rick's constantly falling down. It was several months before one finally said it was a side effect of the meningitis and recognized his hearing loss. They took him to speech correctionist, Miss Grace School, who began work to restore his speech. It was she who recommended the Oshkosh Program for Deaf and Hard of Hearing Children.

56

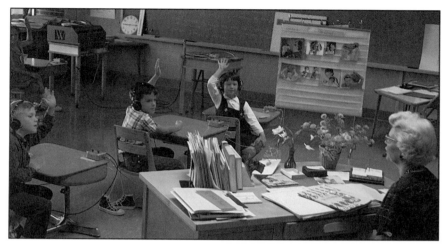

Mrs. Vanita Kiser is teaching a lipreading class. The children are wearing head phones. Patrick is to the left, Mike and Karla.   Photo by James Auer

bulky head phones. Mrs. Mitchler was sometimes hard on me, probably thinking I was not really trying.

Another memory that I recollected is my brother learning how to ride his bike without the training wheels and going into the prickly bushes.

The first attempt at mainstreaming occurred at 9/10 years old at Emmeline Cook School in Oshkosh. There were three other hearing impaired children with me: Cindy, Jolene and Sharon. We were there for half days. We did not have any support of any kind in that class other than sitting in front of the class near the teacher. One memory was having apprehension sitting in the circle waiting for my turn to read out loud.

My next school was the local elementary school at Edison School five blocks away from my house in Appleton. The school placed me in the third grade instead of fifth grade. The logic at that time was to be in the same classroom with my sister who was in second grade—a combined grade.

Two grades, fourth and fifth were completed in one year. Mrs. Zerbe was not willing to let me skip sixth grade to be with my age peers.

Mrs. Zerbe always had me write down new and unknown words for speech therapy training with Miss School. Probably this is where my reading habit was developed and carried to this day. Speech therapy was a lot of fun pronouncing and learning new vocabulary. This kept me abreast with the other kids.

The next school was Roosevelt Junior High School in Appleton. There was a different teacher for every subject during seventh grade. It was something of a novelty to me to keep track of everything. At the beginning of eighth grade this one English teacher had the students placed in alphabetical order.

My seat happened to be in the very back. The teacher thought my hearing was good enough and that I was playing games with her. She made me stay after school as punishment. My mom had to come in to straighten everything out. By then school was becoming somewhat of a bad experience. Question and answer sessions were going back and forth in the classrooms. It was difficult/impossible to keep up.

The speech therapists there were not helping me to keep up my speech. The last speech therapist said that it was NOT NECESSARY for me to come in anymore. Now, looking back, it was obvious that either they did not know or care how to do their jobs.[2] However, most of the teachers were good and gave me the individual attention that was needed when I came in after class.

For high school, my parents sent me to J.F.K. Prep located in St. Nazianz, Wisconsin. J.F.K. Prep was a private, boarding, co-ed, ecumenical, non-graded high school. My brother went there for his freshman year, and my parents perceived that more attention would be given since the average class consisted of 10-15 students. It was a very good school for me. Again here was an opportunity to catch up with my peers. Course work was completed in three years instead of four.

To become acclimated to a large population and environment, my last semester was spent at Appleton East High School. My plans were to go to college as an accounting major. My admission eligibility was accepted by two colleges—Carroll College of Waukesha, Wisconsin and Edgewood College of Madison, Wisconsin. By the end of my senior year it was obvious to me that my heart was not in accounting.

My folks recommended me to try the National Technical Institute for the Deaf in Rochester, New York. At first my reaction was rebellious and full of skepticism, Why would I go to a Deaf School? My dad said, "It's just for the summer. Just go and check it out."

NTID was just like one big family. There were people just like me. People whom I could identify with, people who grew up like me. It was great. Everybody was using sign language and people were getting on my case for not signing. It was easy. I picked it up very quick and never took any sign language classes. It came out naturally and so relaxing. It was (and still is) a pleasant form of communication. During the summer vestibule program, from all the various career exposure and sampling, the civil engineering technology program interested me the most. Today I am a Civil Engineer. The funny thing is—I still like it.

Nobody said it's going to be easy. There are always some form of obstacles to overcome whether they be physical barriers or covert/overt discrimina-

2. Few regular speech therapists, at that time had experience with hard of hearing or deaf children. Today emphasis is placed, not only on vocabulary development and articulation, but also on voice quality, phrasing, stress, breath control and lipreading.

tion. Every deaf and hard of hearing person has to face it. It's a fact of life. You have to try and fight at least twice as hard to get where you want to be.

The world is getting better. Fax machines, and electronic mail are helping. Conversation over the telephone with the relay system. Soon there will be video phones.

Passage of the Americans With Disabilities Act has accelerated the progress towards equality and heightened people's awareness. This does not mean you may rest on your laurels. You still have to fight for your rights.

Communicate with your child the best way you know how. Take a pro-active role in your child's education. If your child is utilizing a hearing aid, keep the child in speech therapy (my opinion). Buy a decoder, a TTY, video tape player, CC tapes, flash cards.

Finally I would like to thank all those people who helped me when I was growing up, especially my mother.

* * * * *

Washington, D.C.

By Heidi Burghardt Guzman
Member of the U.S. Treasury Department

The critical element in helping a deaf child move successfully throughout his growing years is parental guidance and love. Another important element is *Communication*. This is what I learned as I went along in my life . . .

I graduated with a Bachelor's Degree from the University of Maryland. There are many deaf people who have earned Ph. D Degrees. Dr. Robert Davila, a deaf man, was recently selected by President Bush to be the Assistant Secretary for the Office of Special Education and Rehabilitative Services in the Department of Education.

After the historic demonstration at Gallaudet University in 1988, King Jordan became the first deaf president of the University. The U.S. Congress, with whom he is in close contact, holds him in great respect.

In Washington D.C. many deaf people work for the Federal government, some in important positions. There are deaf lawyers, stockbrokers, dentists, business men and women who graduated from Gallaudet University. There is an organization called the "World Federation of the Deaf", where there are deaf leaders from all over the world who meet like those in the United Nations. Those deaf leaders play important roles in our lives and in the deaf generations to come.

I could babble on and on about the success of deaf people, along with a long list of their names, but the point is "deaf people can do anything but hear," which is Jordan's famous sentence and which the world is slowly beginning to realize.

Despite the success of deaf people, there is still a vast amount of discrimination in every part of the world, which is another long story but in the long run, it is a good and beneficial experience for all deaf people to have had to fight for their rights.

I have been profoundly deaf all my life and was two years old when I first learned how to speak and read lips. When I was three years old I attended the School for the Deaf in Oshkosh, Wisconsin. At the age of eight, I was mainstreamed into Appleton public schools. I was one year behind regular hearing students. I graduated from Appleton High School-West and went on to the University of Wisconsin in Oshkosh. Two and a half years later, I went to Gallaudet University as an exchange student. I was planning on staying there for one semester, "to get my feet wet in the deaf world," before returning to Oshkosh to complete my degree. That turned out differently. I ended up staying for another semester—to 2, 3, 4 years. It has been seven years now and I still haven't moved back to the state of Wisconsin.

What have been my experiences as a deaf person? There were advantages and disadvantages. When I was a kid, I wanted to be like other hearing people. I had many hearing friends in my neighborhood and had many cousins I could play with. Those kids always treated me as one of them. Why was that? I believe it was the kind of behavior my parents had towards the kids and adults. My mother told me that when I was a little girl, I once asked her "Are there deaf kids who are also handicapped?" My mother knew then that I didn't think of myself as handicapped. I believe that when other people saw how my parents and family treated me, they felt I was like them, so I had a very healthy childhood and was always a happy kid. I will never forget how, when I had to wear hearing aids to the school for the deaf, I would come home and take my hearing aids off immediately. Why was that? No one in my neighborhood had a hearing aid. I wanted to be like them, and I was determined to be treated like them. I was very ashamed of my hearing aid . . . I hated it! Poor mother would struggle with me every day to wear my hearing aid. She finally gave up when I started going to public school.

While at the School for the Deaf, which was an oral school, I never learned how to sign except for the gestures I made up with my deaf friends. The administration strongly believed that it was important for deaf kids to learn how to read lips and talk. I never learned how to sign until I decided to attend Gallaudet University as an exchange student and their rule was that I had to use sign language to be accepted as a student. As required I took a sign language class in Appleton, but my signs didn't improve until I moved to Washington and started communicating with other deaf students.

After many years of learning about myself and learning from other people re: bilingual, I came to realize the importance of learning bilingual language especially for a deaf child. Why is that? I felt that I missed an awful lot while growing up. I couldn't read everyone's lips like a pro. For example, imagine yourself watching your favorite T.V. National News (ABC with Peter Jennings, maybe?) and turn off the volume. Jennings is looking at you, not moving his head sideways or looking down. Can you read his lips? People who talk softly would be difficult to understand whereas it would be easier to read the lips of people who speak loudly—but do I know what I think they are saying? I couldn't be too sure. With a sign language interpreter (and this I came to realize after years with an interpreter at college and at work), I didn't have to worry about my doubts. Instead I could relax and be able to concentrate on my conversation, rather than concentrate on the person's lips, whether I understood what the person was saying or not. So, my point is, if the parents of a deaf child came to me and asked what I would do if I had a deaf child, I'd say, "Teach him/her sign language from the very beginning." Then if the parents wished, the deaf child could learn to talk and read lips more efficiently when he/she has a natural language of the deaf. I do regret that I hadn't learned sign language early, I wouldn't have had some hardships that I had to face while growing up. I'm not blaming anyone for this matter, I know everyone did what they thought was best for me. But I wouldn't encourage the teachers and administration to continue this method of teaching orally only and prohibiting sign language.

When I learned how to sign and had many group conversations, I became more sensitive about my deafness than I ever was when I was in the hearing world. I began to see how much I had missed. I was more sensitive in family gatherings. Before I went to Gallaudet, it never bothered me to be in the family gatherings and not know what was going on. I just didn't realize what I

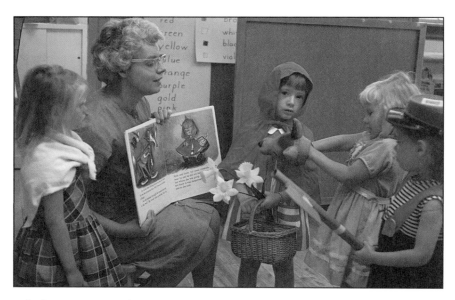

Acting out the stories is not only fun, but introduces creativity, spontaneity, language and better understanding of the stories.
Left to right: Diana as grandmother, Heidi as Red Riding Hood, Deborah as the wolf, and Quinn is the hunter.   Photo by James Auer

was missing. Afterwards, after many gatherings with the deaf people, I started to hate being with other hearing people because I knew I couldn't catch up with them as easily as I do with the people who knew sign language. I then started to resent hearing people. I was going through a hard time with my identity. I even had some anger towards my own family (after all the good things they did for me during my growing up years).

My family has been extraordinarily great—my parents, Bruce and Joyce Burghardt, my sister Cindy and brother Dave along with their spouses Jeff and Cheryl (whom I have grown to look at as another brother and sister.) Their caring, attention and understanding and above all their love have made me the way I am today. I have grown to appreciate them more as I got older. After my Gallaudet days and my second language being sign language, my family kept saying, "I should learn sign language" or "we should have learned sign language earlier." My parents, in fact, took a sign language class shortly after my engagement to Rafael. But the difficult part for them was not being around us as we are 1,000 miles apart and they don't have enough association with other deaf people in order to keep up with their signs. My sister Cindy, who took sign language lessons with me, still signs although not as fluently but impressive for someone who doesn't have daily communication with a deaf person. My brother Dave, who I now see once a year, hasn't learned signs but has always shown his interest in the deaf issues. What amazes me is Cindy, Dave, Jeff and Cheryl have understanding about the deaf even without me explaining in detail.

From what I've heard and seen in other families with deaf children—I would encourage the families to learn sign language as soon as their child is exposed to it in order to communicate more efficiently. I didn't have communication problems with my family on an individual basis but I was lost in their group discussions. I couldn't follow word for word so hence I missed a lot of points in the conversations. I know no one meant any harm but this habit was hard to break—I'd ask, "what is he saying?", someone would say, "oh, I'll tell you later", then forget all the details of some of it later on or they would say in short sentences but not as satisfying for me—with all the bottom lines which I understood but was hungry for more information. I was always filled with curiosity while growing up. My favorite questions were, "why . . ." or "what . . ." or "how . . ." Other deaf children would feel left out, frustrated and angry for not knowing what's going on. So, my bottom line is, *learn to communicate with your child and ensure that your child is part of the discussion but it has to be in his natural language.*

How did I make it through public schools? and why did I go to Gallaudet University? My first teacher in public schools was a very good teacher, understanding and helpful. She actually "paved the way" for all my later teachers in elementary school, who were patient and helpful throughout. I always sat in the front of the class (which I hated but later accepted). I didn't have or want a note taker or interpreter in elementary school. If I needed help, I would ask my teacher later . . . I was determined not to be treated as a teacher's pet. I made it clear to my parents that I wanted to be treated like other students and my parents must have told the teachers because to my knowledge, I wasn't a teacher's pet, and no one made fun of me.

At first my mother met daily, after school, with my teacher in order to help at home with any necessary tutoring. Later, she would meet once or twice a week with my teachers and was always available for special meetings or consultations. Both my mother and father helped me at home to understand my daily class work and this went on all through my public school years.

In junior high school, I had my first difficult weeks. The kids, who came from other elementary schools, made fun of me (and my deaf accent). For a while I hated every minute of it and was frustrated. I would go home all upset and my mom would encourage me to think positive. Her philosophy, and which I came to use in today's society, was to try to have at least one good loyal friend and then nothing else matters. I became fast friends with one to two to three girls in my junior high school classes. They were as sensitive and vulnerable as I was which was why we became fast friends. If other kids made fun of me, I ignored them. To this day, whenever I bump into them at the bars or at parties, they treat me as they treat other friends and they have more respect for me today than they did in junior high school. As the saying goes, teenagers have a hard time growing up.

When I went to high school, most kids were mature and understanding. I made many friends but I was vulnerable the whole time. The only thing that really kept me going was my family who had faith in me and the good friends I had. My mother's philosophy always stuck in my mind. My brother once mentioned that you treat others the way you want them to treat you. I kept that philosophy too. It worked. I was the first profoundly deaf student to mainstream successfully in Appleton public schools. I was busy thinking about having friends and "just making it" through my years at public schools. I also had a childhood friend, Rozelle, who substituted for my sister when my sister was away at college. She was two years and three grades older than me. She, too, helped me make it through my years and is my treasured friend to this day.

Speaking of academics, I did well when I wanted to do well. I did earn A's in some courses and in other courses I received B's but, overall I was a C-average student when I graduated at age nineteen. I had note takers in junior and senior high school. I would carry a tape recorder with me in some difficult classes (math and science) and my dad would listen to it at night and help me with those courses. My mother would help me with English, social science and history classes. The teachers in the Appleton school system were all helpful and understanding and had a lot of patience with me. They cared about me and wanted to be good teachers. My parents continued to meet with the teachers on a regular basis which also contributed to my successful completion of public school.

I followed my sister and brother's steps and went to college. I thought of going to college out of town but I got scared and wasn't sure if I could stick to it. My dad suggested I try Oshkosh and commute which I did. The first semester was not easy. I wanted to make friends but it wasn't easy when I didn't live in the dorms. I made the first semester with the note taker, but I wasn't satisfied. I arranged to move to the dorms the next semester. I made many friends that semester. I would join parties with my friends and go to the bars with them. I stayed at the University of Wisconsin-Oshkosh for two and a half years until I took a social work class with a very understanding professor. She knew my interest in working with deaf children. One day she called me after class and wanted me to make an appointment with her in her office which I did. When I met with her in her office later on in the week, she asked me how I was going to learn about working with the deaf children if I grew up in the hearing world and had no contacts with the deaf people. Of course this was something I had never thought of. I was so engrossed with my own social life and trying to make it through college. She then told me about Gallaudet College (now Gallaudet University) in Washington, D.C. The idea of going to college in another state appealed to me. I loved to travel and found it exciting and interesting.

My professor called the social work professor at Gallaudet and told her about me. The professor at Gallaudet then sent me materials and applications. I applied to Gallaudet as an exchange student immediately. A few months later, I received a letter from the Administration saying I was approved. I was ecstatic, but I had no idea how much it would change my life. In January of 1982, I said good-byes to my family and started on the road which was the beginning of my life in the deaf world.

As soon as I touched the grounds at Gallaudet, I was struck by all the signs flying by other students. I took classes under professors who used sign language. I had a hard time understanding them and had to borrow notes from my classmates. (This was no different from my hearing classes.) Through the orientation for exchange students (which Gallaudet calls special students) I made friends with my classmates who were all hearing students enthusiastic to learn sign language and to learn about the deaf culture. We would get together at the end of the day and talk about our frustrations with other deaf students who didn't trust us. I had a hard time with the deaf students because they called me a "hearing person" in a sarcastic way because they knew I was totally deaf but couldn't sign as fast as they did. Despite the hard times I had, I was deeply engrossed with the deaf culture. I was slowly beginning to understand my identity and after all these years of not accepting my deafness, I was slowly beginning to accept it through the deaf people. They taught me something about being deaf that hearing people could never teach me. As the months flew by, I became good friends with other deaf people. Through them, I was able to understand my frustrations and anger.

My sign language improved a great deal by communication with the deaf people and they came to accept me as part of their world. I was very happy.

When the spring semester drew to a close, I knew I wasn't ready to move back to Wisconsin. I had to stay a bit longer and learn more about myself. In order to support myself throughout the summer, I applied for and got a job as a summer-aide with the United States government.

As the summer drew to a close, I knew I had to pack my suitcases and go back home. Then, all of that changed when my boss talked me out of it. He wanted me to remain and continue school at Gallaudet University. That was another decision I knew I had to make. I weighed the pro's and con's and came up with more pro's for staying in Washington, D.C. Why was that? I wanted to stay in the deaf world, I loved my job which turned out to be glamorous and exciting (I was able to go into the White House on errands which I loved). I loved big cities. I then called my parents and told them my decision, wrote a letter to the wonderful academic counselor at University of Wisconsin-Oshkosh and told her that I wasn't coming back at all. I applied for another semester as an exchange student at Gallaudet and was again approved. Things were falling into place and I was happy with my decision. My friends were happy to have me around longer. As the semester went by, I wanted to transfer my credits from the University of Wisconsin to Gallaudet but due to their different systems I would lose a lot more than was necessary so I then decided to transfer to the University of Maryland where most of my credits from Oshkosh were accepted. My job was still exciting and the people I worked with were understanding and fun to be with. I was very proud to be part of the U.S. government family and still am. I later was promoted to a full time job which was when I dropped out of school. (I was having a hard time running back and forth to school and my job.)

A few years later I realized that I just couldn't go on with my life without a college degree so I went back to the University of Maryland as a part-time student. During my last one and a half years at Maryland, I decided to go full-time (to hurry and get my degree) and also remain in my full-time position. It worked out well and in 1988 I earned my bachelor's degree at University of Maryland with a psychology major.

Upon receiving my degree from the University of Maryland I applied for and accepted another position within the Agency. My work continues to be exciting and challenging.

I am currently involved with the deaf community especially at a local deaf club. I was the Publicity Director last year and was Secretary to the President of Metropolitan Washington Association of the Deaf (MWAD) a deaf club in Washington D.C. It all got started when MWAD sponsored my participation in the Miss Deaf Maryland Pageant in 1987. I was Second Runner-up and voted Miss Personality in the Pageant.

Altogether, my life thus far has been rich with experiences. There are still frustrations and anger, but I am still learning and will continue to learn for as long as I live.

Someday, I hope to fulfill my dreams and work with deaf children and encourage them to meet their dreams and to enjoy their lives in both hearing and deaf worlds. My goal would be to see deaf children become more successful than we deaf adults are in today's society. By the time they get older and on their own, there should be less discrimination in their society and they will have even more opportunities than we have had.

I agree with King Jordan . . . "Deaf people *can* do anything but hear!"

Father's Comment

Heidi wrote the above in the summer of 1988 just before her marriage to Rafael Guzman. Heidi and Rafael, also deaf, met while she was in Puerto Rico on business. Rafael is employed by the Department of Justice in Washington D.C. Their first child, Jessica Marie was born in February of 1992 in Washington, D.C. Jessica is hearing and is learning to communicate with both signs and voice.

* * * *

V

PARENTS CAN MAKE IT HAPPEN

1961

Parents Can Make It Happen

It was early spring of the year I returned to teaching that the Parent Teachers Organization made a scholarship available for a high school graduate that would be interested in becoming a teacher for deaf and hard of hearing children. I spoke up and suggested we should wait until the student was in the junior year at college and ready to choose a major. In short time the parents told me that there was only one student graduating in Deaf Education at the University of Wisconsin-Milwaukee, the only school in the state offering that program. The need for teachers was desperate and we should help a young person from our area.

The following year our college professor, Alice Streng, wrote to the day classes in the state that Senator Alexander Wiley of Wisconsin was sponsoring Public Law 87-276[1] which would set up an appropriation of $3,000,000 for scholarships to train teachers of the deaf over the next two years. These funds would cover tuition and living expenses for young people who might otherwise find it impossible to take the training in this field.

I thought about this and came to the conclusion that "the government giveth and the government taketh away." The needs of the profession were on-going. We needed to solve the problem of encouraging "many young people" to become teachers over the years. We had a good school in Oshkosh which serviced hearing impaired children from ten counties. We could demonstrate the career to Future Teachers and college age students in this large area. We were frequently giving demonstrations to organizations. Certainly they would donate toward such a good cause.

I presented the plan at the next Parent Teachers Organization and 12 parents joined the enterprise. Deaf Education Aid Fund, Inc.—D.E.A.F. Inc.— was born and existed for 12 years. We assisted 19 students to become teachers of deaf and hard of hearing children. Several on our Oshkosh staff ·were recipients.

Parents and teachers spoke to civic organizations, church circles, lodges, career days, and many other school meetings. Wherever people gathered, we

---

1. P.L. 87-276 did pass September 1961 and was followed by several more laws that included training teachers in all the special education fields. President Kennedy signed a new bill—Public Law 88-164 on June 30, 1964 saying ". . . no law providing facilities can be effective so long as there is a persistent and nationwide shortage of qualified personnel to instruct the handicapped." At this time he also announced the establishment of a new division in the United States Office of Education to administer the teaching and research program under this Act— called the Division of Handicapped Children and Youth and will be headed by Dr. Samuel Kirk, who is now Professor of Education and Psychology and the Director of the Institute of Research on Exceptional Children at the University of Illinois. (Dr. Kirk was the Director of Exeptional Education at Milwaukee State Teachers College when I attended there.)

spoke. We wrote letters, we held dances to raise funds, we put displays in store windows, and at libraries. We wrote newspaper articles. We contacted high school and college advisors and counselors. We were on television and radio. We wrote to foundations and businesses in our area. And gifts were generous.

One person could not have accomplished this. The parents, many in addition to the original volunteers, grandparents, friends, all helped. Parents made it happen.

* * * * *

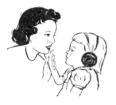

Deaf Education Aid Fund, Inc.

Recruiters of Teachers of the Deaf
A NON PROFIT TAX EXEMPT ORGANIZATION

CORPORATION MEMBERS

Leonard F. Becker
Thomas T. Evans
Mrs. Thomas T. Evans
Mrs. Garwood Ferris
Mrs. A. Charles Kessler, Jr.
Mrs. Maynard Mathison
Henry Pauli, Jr.
Mrs. Henry Pauli, Jr.
Mrs. Raymond Pfeiffer
Donald E. Rawson
Mrs. Donald E. Rawson
Mrs. Harry Roley, Jr.
Mrs. Donald Theisen
Averill Wiley
Mrs. Averill Wiley

HONORARY DIRECTORS

John W. Melcher, Director
  Bureau for Handicapped Children
  Assistant State Superintendent
  Department of Public Instruction
  Madison, Wisconsin

Samuel D. Milesky
  Bureau for Handicapped Children
  Supervisor of Schools for the
  Deaf and Visually Handicapped
  Madison, Wisconsin

Maxine Bennett, M.D.
  Professor and Chairman
  Division of Otolaryngology
  University Hospitals
  Madison, Wisconsin

James S. Veum, M.D.
  Pediatrician
  Appleton, Wisconsin

Alice H. Streng, Professor
  Education of the Deaf
  University of Wisconsin—Milwaukee
  Milwaukee, Wisconsin

Philip J. Schmitt
  VRA Fellow
  Institute for Research
  On Exceptional Children
  University of Illinois
  Urbana, Illinois

Judge James V. Sitter
  Winnebago County Court
  Branch 3
  Oshkosh, Wisconsin

Perry A. Tipler, Superintendent
  Oshkosh Area Public Schools
  Oshkosh, Wisconsin

Mrs. Ted Hoyer, President
  Ted Hoyer and Company Inc.
  Rehabilitation Devices
  For the Handicapped
  Chairman, Governor's Committee
  On Employment of the Handicapped
  Oshkosh, Wisconsin

Peter J. Owsley
  Assistant Headmaster
  Pennsylvania School for the Deaf
  Philadelphia, Pennsylvania

Rolland C. Nock
  Director of Special Education
  Appleton Public Schools
  Appleton, Wisconsin

Robert E. Rucks
  Director, Pupil Personnel Services
  Joint School District No. 1
  Fond du Lac, Wisconsin

Helen V. Halpert, Director
  Speech and Hearing Clinic
  Wisconsin State University—Oshkosh
  Oshkosh, Wisconsin

Harold Homann, Ph.D.
  Assistant Professor
  Speech and Hearing Clinic
  Wisconsin State University—Oshkosh
  Oshkosh, Wisconsin

751 London Street
Menasha, Wisconsin
October 1965

To GUIDANCE PERSONNEL
  Of Public and Parochial
  High Schools and Colleges:

Deaf Education Aid Fund, Inc. was organized to interest capable young men and women in the very challenging field of Education of the Deaf; and to offer scholarships to those in need of financial assistance at any time during undergraduate study.

In the *HANDBOOK OF SERVICES* published by the Wisconsin Bureau for Handicapped Children, March 1964, the following guidelines are offered for recruiting teachers of handicapped children:

  1. All the qualities of a good teacher but to a greater extent
  2. A mature personality
  3. Tolerance for frustration
  4. Professional competency

The Teacher of the Deaf is a specialist in the Communication Arts. The applicant must have normal hearing and dentition, good diction, and a creative and lively interest in spoken and written language. Therefore, the scholarship committee requires a comprehensive evaluation of the applicant's oral and written language ability by his present English instructor.

Guidance Personnel are urged to encourage the sensitive, outstanding students to explore all areas of Exceptional Education, to visit classes, to assist in church and recreational activities for the handicapped children. Students should gain some meaningful experience before making a decision to teach the deaf.

University of Wisconsin-Milwaukee is the only training center in the state for teachers of the deaf; therefore, the students should plan to attend Milwaukee as soon as possible. To delay until the Junior year will require two additional summer sessions.

Sincerely yours,

Margaret H. Ferris

Mrs. Margaret Ferris, President
Deaf Education Aid Fund, Inc.

VI
RUBELLA EPIDEMIC
1964

Rubella Epidemic Runs Its Course
1964-65

In June 1964 the Board of Health reported in the Appleton *Post-Crescent* that the Rubella epidemic, also known as German Measles, had run its course. Dr. Laird said that during the course of the German Measles outbreak, "there were no serious side effects reported".

In March prior to this report, I broke out with German Measles. If I at age 44 had the measles, how many young pregnant women were infected? I foresaw, in bold headlines, the tremendous increase of hearing impaired children.

And so it was. German Measles, also called Rubella, a three-day mild disease can cause havoc in the first trimester of pregnancy. A child can be born prematurely, have a heart condition and cataracts, and a hearing loss. Where my preschool class might have three or four new students a year making a class of eight toddlers, three years later the enrollment was 26 as a result of many mothers having had Rubella.

This large number of preschoolers required program adjustments. As no class could accommodate more than eight preschoolers, some came Monday, Wednesday, and Friday mornings, others Tuesday and Thursday, and several afternoon sessions had to be established.

And this was the time I encouraged the mothers to attend so they could learn how to continue the speech and lipreading at home. It was still an oral program.

Congenital Rubella Syndrome—C.R.S. 1993

From the April 1993 issue of the Diocese of Green Bay the following report appeared.

Rubella, most often referred to as German Measles, can be avoided through the use of vaccines. This was not always the case. In the mid-sixties an estimated 20,000 to 30,000 children were affected by a nationwide Rubella epidemic.

The Helen Keller National Center-Community Education Department has been maintaining records in regards to the issue of late onset manifestations which are occurring in young adults with C.R.S. Medical conditions such as diabetes, glaucoma, thyroid dysfunction, drastic weight gain and other symptoms are being reported by individuals, families, and caretakers around the country. Anyone interested in learning more about these records and the family-to-family network developed by HKNC should write to:

C.R.S. Late On-set Survey • c/o Ms Nancy O'Donnell • HKNC/Community Ed. Dept. • 111 Middler Neck Road • Sands Point, NY 11050

Please send $2.00 to cover postal charges.

While all post rubella children will not develop these symptoms as young adults, there is cause to be aware of the possibility. Regular health care check-ups are recommended.

. . . . .

Neighbors

The Redmond family with several children lived across the street from my home in Menasha. The spring that I had German measles, Mrs. Redmond had caught it from her children. However, she was in the first trimester of pregnancy. And Jim was born with a profound hearing loss.

I learned of her infection some time later. Because we were apprehensive that Jim would be deaf, I began holding and playing with Jim and showed Sally Redmond how to help him. Jim was the youngest child to be tested and fit with a hearing aid at that time.

Mrs. Redmond brought Jimmy to school. One morning her older boys ran home to tell her Mrs. Ferris had a bear. She said they had to be mistaken. However, when she and Jim entered the classroom, there stood the mounted bear cub. It was a gift from other parents and had been in a granary for years.

We often visited the small zoo in the park, but now we could touch the bear. How much more interesting—to feel its fur, see its claws and talk about how it lived.

1984
Jim writes: I graduated from Oshkosh North High School in 1984. I worked at a bakery and a wood working place until I got my job at Oshkosh Post Office. I am a postal clerk there and I am happy with my job.

I bought a new truck and I drive 50 miles round trip everyday.

That is not all that Jim is happy doing. He is married to a hearing young woman and they bought a home south of Oshkosh. His wife Paula has graduated in Exceptional Education from the University of Wisconsin-Oshkosh and is teaching handicapped children. They went together for seven years before marrying. Paula has good signing skills and is accepted by the deaf community. Both young people continue to have friends in both cultures. They have the best of both worlds.

Now, several years later they have a hearing infant.

Author's Comment
Jim Redmond's sister, Lynn, 18 months older, was his companion and learned to sign at an early age. Lynn Behnke became a Registered Interpreter.

She says her little girl Nicole is learning to sign so she can visit with her Uncle Jim. This family shows the dedication that assures a successful life for the hearing impaired member of the family. Understanding and action, not tears, with a wholesome outlook is every hearing impaired child's birthright.

· · · · ·

Questions Parents Ask

A formal visit a teacher makes to the home of a student does not reach down into the real concerns a parent has. Even for the mother who accompanied her child to class, it was some time before she could express her feelings.

Through the years, in each of the several classes, the same questions were asked. The hearing impaired child was usually not the first child in the family, but the training that had worked for their other children did not always work for the hearing impaired child.

The mothers, and often grandparents, aunts and uncles, and siblings— even neighbors, came to school with the children. Gradually the barriers fell away and they sought each other as parents who shared a problem and looked for help, not only from me, but from each other.

In the early years the department for the deaf and hard of hearing children had a strong Parents Organization. At these meetings the parents of the little children could benefit from conversations and programs concerning the older children. However, these parents of mostly post-rubella children were the first to be enrolled with their children.

Slowly the questions emerged.

What do we do with the child who constantly gets out of bed during the night or very early in the morning? The child who will not settle down?

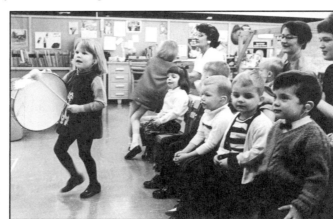

Preschool children and mothers

Photo by
Oshkosh Daily Northwestern

73

Together we struggled for solutions. A hearing child can hear the family moving around, hear the T.V., hear the voices of mother and dad. The hearing child knows the family is there. However, the hearing impaired child is completely shut away when he is in the bedroom. So he constantly comes out to see if the family is still there.

Our hearing impaired child needs a night light.

Leave the door open.

Can have favorite toys and stuffed animals in bed.

Go in frequently and tuck him in, hug him, but make it plain that he is to stay in bed.

A warm drink of milk at bed time is said to induce drowsiness.

Under no circumstances give the child any sweets in the evening as sugar is a stimulant. Pop leads to the need to go to the bathroom.

Does not go to bed until the family goes to bed.

No family wants a whining, over tired child around all evening.

Start to bed a few minutes earlier each night. Eventually get the hearing impaired child ready earlier. Make a show that the other children are taller (that is how children determine ages) and can stay up a little longer. Dad has to read the paper.

Mother has to do some task.

This will take time to establish the new habit. But keep at it.

Eating during the night.

Many reported that the child got several bowls of cereal during the night. Parents left a glass of milk in the refrigerator. They said it was better than having the child try to pour milk from the bottle. One mother bemoaned the fact that her child got ice cream out of the freezer and left it on the table— the whole gallon—to melt, or ate a whole can of chocolate syrup.

Put a loud sounding bell on the refrigerator door that will wake you if the door is opened.

One parent suggested a bell on the child's bedroom door, but we thought this door should not be closed. All bedroom doors should be left open so the parents can hear any child who is sick or moving about at night.

Another mother put a couple of sets of metal measuring cups along the hallway floor. In the morning the cups were neatly stacked! Another mother woke to the smell of cooking. Her young son was frying an egg! This same mother reported later when her son was seven that while camping he was missing when they got up. They rushed to the lake and met him coming back with a string of fish. He had even taken the row boat out. So this restlessness and difficulty recognizing danger extends beyond the toddler stage.

Mothers were worried about the medicine cabinet and the cupboard under the sink where dangerous products were kept.

Buy cupboard locks at the hardware store. Certainly these should be put on the medicine cabinet and the cupboard under the sink or wherever dangerous products are stored.

Even the vile taste of dangerous products does not deter any child from taking a drink. One mother called me early one fall evening to say her child had drunk bleach from a bottle in the rubbish at the curb. I said take her to the Emergency Room immediately. She said they were waiting for the cab to do so. (To this day I cannot imagine even thinking about the preschool teacher, much less calling her, at such a stressful time.)

Wants to get in bed with parents every night.

We all agreed you had to stand firm on this. This was before the study that says the family bed is acceptable. We did not think it was a good idea as it could cause parents to miss getting their rest as children are restless sleepers. And allowing it only prolongs the time for the child to mature.

Until the time my girls were two and four years old, there were French doors between our bedrooms that we left open. When we moved into our next home, the children slept upstairs and were fine. We did not have the bed time problem.

I was not aware that this was so pervasive a problem with even normal hearing children until one of my own daughters had this problem with her middle child. The third baby was born when Katy was only two years old. Katy would sit on the arm of her mother's chair while she nursed the baby at bed time, and scream if put in bed. My son-in-law would lay down with her, but it took a long time before Katy could go to bed on her own. Breaking that link with mother was difficult to do, especially when still a baby herself. You can't reason with a tired hearing toddler, nor with a tired hearing impaired toddler.

Bed wetting up to age ten.

One mother had this problem with the older hearing children. She did not want to go through this again with her hearing impaired child. We reasoned that if this happened there might be a physical reason and she should consult a physician.

Do not shame the child.

No liquids in the evening—not even the warm milk.

Toilet training.

As one of the mothers had four other children before the hearing impaired one, she would not put up with "late development of toilet training". She reasoned that there was nothing else wrong with her son and he could learn to go to the toilet just as her other children had learned. It took more persistence, but she won the day.

Eats only ice cream and peanut butter.

Fortunately both are good for the child, but not enough even with vitamin pills.

One mother used the technique of saying "Mrs. Ferris says to eat your vegetables and meat." However, this back fired as the child answered, "Ferry (Ferris) no meat."

Fortunately lots of play and good exercise encourages a good appetite.

Again my own experience was that one daughter liked only radishes, olives and mustard. (These items must have more nutrients than we thought.) I had to be careful to put relishes on the individual salad dishes. Hid father's extra ones under the lettuce leaves.

Spoon fed the children until they were five years old.

We doubted if a child would starve if expected to use his spoon. I am sure you have seen the remarkable scene in the movie or play, "The Miracle Worker" where Annie Sullivan fought with Helen Keller to use her spoon.

North High School in Oshkosh put on the play and one of our hearing impaired high school students was Hellen Keller. The fight was so strenuous the spoon flew off the stage. One of the members in the audience had to throw it back on the stage so that Annie Sullivan could get Hellen Keller to use the spoon.

Temper tantrums: Throws self on the floor constantly at school and at home if he does not get the bike, the red pencil, or be first.

This can happen at the super market, on the playground, at home or at school. Both boys and girls have tantrums. If the child is not in danger—not in the middle of the street, walk away and ignore the behavior. (Hard to do in the supermarket!)

The child wants attention. Many of these behaviors happen in all families with normal children. Deafness should not be an excuse for allowing the children to take advantage of you.

One lad in the preschool class would sling a heavy oak chair when he did not win or get his way. He had to sit in the hall briefly to calm his feelings. One day he threw the chair half-heartily and then went into the hall by himself. That was the last time he threw a chair.

Scratches and hits and bites other children at school and at home.

Separating the children helps. Isolate the naughty one. This eventually will carry the message that such behavior will not be allowed.

Bangs the table to get more or get attention.

"More" is an easy word to say or sign. The child can learn this general term before he learns the names of food. Say it each time you give the child more. (In speech or in sign.)

Throws the food which he does not like on the floor.

Put him down and away from the table. (Read Kristine's Life). Ignore his tantrum. Deaf parents' deaf children throw their food on the floor only once as these parents know that deafness has nothing to do with this behavior.

Fights with siblings.

One mother reported she could not leave the baby alone in the room with her deaf preschooler as he would bang the baby's head on the floor. We all agreed this was jealousy and parents have to give extra love to all the children.

Simply refuses to do things: come to eat, get dressed or undressed: go to school or go home.

Again, a good dose of ignoring will eventually bring the child around. However, if the school bus is waiting, you have to firmly dress the child.

When to spank. When to isolate the child. When to set him on a chair. (Getting him to sit there is another matter.)

We all realized that you cannot reason with a hearing impaired toddler and if he runs into the street, a swift swat on the seat of the pants is necessary. Spanking for all transgressions becomes ineffectual. Save punishment like that for really serious situations. And it must be done immediately in the situation. To bring the child back into the yard or into the house will not have the desired effect as if done at the scene.

Little children have short attention spans. It is doubly true of our hearing impaired toddlers. And one does have to understand that many of these children have additional handicaps. If so, it may take longer for the child to understand and learn.

Uninhibited behavior.

Our children miss the interplay of social relationships. Here our facial expressions have to stand in place of the tone of our voice.

All animals and birds have warning signals for their young. Normally we convey danger, the limits of acceptance by the tone of our "no". Or we divert the attention of the toddler by saying, "Look out the window and see if Daddy is coming." We use language to inform, bribe, influence, cajole, warn, amuse, teach, motivate—all these things are impossible until the child has some grasp of language—whether it is oral or sign.

A hearing impaired child does not recognize danger. He goes right ahead with what interests him—out in the street, up the ladder, into the lake. Pushing others, taking their toys, whatever he wants to do or get. I recall visiting in one home when my kindergarten student climbed up on the kitchen cupboard. She wanted to show me the new dishes her mother bought. How else could she tell me? Today with Total Communication she would have the sign language. However, she still would have to climb up there to show me the dishes.

How much responsibility must our other children have for watching the hearing impaired one?

If the other children are asked to watch him, a time limit must be set— while mother goes to get the clothes out of the washing machine. Limits must be set—not to go outside or into the kitchen. Stoves have a fascination for all toddlers.

The other children become very aware if the deaf child seems to "get away with actions". Under no circumstances should you say or convey the feeling that the hearing impaired child must be catered to or excused for his behavior.

All the children must have duties. This is so for the hearing impaired child. This child can set the table, feed the dog, get dad's slippers. Help wash the car, but it is recommended that the windows be rolled up! One mother was not quick enough to catch her daughter sprinkling the car with the hose. It took some time to dry the seats.

Teasing.

Even siblings are guilty of this as well as other children. Only patient explaining about the problem and the hearing aid helps. T.V. is filled with people wearing mikes and head sets. Radio Shack has inexpensive mikes and head sets that you can purchase and have the other children experience listening through the ear phones. What family today does not have a Walkman radio with ear phones?

This is the time one can encourage other children to include the hearing impaired child in play. Have lots of play equipment in your home and yard and direct play to teach taking turns and sharing. Sharing does not come naturally for any child. It is something the children learn by doing and being praised.

The child needs to wear the hearing aid at all times.

There is insurance for hearing aids—even adults lose and break theirs. Do not put the hearing aid away at home. The child needs it when he plays. *Play is what children do.* It is in play with other children that he learns how to get along, and to take turns. *He needs to hear a car horn.*

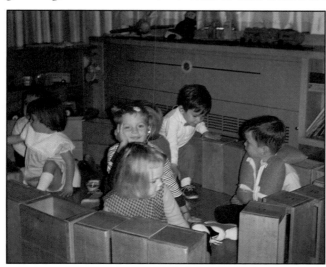

Toddlers in a boat. One child is wearing a life jacket.

"We are off on a cruise."

78

All remark how stubborn the hearing impaired child is.

Before he can tell what he wants or feels, he stands pat. It is his way of protecting his inner being. He has yet to learn how to express his feelings and needs.

Why does it take so long to learn to talk?

This was still an oral program. (Even if sign language was used in school and the parents were learning to sign—the toddler would have a limited vocabulary.)

One mother of a two-year-old said she had not thought that the deafness caused by meningitis would affect her child's speech.

If the child gets no feed back, the speech fades in weeks.

A father suggested that when the child learned to read would he not understand. As though a deaf child could learn to read or talk without language.

Sign language has no relationship to spoken or printed words. A deaf child can be a proficient signer and understand all that is going on around him—but he will not understand the printed word. He has to be taught. Our normal six-year-old children have to learn how to read and they come to school with a wealth of concepts, a huge vocabulary that they understand and use. They learn to sound out the words. But our hearing impaired child has a much more limited vocabulary and is just learning the English language.

What do the older students do?

This was before our department for the hearing impaired had an integrated high school program.

These very parents along with the teachers developed such a program at North High School. This story deserves a separate chapter.

Today our students graduate from high school and many attend technical schools and colleges. Others learn on the job. They all find work in the community, marry, have children and are contributing citizens.

· · · · ·

Kristine's Life
1979

By Phyllis Clarke

I'd like to share some of my feelings and problems with you on raising a deaf child.

My daughter, Kristine, is now almost thirteen and growing into a nice "calm" young lady.

When Kristine was two and a half years old, she contracted spinal meningitis, which left her profoundly deaf. She has no residual hearing which every deaf child is supposed to have and has never registered on an audiogram.

She has always been a very active and curious child.

She had quite a lot of speech before she became deaf, but then lost everything.

There were many exasperating moments when she came home from the hospital—she couldn't understand me and I couldn't understand her, which led to many temper tantrums.

Once it took me an hour to get Kristine to not come to the table with her winter coat on when it was 96 degrees. I would send her back upstairs to take it off and she'd appear with it on. Then I would scold her and she'd throw a chair down the stairs and this went on for almost an hour. Finally she appeared at the table without her coat.

Sometimes she'd get so mad and frustrated she'd run up to her room and slam the door and the door knob would go through the plaster board.

At that time I knew no signs and she knew none. We communicated by pointing and facial expressions so I'd let her get away with more. Then her brother and sister would say I babied her because she is deaf. Then I'd yell at them for talking to me like that. Then we would be into another family argument.

It was very easy to feel depressed once in a while.

I didn't really know anything about deafness and was surprised to find out that her deafness would effect her speech, language, education, understanding and sociability. I thought she'd keep all the speech and language she had, but she didn't. Sometimes if she was upset, a perfect phrase would come out and then I'd try to get her to say it again, but nothing happened.

Today with all our modern advances there are still many misconceptions about the deaf—even among professional people and media.

It upsets me when people come up to me now and say Kristine won't have problems because lipreading is so easy. As if the deaf can take a six weeks crash course in lipreading and all their problems will be solved.

Kristine had problems with fluid in her ears and ear infections. When I'd take her in, the doctor would talk to her (he also had a long mustache). When Kristine couldn't understand, I'd interpret for her and he snapped at me— "Maybe if you didn't sign for her she would be able to lipread and talk."

Just recently I took her to her orthodontist and he is super nice to Kristine and invited her to go sailing this summer, but only if she'd take a lipreading course and learn to lipread better.

They don't understand that if you don't have the language or vocabulary, you won't be able to lipread it anyway. Only 25 percent is lipreadable.

I think much of the public thinks of a deaf person as hard of hearing or that they have all the language background and understanding, but that they just can't hear. A lot of them assume that she is up to her normal age level in everything.

Safety

I've felt concern for Kristine's safety at times. When she was three, she walked away once, so we got her an I.D. bracelet and it came in handy several times.

When she was seven, I was going to the store at 6:30 p.m. I told her good bye. (She was at the neighbor's swinging.) I had returned home for a while and saw a squad car pull in the driveway. He came in and said, "Your daughter is lucky to be alive. She just missed getting hit by a train and a car. A man brought her to me." She was going into town to tell me to remember candy.

Swimming at South Side Beach in Oshkosh, Kristine almost drowned. I would panic and yell at her, which of course did no good. Then I put her over by the chinning bars and she fell there and cut her lip and was bleeding all over. A man who ran to help her, couldn't understand her.

It's frustrating to always have to run up to her to tell her something instead of just calling to her.

One day I saw her bike at the edge of a lagoon behind our house and I had to go looking into the woods near-by before I found her.

Kristine has gotten good about looking both ways when she crosses the street, but crossing alleys, driveways, or parking lots scare me at times.

Once we were walking out of the Ponderosa restaurant and she ran ahead and a car was backing out, and she ran right up to the back of the moving car. Again I screamed, but it didn't do any good.

Leaving church we all climbed into the car and the usual fight to see which child would sit by the door. Well, it was Kristine and she didn't hear that the door didn't shut tight and she fell out when we went around a corner.

I never used to think much about Guardian Angels, but I think there must be one with Kristine.

I've had problems of *sociability. When she was very young, the language barrier didn't seem to be such a problem, but the older she got the more evident the problems became.*

I also feel that any handicap puts a strain on the family.

81

Just before the punch line comes on an interesting T.V. program, Kristine will turn to everyone and say, "What? Why the boy sad?" And someone will say with a scowl, "If you'd watch, you'd know." Then I'll get mad because everyone is scowling at Kristine and all of a sudden there's an argument going on.

She sees her brother and sister going to the YMCA, listening to records, talking on the phone, and listening to T.V.

When we are on a trip and traveling at night and it's dark and we're all listening to the radio and talking and there's Kristine just sitting there. I am sure that instances like that must be very boring.

One time Kristine was playing with a neighbor friend and all of a sudden she came home early and I asked her why and she said, "It was boring." Later the mother phoned and said another girl came on the scene and was laughing and making fun of the way Kristine talked.

Then Kristine would cry and ask, "Why do I have to be deaf?" There are some heart breaking times, but I feel she must learn to accept her deafness if she is ever going to be happy.

Sometimes, when at the table the whole family is together, we're all laughing and talking and then I remember that Kristine is getting nothing unless I interpret it. She must feel very left out at times.

It got to be that there weren't a lot of friends for Kristine right in Oshkosh, and she wanted to visit Delavan (The Wisconsin School for the Deaf), because she had heard about it from some of the kids at Lion's Camp. So we went down to Delavan last May to visit. She liked it so much that she got mad that she had to come home with us.

She now likes it very much at Delavan. She has made lots of friends and has joined Girl Scouts and other social activities.

I feel that she's developed more self-confidence by being accepted as a deaf person and not always having to compete with the hearing. Parents' Day example—father taking her back, he said, "There's something to be said for being in the majority."

Once I had not heard from Kristine for three weeks and I had crying jags and chest pains so I went to the doctor and he said I was having some trouble adjusting to the fact that Kristine could get along so well without me.

I don't mean to sound like everything has been negative. I have met many wonderful and interesting people through Kristine. I have a nice job as an interpreter for the deaf students at school. There are more programs and church services being interpreted—more improvement in hearing aids and TDDs. Good library services are being offered. Kristine's brother and sister have more empathy. I have found out how wonderful people are when you have problems.

• • • • •

Kristine Clarke

I lost my hearing when I was two years and five months from Spinal Meningitis. I am profoundly deaf. I started learn sign language when I was three years old. I went to Public Lincoln School. When I was young, I didn't accept that I am deaf. I was unhappy sometimes, even though I have a wonderful family. My mother is interpreter and my family knows sign language too.

I went to Lion's Camp when I was eight or nine years old. I never forgot that I was very shocked and thrilled to see *many* deaf children (about 150 deaf children included boys.) I met many deaf children who went to the Wisconsin School for the Deaf (W.S.D.). I told my parents about that. They decided to send me to W.S.D. when I was twelve years old. I was surprised to see several deaf teachers work there. I was really looked up them. They are the best role model for the deaf. I was very *happy* at W.S.D. because I felt so normal and not felt isolated anymore. There were so many activities that I could participate such as Girl Scout, drama, sign song dance, sports, Jr. N.A.D (National Association for the Deaf). I was vice-president for Jr. N.A.D. and class of 1985. Also, I was secretary and treasurer for Student Body Council. I involved volley ball team for four years, cheer leader for boys basket ball for three years and track and field for four years. I learn a lot from W.S.D. They really taught me many things. My personality growth a lot too. I graduated from W.S.D. in 1985.

I enrolled Gallaudet University in 1985 fall. I was so culture shocked out there because there are so many deaf students (about 3500) and also, many deaf staff and faculty.

I really love Gallaudet University so much. There are various—hard of hearing, oral, and deaf. It is really interested to meet many different people. I involve some activities such as Student Body Government and jobs. I worked

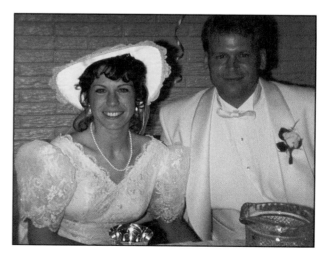

Kristine married John Misko in the summer of 1993. They are living in Warren, Michigan. Kristine has enrolled in a local university to complete her work for her degree. John, also deaf and from a deaf family, works in the post office.

as student Resident Assistant for two years. Then I work as Peer Advisor for freshman dorm for one year. Now I am working at Abbey (snack bar). My major is Psychology. I will graduate from Gally in 1991 then I will study Parents Infant in Master Degree.

• • • • •

"No room! No room! They cried when they saw Alice coming."
—Alice's Adventures in Wonderland

Parents Need Love Too

Pam sat quietly in the back seat of the family car holding a piece of paper on which her mother had written, "We will go home and pack a picnic lunch and then come back to the park to eat and play." A pleased expression played across Pam's pixie features. Pam, a five-year-old profoundly deaf child could lipread simple sentences, but to be sure Pam understood her mother wrote the message. As soon as they entered the house, Pam ran to the cupboard and got out the picnic hamper.

It had been a cold, bright Monday morning, February 14, 1966, that Pam's parents brought her to my nursery class of deaf and hard of hearing children. Pam had delicate features, bright blue eyes that did not always focus, and an unsteady gait. She was three years old. She was not toilet trained.

Her parents feared this would mean she would not be accepted. However, every day of every month of a toddler's life is the optimum time for comprehending spoken language and learning to talk.

It was arranged that she would come to school in the van with other little children from Appleton.

Our class was in the old Longfellow Elementary School. We had a basement room six steps below street level, across from the gym, a boys' bathroom, and the boiler room with a huge coal fed furnace and boiler.

It soon became evident that the first task was to keep Pam in the classroom. The class now had eleven small children. Even constant vigilance on my part and that of my aide, Mrs. Ruth Beck, was not enough. So we put up a gate across the doorway. Surprisingly, the other children did not resent it. They could all work the latch, and they seemed to understand it was for Pam. She was not the youngest child in the room but the smallest.

Any attempt at a group activity did not hold Pam's attention. We could all be marching around with paper hats to a drum and fife record, and Pam would wonder off. I was never sure she looked at me. She looked above me, through me, and at far away places only she could see. When we sat at the table to do some activity, Mrs. Beck sat beside Pam with her arm around her to direct her attention.

Early May of Pam's first year was unseasonably cold. One noon the van was very late and as we waited for it, I pushed the children on the swings and we played games to keep warm. We kept expecting the van any minute, but it was a half hour late.

It took Mrs. Beck and me another half hour to put the room in order and arrange for the next day. When I arrived home some twelve miles away, my husband said to call Pam's father immediately at the hospital in Appleton.

The surgeon wanted to know how Pam was when she left school. By this time she had a tracheotomy. Nothing was found in her throat except mucus. Perhaps she had gotten chilled while we waited for the van. Her breathing was maintained by an artificial respirator, and she did not breath on her own for 24 hours. She suffered her first deep epileptic seizure.

It seems Pam slumped over in the van, but the little children often fell asleep on the ride home. The driver had noon day traffic and as long as the children were quiet, he did not notice anything unusual. But when Pam's father lifted her out of the van, he realized she was not breathing and was turning blue. Fortunately, they lived directly across the street from the hospital. He ran with her to the Emergency Room. As it was noon, several surgeons were still in surgery and could act immediately.

Following Pam's recovery, the Appleton school system would not assume the responsibility for transportation. They would pay for it, but would not do it. She stayed home the last few weeks of school.

The following fall Pam's mother drove her to school each morning, but by this time she had three month old baby Missy. One morning Mrs. Johnson arrived in tears. It was just too much to make two round trips through the traffic of three cities and the country road into Oshkosh.

The possibility of finding a baby-sitter for Missy had not been successful, so she had been brought along.

The solution was simple. Bring a play pen and spend the morning. Why it took so long for me to realize the mother could be part of the learning

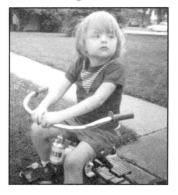

situation still puzzles me. One other mother had made long round trips, so I thought, until I found her and a younger child slumped over in their car in the park where our class went to see the small zoo. They were just asleep, but it frightened me. Another mother got a business going in Oshkosh. Up until this time with Pam the parents had attended a summer session covering the school and home problems of hearing impaired children directed

Pam — August 1966

85

by our principal, Peter Owsley. And I held monthly parent meetings.

Baby Missy was happy watching all the activity in the classroom, and she became the source of natural language. Many of the children had a baby at home. One day we gave Missy a bath. Everyone helped wash, dry, and powder her. We talked about her diaper, her pink dress and sweater and shoes and socks. Missy was our baby.

In the beginning of that second year I thought Pam was not ready for beginning reading, but her mother insisted she understood. So I started her on basic reading of commands, and simple words like "mother, daddy, baby, dog". We had family pictures to relate to the words. Then one day I watched her point to the printed names of wild animals in a book. I put twelve ovals on a large piece of tag board and printed the names in the ovals. Without hesitation Pam placed the natural colored plastic animals correctly in each oval. It was not I who taught Pam to read, she taught me she could read. After that she moved rapidly into language and reading.

Speech development moved very slowly as her cerebral palsy did involve facial muscles. But her lipreading was good.

Pam then moved to the primary department in another building. When she met with problems there she was returned to my preschool class. We too had changed locations, and were now in a new building with a sunny kindergarten room. We had our very own bathroom, and our own safe play yard. We had lots of cupboards and a sink, and plenty of room for our jungle gym, large blocks, and still a large play area. The superintendent was so pleased to move me to this ideal setting. He was only sorry that there was not a see-through mirror so parents could watch the activities in the room. But by this time I wanted the parents right in the room to be part of our activities.

The plans proved difficult to put into practice because it was the time of the influx of many post-rubella hearing impaired children—a class of 26 that fall. So we had to break up into sessions with no more than eight at a time. Some parents did not have transportation, so they came in the van with the children. In no time the state supervisor for the hearing impaired from the Bureau for Handicapped Children visited my room. "Who do you think is paying for all these rides?"

When the program was explained, he patted me on the shoulder and said, "Keep up the good work."

Pam and one other older lad not yet ready for the primary department came every morning. Pam's mother thought that even though it was only a morning session she could work with Pam afternoons. At least by this time the school system of Appleton had accepted responsibility for transportation. It was one of the problems the state supervisor ironed out on his early fall visit.

The following year the Deaf Department in Oshkosh established a primary multiple handicapped program and Pam entered this class. The children were taught sign language and fingerspelling with no effort made to develop speech. I did some speech work with Pam during the summer, but once a week lessons were not sufficient to make a difference.

Some years later the family moved across the state. Letters indicated that Pam's needs were not being met. A part of a year at the state residential school at Delavan, Wisconsin also was not able to help. So the family had arranged for Pam to return to the Oshkosh program. And they were pleased that I was then teaching the high school class for the multiple-handicapped hearing impaired.

A boarding home had to be found. This presented a problem as Pam could not go home every weekend as was the usual practice. She would stay with the boarding family a whole month at a time. The family who accepted her lived some distance from the high school which meant she would have to take the city bus. Pam tended to be a dreamer and the family, rightly so, feared she might not get off at the right stop.

In the past when the city children and boarding children had to learn to ride city buses, the social worker or aides took over teaching that skill. The students had to be taught that they pulled the bell cord to alert the driver to stop. They did not hear the bell, so did not understand the connection without illustrations and much experience. When I phoned Social Services to see who could help Pam the office informed me that her social worker worked part time and not afternoons.

At that moment my problems began with Social Services, and worked to the breaking point. So for several days I followed Pam's bus in my car to check that she got off at the right stop.

For whatever reasons, Pam did not make a good adjustment in the boarding home. The morning of Thanksgiving Mrs. Johnson phoned to say the boarding family would not be home until late Sunday evening. She was uneasy about having to drive across the state at night in uncertain weather. I said for her to come early Sunday for dinner and Pam could spend the night with me. While at my home that Sunday Pam's mother phoned several people. One call was to the social worker at her home. Meanwhile on Thanksgiving I immediately wrote to the secretary of the school where I was to go for a meeting that Monday after school to ask if she could arrange to have an aide sit with Pam while I attended the meeting.

What followed that Monday was a series of misfortunes. Four attempts during the day to reach the boarding home failed. I hesitated to send Pam home if I did not know if someone was there. The secretary at the other school was ill and her mail had not been opened. Pam sat quietly with us through the meeting, and then I drove her home.

The father was furious. "Do you know how worried we have been? Don't ever do that again. Why didn't you phone me at work? The social worker is going to hear about this. Our son ran back and forth from the bus stop and he called me. We have been looking for Pam for an hour." and on and on.

There was no telling him that I too was worried. I had called their home before leaving high school and again on arriving at the other school. He could have called the high school office. It was an unfortunate situation for everyone.

Now I was at odds with the boarding family. They not only wrote to the social worker, but to the principal who directed our program, to my high school principal, and a long letter to me listing the wrongs I had committed.

By Christmas a new boarding home was sought. One was never found.

Pam sat at home until the following fall when her school district made arrangements for her education.

During this time I made every attempt to locate a boarding home. I found two possibilities which I reported to Social Services and was immediately told not to interfere. Finally I wrote to the Assistant Superintendent, Department of Handicapped Children. I had been in college with him many years ago and on other occasions had made my needs known and sought guidance and direction from him.

Much to my shock he wrote back that their office could not interfere with the work of another agency. And because I had written on official school stationery, his answer went to our supervisor, my principal, the director of special education of our system and that of the city where Pam lived.

Shortly following that letter, I was asked to meet with my supervisor and a man from the Madison Bureau for Handicapped Children and told not to interfere with problems that were not classroom related. I was given a booklet on Boarding Homes, the rules and regulations.

Despite the thwarted efforts to help the family, my steadfastness through this time did give them moral support to pursue help in their own community.

* * * * * *

The Tea Party
Only Half A Cup

Did I imply that Pam's home town would work out a program for her? Let us follow the story:

October 25, 1977
To quote from Mrs. Johnson's letter:

Last Thursday we called Dr. Thompson, Superintendent of Schools in Wisconsin. She said she would not be able to do the investigating herself, but would turn it over to one of the assistants. Yesterday Mr. Contrucci called, said Dr. Thompson had turned it over to him and he wanted to call and let us know he was now on top of it. He said it seems some adults have been remiss in doing their duty in seeing that Pam gets an education, and it seems that the truancy law is being broken. He said he was the person responsible for her education. I told him this in itself was a breath of fresh air, because no one up to this point would take responsibility for anything.

November 5, 1977
We had an M-Team meeting yesterday and have the recommendation for La Crosse, and for now, an itinerant teacher for, would you believe, two hours a week—Tuesday and Thursday from 7:30 to 8:30 a.m. I was not too happy about that, but that is all they had here in Eau Claire. Would you write a letter to the teacher and tell her what Pam was doing in class. She said it would take her six weeks to figure out where Pam was.

November 20, 1977
Pam had her first hour at school this Tuesday. All went well until it was time for her to get on the bus at 8:45 to come home. When she got home she was very upset, "Go get Missy. Missy is at school." She had expected to stay all day as Missy did. If not, then Missy must come home.

It happened that our lawyer called four days after our M-Team meeting here. This was before Pam had the hour at school. He wanted to know if we had anything new to report. I told him about the two hours a week in a way that he could not know my feelings. He was quite upset and thought it might be worse than nothing. Dave called him after Pam's day at school and told him her reaction. He was not surprised and told Dave to call our Director of Special Education. As it turned out when Pam did not want to get on the bus at school, the problem had been reported to him. It was just today that Dave talked to him and told him if they could do no better for Pam, we could not send her for one hour and have her upset until 4 p.m. when Missy came home. He said okay that he would call the teacher and tell her that Pam would not be coming again.

All the news concerning Pam is not bad. On Thursday, November 17, Dave, Pam and I went to La Crosse and met Mr. Buisse and then we all went to the prospective boarding home. Mrs. Knutson, whose family is raised and gone, lives alone with her dog. She has been caring for unwed mothers, and is state certified. We visited for two hours. It was a very comfortable meeting. She seemed very understanding. We discussed the problems Pam had before, that the people who had her said she clomped around making so much noise, about being put to bed with a guard, and the fights over when the work was to be done. We told Mrs. Knutson that we expected Pam to help around the house, do dishes, make her bed, and keep her room clean.

The lady's response was, "What are her hobbies? Does she crochet? I can teach her that. Will she make herself at home? Will she find something to eat for herself when she is hungry between meals?"

She raises rabbits to sell for meat—has eight now and two, I think, are ready to have babies. Pam liked that since we have a rabbit. One concern of

Mrs. Knutson and Mr. Buisse was that she can't sign. We both, David and I, said if she will accept Pam as she is and try to understand what she has been through the last year and help her adjust to her new situation, that was more important than being able to sign. All she needed was a blackboard.

She said, "I will probably learn to sign when she comes, just being with her."

We got good vibs, as we did from Mr. Lowry and Buisse the first time we met them. We will be taking her down for an over-night November 30. We will stay in La Crosse too, and pick her up the next day. If it works out she will start school on December 5th.

Thanks for all the information you sent about Pam. As it turns out it is good you sent it to me rather than her teacher in Eau Claire. I will give it to the teacher she will be having in La Crosse, Miss Joan Pitzner. She joined the Tripod Committee last year when we were in Madison at the Governor's Committee. She took over my job as secretary with Tripod. She also belongs to WWRID (West Wisconsin Register of Interpreters for the Deaf) that I joined this summer. It is just a group of people who are interested in the deaf—not certified RID. Some have sign language and some do not. Miss Pitzner does not sign as yet, but has a half-day aide who does and all the kids do. La Crosse, as you probably know, is quite oral. Had signs added just three years ago. Pam will get speech therapy. They don't expect anything more than an attempt at speech. But I think Pam will like that.

The Director of Special Education there, Evan Loury, was a boarding home parent for deaf kids for years—had one child from eight years old until she graduated. So he understands our kids better than most administrators. I really feel good about people in La Crosse—am thinking good thoughts. And the social worker, Mr. Buisse—as you know, I feel good about him.

And Now

Pam finished school in La Crosse. She spent two years at Mrs. Knutson's home and then lived with a family where the husband was deaf and the family used sign language.

For a while Pam lived in a Group Home in Eau Claire, but for the last two and a half years she has lived at home. She works in a Career Development Center. Recently her medication has been changed so that she does not experience mood swings.

She is being fit for a hearing aid and wants to start speech lessons. Her therapist cautions that it might not be too successful at age thirty. However, Pam has always wanted speech lessons. Her desire to learn, now as an adult, may well bring her success.

It has taken a long time for Pam to exert her right to get the services she is entitled to receive.

· · · · ·

Bureau for Handicapped Children

Madison, WI
July 25, 1965

Dear Mr. Milesky:

While you were trying to call me, I was making home visits. However, I am planning to spend the entire session of the Parent Institute at Delavan.

May I say that this traveling about the state in our own area has given me a small idea of the tremendous task you have in covering the entire state! You wrote in the *Amplifier* about the Department needing a Social Worker. I would think you would need a whole staff of them! Those who would be versed in childhood problems and then ones who could give vocational guidance to the adolescents.

Even though I have always included home calls for nearly all of my students, this is the first time I have gone about it in such an organized way. A curious and most wonderful thing happened time after time. The first hour would go with casual conversation and exchange of ideas, and then an imperceptible change would take place, and I found myself in the real world of the parent of the deaf child, and the real concerns. The true picture of the child emerged. Perhaps it was the response of the child (and I always included all the children in the family as they are the ones who can do the most in the hour-to-hour and day-to-day help) that assured the parents that I was sincere and knowledgeable, and for once they could speak their real thoughts and worries. I did not elicit this—it just came about.

Long experience with parents new to this problem of deafness tells me that facts and figures, advice and demonstrations fall on "deaf" ears. They cannot begin to comprehend the total impact until the child has been in school several years. I always know that when the child has finally started to school, they expect a great deal more and immediately! The tiny deaf child exists in a "shallow" world, few associations, little depth of emotion, and always spoiled and given in to. Changes to be made in this area the parents recognize and are grateful for help. Nearly every parent has asked me, "Will my child ever be able to go to regular school?" Isn't that a difficult question to answer truthfully!

I myself would grow faint of heart if I could not frequently sit for an hour or so in Mrs. Sitte's class where my students have moved. Then I can see how well they are progressing.

I do want to address the "gray children"—the children whose slight hearing loss is such that they are not eligible for our program until they are *eight years old*. What our audiologists fail to comprehend is that a hearing loss that is not great is not a handicap when the child is sitting at a table in a quiet room perhaps three feet from them. But in a noisy classroom this is a major

91

handicap—even with a hearing aid. And what makes me so heartsick about the "gray children"—they are the ones for whom we could do the most.

We have been singularly unsuccessful in integrating our students. It has had to be on a sink or swim basis. The parents have been resentful and the regular teachers resentful. And none of this needs to be with proper orientation and using a gradual approach. As individual teachers of the deaf we cannot go barging into regular classrooms. The authority for the program has to come from the top.

We will have time to talk at the Parent Institute.

Sincerely,

Margaret H. Ferrier

. . . . .

Every Child Is Different

In my beginning days of teaching hearing impaired children I said, "A deaf child is normal in every way. He just does not hear." I not only said it, I firmly believed it. But then children were enrolled in my preschool program who did not fit my theory. Some had physical handicaps, others unusual health problems, and most difficult to manage were those with emotional problems or who were hyperactive.

I returned to college for classes in teaching the Exceptional Child at the University of Wisconsin-Oshkosh. At first I sought classes that addressed the specific problems I was meeting in my preschool class, then the Director of the Department of Exceptional Education advised me to work toward a Masters Degree so that my studies would have continuity. I attended night classes and many summer sessions completing my work in 1974.

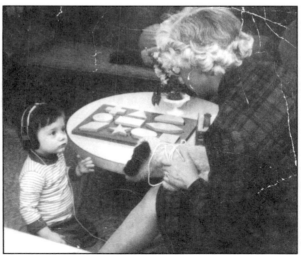

While speaking to a PTA meeting about my teaching, I noticed a couple in the audience were crying. I spoke to them after the meeting and arranged to visit their home. April 1967.

This is the first time Kurt wore ear phones and could hear voices. He entered my class shortly after this visit.

92

VII
AUDIOLOGY

The Changing Profession of Audiology

By Jack E. Kile, Ph.D.

Professor and Clinical Audiologist
Center for Communicative Disorders
University of Wisconsin-Oshkosh
Illustrations by Carol Kile

Historical Perspective

In the 19th century, a number of hearing tests and instruments for assessing hearing were developed due to the joint efforts of professionals in Physics, Physiology, and Otology.[1] The profession of Audiology is relatively new, having existed since World War II. It is the offspring of Speech-Language Pathology, then known as Speech Correction, and Otology. The former deals with diagnosis and treatment/management of speech and language disorders and the latter is a medical discipline involving the diagnosis and treatment of diseases of the ear. The speech correctionists, who worked with hearing-impaired veterans in rehabilitation centers, had the added burden of developing and administering hearing tests, hearing aid evaluations and programs for hearing rehabilitation. The otologists, in addition to addressing their patients' medical needs, were actively involved with the assessment of hearing. The need for another profession, specifically devoted to hearing, was recognized and Audiology came into being in 1945. Raymond Carhart, a speech correctionist recruited by the army to do hearing rehabilitation, and Norton Canfield, an otologist, typically are credited with founding the profession of Audiology.[2] Over the past 48 years, tremendous strides in the diagnosis and treatment of hearing disorders have been made.

Today, audiologists are professionals who hold a minimum of a Masters degree, and have earned the Certificate of Clinical Competence in Audiology (CCC-A) from the American Speech-Language-Hearing Association (ASHA). Audiologists are trained in the prevention, identification, assessment and management of hearing disorders. Many dispense hearing aids and are actively involved in hearing rehabilitation. Employment opportunities for audiologists are numerous and varied. Some work settings include hospitals, schools (Educational Audiology), rehabilitation centers, industry, private practice, medical clinics and university clinics.

Personal Perspective

In the fall of 1966, I came to the University of Wisconsin-Oshkosh to start an academic program in Audiology and to develop an Audiology Clinic which would serve as a practicum site for students. One of the first professionals that I met was Margaret Ferris, who was a preschool teacher of hearing-impaired children. There was an instant professional rapport and the beginnings of a lasting friendship. The first sizeable group of hearing-impaired children we saw followed the German measle epidemic of 1964-

1965. That epidemic was the beginning of a specialization in Pediatric Audiology, which constitutes more than 90 percent of our practice today.

A large picture board, hanging in our clinic, displays photographs of some of the youngsters we have served over the years. As I scan the board, I see a Deaf Olympic Champion shot putter and discus thrower with a college degree from a major university, an electrical engineer, a computer programmer, a dairy farmer, a teacher and even an audiologist. Margaret and I continue to share many wonderful experiences with these individuals and their families.

Strides Made In Pediatric Audiology Over the Years

I have chosen to discuss some of the strides made in Pediatric Audiology over the past 27 years and what the future might hold. I have attempted to avoid technical jargon and hope the information is understood by the lay person.

Strides In The Early Detection of Hearing Loss

In the past, youngsters with congenital sensorineural hearing impairments were often first diagnosed after two years of age because they were not talking. (Note: Sensorineural in our discussions will refer to those permanent, medically irreversible hearing impairments due to an abnormal condition of the cochlear part of the inner ear which contains the delicate sensory structures for hearing) [Figure 1]. Earlier identification and management would have better realized these youngsters' learning potential.

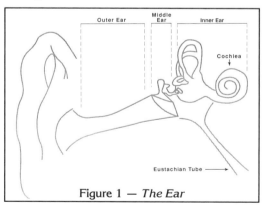

Figure 1 — *The Ear*

In 1982, risk factors for hearing impairment in neonates (e.g., family history of hearing loss, low birthweight) were developed by the Joint Committee on Infant Hearing (JCIH).[3] It was estimated that these factors identified about 50 percent of those children with hearing impairment.[4] The revised high risk register (JCIH, 1991),[5] which also includes risk factors for infants (e.g., parent/caregiver concerns, factors associated with progressive hearing loss), might facilitate earlier detection of hearing impairment. Most recently, a conference sponsored by the National Institute of Health recommended that all newborns, including those not at risk, have their hearing screened before being discharged from the hospital.[6]

Today, no child is too young to have his/her hearing evaluated. For babies under five months of age and for some children who have developmental disabilities, auditory brainstem response (ABR) can be used as an objective means to estimate hearing sensitivity. This technique is a computerized EEG-type of test from which auditory evoked responses are extracted. Electrodes are taped to the head. While the child is asleep or in a quiet state, auditory signals are presented through earphones with each ear tested separately. Neural responses to auditory signals, generated at the brainstem, show up as waveforms which are collected by a computer. The waveforms are identified [Figure 2], and the intensity levels of the auditory signals are reduced until no waves can be observed. The lowest level at which a repeatable response occurs is referred to as threshold and gives an estimate of hearing sensitivity. ABR can also be used as a screening procedure which is recommended for all infants at risk for hearing impairment prior to discharge from the newborn nursery.[7]

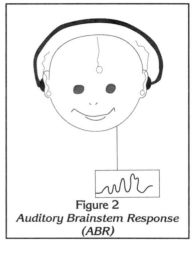

Figure 2
Auditory Brainstem Response (ABR)

A new technology, called otoacoustic emissions (OAE), is being developed to assist in the identification of hearing loss.[8*9*10*11] Otoacoustic emissions are soft sounds generated by the outer hair cells of the cochlea. Typically, one is not aware of the OAE's for the auditory signals that activate them are louder and generally go unnoticed. The OAE equipment includes a probe assembly connected to a computerized analyzer. The probe includes miniature loudspeakers, from which auditory signals are transmitted, and a small microphone which picks up the OAE's. Otoacoustic emissions are sensitive to even small degrees of cochlear damage. For those having sensorineural hearing impairment greater than mild-moderate in degree, OAE's are generally absent. Thus OAE holds promise as a screening tool for differentiating between normal ears and those with hearing impairment.

Visual Reinforcement Audiometry (VRA) has been shown to be an effective behavioral technique for assessing hearing in infants as young as five to six months of age.[12] This procedure employs a head-turn to an auditory signal followed by a visual reinforcer. In our clinic, we generally have the child seated in an upright position on mother's lap between two loudspeakers in a sound-treated room. The child is distracted to one side by toys or hand puppets held by an observer. An air-conducted auditory signal is presented to the other side. If the child responds with a head-turn to the sound source, he/she is visually reinforced with an animated toy which is positioned to the side of the loudspeaker. The audiologist determines the lowest intensity levels that a child responds to speech and to tones that are critical for hearing and understanding speech. For youngsters who will wear earphones, each ear can be assessed. In addition, for those children who will accept the bone conduction transducer, type of hearing impairment can often be determined.

Air-conducted auditory signals, presented through free field loudspeakers or under earphones, are transmitted to the outer ear, middle ear, inner ear [Figure 1, see page 95] and then travel up the auditory nerve to the brainstem and ultimately to the brain. When a hearing loss is suggested by air conduction, the type of hearing impairment is unknown until bone conduction testing is completed. Bone conduction testing assesses the sensitivity of the cochlear portion of the inner ear. For this test, a small transducer is placed on the bone behind the child's ear and held in place with a headband [Figure 3]. For example, if there is a hearing loss by air conduction but not by bone conduction, a conductive impairment is suggested and the involvement is in the outer ear (e.g., earwax) and/or middle ear (e.g., middle ear infection—otitis media). However, if the degree of hearing loss is the same both by air and bone conduction, a sensorineural hearing impairment (e.g., noise induced) is indicated. While conductive hearing impairments are generally correctable with medical intervention, sensorineural losses are generally not. Finally, mixed hearing impairments involve a combination of conductive and sensorineural involvement.

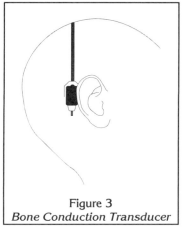

Figure 3
Bone Conduction Transducer

To determine changes in age of detection of childhood hearing impairment, we recently reviewed clinical files of 244 children with congenital sensorineural hearing impairment seen in our clinic from 1966-1992 for three time intervals: 1966-1972, 1973-1982 and 1983-1992.[13] For each interval, an inverse relationship existed between average age of detection and severity of hearing loss. As the severity of hearing loss increased, the average age of detection decreased [Table 1].

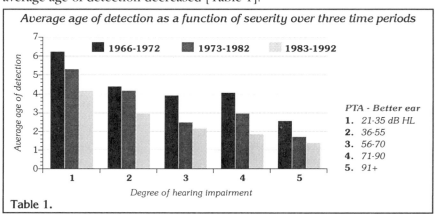

Table 1.

In 1966-72, the average age of detection for children with mild hearing impairment occurred at 6.27 years and was 2.58 years for those having profound hearing impairment. Thus, during this time period, children often did not have their mild hearing impairments detected until they reached school age, while others had their profound hearing losses identified about the age when concerns were expressed about speech and language delays.

In 1973-82, the average age of detection was lowered about one year to 5.35 years for those with mild losses and to 1.75 years for the profound hearing impairments. This earlier identification could have been related to new audiologic testing procedures (e.g., ABR, VRA) which became available clinically during this time interval.

In 1983-92, the average age of detection of mild hearing impairments was lowered about another year to 4.19 years and profound losses to 1.36 years. While the impact of the High Risk Register could have contributed to lowering the age of detection, it still was not lowered to acceptable limits based on today's technology.

The data on average age of detection of hearing impairment for children being seen in our clinic, although not acceptable, are lower than reported nationally. A 1989 report to Congress and the President by the Commission on Education of the Deaf indicated the average age of detection of childhood deafness in the United States to be 2.5 years.[14] In 1990, Surgeon General C. Everett Koop recognized the deleterious effects of late detection of childhood hearing impairment and set a goal for identifying 90 percent of children with significant hearing impairment by the year 2000.[15]

If technology is available, why aren't hearing losses being detected sooner? The following factors are suggested as possibly contributing to late detection of hearing impairment:

1. Increased incidence of medically fragile children with hearing impairment;
2. Inadequate follow-up services;
3. Not determining at-risk status;
4. Lack of methods for following low-risk infants who have or might develop hearing impairment;
5. Uninformed primary health care providers;
6. Inordinately long periods of time to diagnose hearing impairment.

By today's standards, congenital hearing impairments can be diagnosed, amplification introduced and an early intervention program initiated when the baby is six to eight months of age. With the benefit of amplification, these youngsters will often babble more as they hear their vocalizations for the first time. Frequently, with extensive auditory training, some learn to make good use of their residual hearing as they develop speech and language skills. Further, there is greater emphasis on early identification of hearing impairments in developmentally disabled youngsters. For example, in children who have Down Syndrome, the incidence of hearing impairment is about fifteen times that of the general population of children.[16]

Due to advances in medical technology and treatment, many high-risk babies, including those having birthweights under three pounds, are surviving today. Neonatal intensive care clinics are providing invaluable services in saving and maintaining the lives of many of these infants. The development of identification, assessment and intervention techniques in high risk infants has given physicians, particularly pediatricians, a greater awareness of intervention strategies.[17]

Strides in Acoustic Immittance Measurements

Behavioral testing can miss some middle-ear dysfunctions such as pressure problems and otitis media (any infection of the middle ear accompanied usually with fluid). While some cases of otitis media are symptomatic (e.g., pain, discomfort), many others are asymptomatic. In the past, these conditions were more difficult for the audiologist to identify. While some youngsters had conductive hearing losses due to otitis media, others had otitis media, but normal hearing sensitivity. Since the behavioral test results did not identify the condition and because of the insidious nature of the problem, no medical referral was made.

Acoustic immittance measurements (tympanometry and middle ear reflex) have been used clinically in the United States since the early 1970's to objectively assess the condition of the middle ear. When tympanometry is done, a small probe is inserted into the entrance of the ear canal. Differing pressures are presented and transmitted to the eardrum. In the normal air-filled middle ear, the eardrum should move freely with changes in pressure. These movements are recorded on a graph called a tympanogram [Figure 4]. If the middle ear has fluid, which is noncompressible, the eardrum will not move and the tympanogram will be flat. In the case of negative middle ear pressure, the Eustachian tube, which supplies air to the middle ear, is not working properly. Otitis media and abnormal middle ear pressures are quite common in infants, toddlers, and pre-school children.

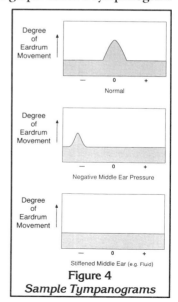

Figure 4
Sample Tympanograms

Another acoustic immittance measure is the middle ear reflex. Often when there is a loud sound, a small muscle within the middle ear (stapedius) will contract, stiffening the middle ear system and reducing the amount of sound arriving at the inner ear. The presence or absence of these muscle contractions provides information about the condition of the ear.

Tympanometry and middle ear reflex measures, in conjunction with standard behavioral audiologic results, are often useful in diagnosing other types of middle ear dysfunctions not related to otitis media or pressure problems, such as disconnected or fixated middle ear bones. Today, most audiologists routinely make acoustic immittance measurements on all patients seen for diagnostic evaluations. When screening hearing of children in schools, it is recommended that both pure tone screening and tympanometry be employed.[18]

Strides in Hearing Aid and Earmold Technology

The choice of hearing aids in the 1960s was limited. Often preschool hearing-impaired children were fit with body-style hearing aids because the ear-level style was too large and cumbersome or not powerful enough. Whether to fit with one or two hearing aids was often debated among audiologists. It was not uncommon to fit a youngster with one body-style hearing aid with a Y-cord with one branch going to each ear [Figure 5]. While providing amplification to both ears, it did not result in binaural hearing and did not assist in localizing to the sound source. Binaural body style hearing aids were cumbersome and bulky when worn by small children. In that their microphones were not ear level, it was often not possible for these children to localize to the sound source. [Figure 6].

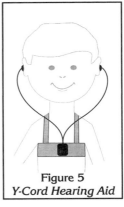

Figure 5
Y-Cord Hearing Aid

In the past, there was minimal concern within the profession concerning handicapping conditions resulting from mild hearing impairment and also one-sided (unilateral) hearing losses in children. Few of these youngsters wore hearing aids and most that did received less than optimal amplification. This was often due to inappropriate frequency responses, excessive amplification and limited variety of earmolds.

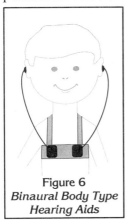

Figure 6
Binaural Body Type
Hearing Aids

Due to technological advances in microelectronics, hearing aids are now smaller, have greater versatility and are more efficient amplifying systems. Most infants and small children can be effectively fit with ear-level hearing aids [Figure 7]. When compared to the body type, ear-level hearing aids provide better sound quality and the microphones are in a more

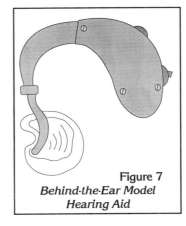

Figure 7
Behind-the-Ear Model
Hearing Aid

favorable location for the reception of speech signals.

While in-the-ear model style hearing aids are fit on the majority of adults, they are generally not appropriate for infants, toddlers and small children. These youngsters'ears are often too small to retain this style of hearing aid. Further, as their ears grow, the hearing aids require re-casing at considerable expense. In addition, these hearing aids generally do not have telecoils or have capabilities for coupling to FM units.

Currently, there is considerable support by audiologists for the fitting of binaural hearing aids on all children with symmetrical hearing loss and also for many whose hearing differs appreciably in each ear. To illustrate the latter, we have been following a six-year-old youngster with a bilateral asymmetrical hearing loss since he was about one year of age. Initially, he was fit with binaural ear-level hearing aids. In his better ear, he has a moderate to severe hearing impairment, with a severe to profound hearing loss in his poorer ear. He is an extremely bright youngster who makes excellent use of his residual hearing and has intelligible speech. Recently, auditory word recognition testing showed that in his better ear, speech discrimination was moderately reduced. In his poorer ear, amplified sound was so distorted that he was unable to discriminate any speech. He was asked to make a comparison between wearing a hearing aid in his better ear versus wearing both hearing aids. He reported a strong preference for wearing both hearing aids which enable him to better localize to the sound source. This suggests that hearing impaired children with asymmetrical hearing impairment should not be precluded as being good candidates for binaural hearing aids.

It is now being recognized by many audiologists that one-sided hearing losses may result in educational disabilities in children.[19] Many of these children may benefit from amplification and/or support services in school.

Because hearing aid performance is affected by interaction with the earmold, the importance of the earmold cannot be underestimated. Because of advances in earmold design and fabric, it is common practice today for the audiologist to select the earmold for the hearing impairment and the hearing aid for the earmold. As the result of research in earmold acoustics, there are now many more successful hearing aid fittings. Earmold modifications can significantly alter the power and frequency response characteristics of the hearing aid.

Presently, research is being carried out to develop and perfect a digital hearing aid.[20] The digital hearing aid is controlled by a microprocessor, a wearable computer, which is used with an ear-level type hearing aid. Most hearing aids on the market use analog electronics. Analog signals are continuously changing.

Digital devices, however, can change speech signals from their analog or continuous state to a digital state using a series of numerical values. In this digital state, the signals can be modified to compensate more accurately (or precisely) for the person's hearing impairment. After modifications, the signal can be transformed back to the continuous state. The hearing-impaired individual's specific needs for amplification can be programmed and placed on a microchip. If hearing changes in the future, the chip can be reprogrammed or replaced without changing the hearing aid. A further advantage of the digital hearing aid is the selective filtering of various types of background noises which significantly improves speech discrimination of most hearing aid users. Also, the digital hearing aid will enable some to hear sounds often not heard using conventional means of amplification. While a true digital hearing aid is still not commercially available, programmable digital hybrids are now being dispensed with some encouraging results.

Strides in Hearing Aid Evaluation Procedures

Adequate evaluation procedures to objectively assess the performance of hearing aids worn by infants and children, as well as adults, have been lacking.

Now, commercial equipment is available for measuring amplified sound arriving in the ear canal, near the eardrum. The essential feature of this equipment is a small probe tube microphone, placed in the ear canal. This microphone measures the amount of amplified sound of different frequencies in the ear canal. This is referred to as Probe Microphone Real Ear Measurement (PREM). Such measurements have the potential for providing information to assist in selecting appropriate hearing aid characteristics.[21] The data reported on conventional hearing aid specification sheets give power and frequency response characteristics which more closely approx-imate adult ears. Following these specifications can result in over fitting children, and excessive amplification might contribute to additional hearing loss.[22] PREM accounts for each ear canal and earmold individually. Com-puter programs have been developed to assist in determining how much amplification a hearing aid should provide. One such program, specifically designed for children is called the Desired Sensation Level (DSL) program. [23]

Much more research is needed to further define effective methods to test the adequacy of hearing aid fittings. Although progress has been made in this area, there are still large gaps in our understanding of what constitutes optimal amplification for an infant or child who has never heard normally.

Strides in Alternatives to Traditional Amplification: Vibrotactile Aids and Cochlear Implants

For children with little or no residual hearing, who are unable to benefit from amplification, few alternatives had been available to give them sensory stimulation. While the use of vibrotactile training has long been recognized as effective for use with the deaf, the lack of wearable units made use impractical. Today, wearable vibrotactile aids, utilizing two or seven vibrators, each passing a different band of frequencies, are being produced by some manufacturers.[24] [Figure 8, see page 103.] A small amplifier unit

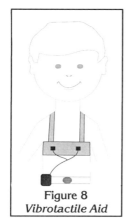

Figure 8
Vibrotactile Aid

can be attached to the trousers, with the vibrators (similar to the bone conduction transducer shown in Figure 3) being placed on the chest, wrist or hands. Any hearing impaired child, using body-worn vibrators, can perceive vibrations generated by sound regardless of the severity of hearing loss. While not a substitute for hearing, vibrotactile training often facilitates the development of sound awareness and in recognizing the rhythmic aspects of speech. Deaf children may be more vocal when wearing vibrotactile aids. Further, speechreading may be enhanced when able to combine visual and vibrotactile clues. Recently, we saw an eleven-year-old youngster deafened as the result of meningitis. Her brother's names, Scott and Todd, looked similar on the lips; however, with vibrotactile clues the two names could be discriminated.

The cochlear implant is another technological advancement which has had an impact on children with profound hearing loss. This device has enabled some persons with profound hearing loss, unable to benefit significantly from hearing aids, to receive some sound awareness. The actual cochlear implant is just one part of the total implant system [Figure 9]. Some parts of the implant are positioned externally: a microphone, a transmitter coil and a speech processor. The cochlear implant, which is placed surgically, consists of a receiver-stimulating device (internal coil) under the skin behind the ear and a series of electrical contacts (electrodes) placed in different areas within the cochlea. The electrodes stimulate different frequencies. The first cochlear implants used a single active electrode while today's implants utilize as many as 22 channels.[25] Sound is picked up by an ear level microphone and transmitted to a speech processor, often worn at pocket level. While not an amplification device, the speech processor selects certain sound elements which can enhance identification. From the speech processor, electronic signals are sent to the transmitter which pass through the skin to the receiver-stimulator. Finally, these signals are transmitted to a series of electrodes which are programmed to deliver sounds varying in pitch and loudness. In this manner, remaining nerve fibers are stimulated and neural impulses are transmitted. While the cochlear implant generally enables these people to hear sound within conversational levels, speech sounds are distorted and difficult to distinguish.

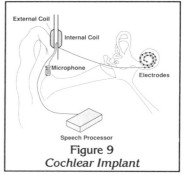

Figure 9
Cochlear Implant

Today, while more people are undergoing this procedure, including some with congenital deafness, the best candidates continue to be those who have acquired their deafness after developing speech and language. They generally make better use of distorted auditory clues than do those born with deafness. Speech recognition can often be improved with training. While some of these people can understand some conversational speech by only utilizing auditory clues (e.g. telephone), they often understand more with the addition of visual clues.

A conservative approach is generally taken with small children in determining candidacy for cochlear implants. It is important to know with certainty that profound hearing loss exists so that the implantation does not result in the loss of hearing that could best be fit with traditional amplification.[26] Even if a profound hearing loss is indicated, a trial period with hearing aids is generally suggested prior to implantation. Then, if the youngster does not respond to that amplification, a cochlear implant might be considered. While the expense of the cochlear implant, around $30,000, often makes it cost prohibitive, the Food and Drug Administration has approved cochlear implants for children and some insurance carriers do cover this procedure.

We have worked with a youngster who was deafened at 21 months of age from meningitis. No auditory responses were obtained using behavioral techniques. Neither were there any responses with objective assessments. Subsequently, he was given a lengthy trial with hearing aids. Since it was determined that he did not benefit from conventional amplification, he was fitted with a vibrotactile device. He was aware of conversational level speech and vocalized more when wearing it. Eventually, he was also referred to a major medical center to determine his candidacy for a cochlear implant. At four years of age, he underwent the implantation. Following the procedure, he received extensive auditory training to teach him to make maximal use of his new hearing. He became aware of soft conversational level speech and could discriminate between his parent's voices. Also, he could distinguish many environmental sounds and differentiate between single vs. multi-syllables in speech and between some vowel sounds. Further, he imitated a wider range of speech sounds.

Today, at nine years of age, this child, with the cochlear implant, is able to discriminate some speech when using auditory clues alone and is also able to speechread more effectively. To illustrate, on a formal test of word recognition (multiple choice picture test), he was recently able to correctly identify 52 percent of the stimuli with auditory clues alone and 88 percent when combining auditory and visual clues. Further, on a forced choice listening test, consisting of five speech sounds going progressively from low to high frequencies (*oo* as in b*oo*t, *a* — f*a*ther, *ee* — m*ee*t, *sh* — *sh*ip, *s* —*s*eat) he identified all of the sounds.[27] His speech utterances are, for the most part, intelligible and reflect excellent use of hearing with the cochlear implant.

Strides in Development of Assistive Listening Devices
The hearing-aid user profits optimally when spoken to from close

distances (less than 10 feet). When the primary speaker is further away, the speech signals arrive at the listener's ears at soft levels which, even when amplified, may not be adequate for him/her to hear conversational speech. In addition, background noise levels need to be considerably softer to optimize the understanding of speech. The traditional recommendation of preferential seating in the classroom for hearing-impaired children has often been ineffective. Frequently, the teacher does not remain in one position but rather moves about the sometimes noisy classroom. As a result, the youngster, even with optimally fit hearing aids, may not hear much of what had been said.

Initially, group amplification systems were used which were wired to the children's desks limiting their movements [Figure 10]. Later, loop systems were employed [Figure 11]. With this arrangement, the children received

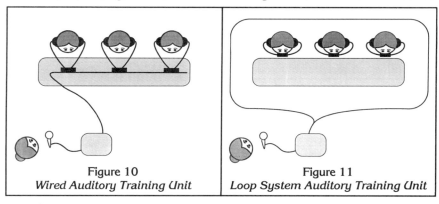

| Figure 10 | Figure 11 |
| *Wired Auditory Training Unit* | *Loop System Auditory Training Unit* |

amplified sound through their wearable hearing aids as long as they moved within the loop. These auditory training units operated in conjunction with the telecoils of the children's wearable hearing aids. *(Note: The telecoil is a coil of wire within many wearable hearing aids that enables some hearing impaired to hear on the telephone)*. The electromagnetic field generated between the telecoil and the loop of wire results in direct transmission of amplified sound. However, there are some problems with the loop systems. First, the loop depends on the children's hearing aid to be functioning

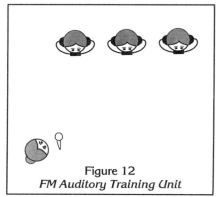

Figure 12
FM Auditory Training Unit

optimally. Second, there can be loss of power associated with loop systems as well as changes in the frequency response of the individual hearing aids when using this mode.

The use of personal wireless FM systems now enables many hearing-impaired children to hear well in the classroom [Figure 12]. These use radio waves in the same way as a radio station. They broadcast signals that can be picked up by a radio receiver provided they are within the limits of the radio transformer. Each operates on an authorized channel approved by the FCC for use by the hearing impaired. Therefore, there should not be overspillage from nearby commercial radio stations. The teacher wears a wireless microphone and the child receives the FM signals through receivers (e.g., button, behind-the-ear and/or walkman headset). For some, the FM receivers can be directly coupled to their hearing aids. In that the loudness of the teacher's voice is being amplified and not the background noise, favorable listening situations are created. The child will hear the teacher's voice at a constant loudness regardless how far away he/she is from the teacher. Many hearing-impaired children in the same classroom can wear FM units with the teacher wearing a transmitter tuned to a single frequency. At times, there can be problems with FM units resulting from outside interference (e.g., beepers, PC terminals).

A convincing case for FM systems can be presented for all youngsters with educationally significant hearing impairment whether mainstreamed or enrolled in special classes. Wireless systems are extremely versatile and can be adapted to almost any listening environment. Many meeting places such as churches and theaters now have group assistive listening devices for their hearing impaired.

In addition to the use of FM systems for individuals having hearing losses, consideration is now being given to fitting systems for those children who have so-called auditory processing disorders. While able to hear well in quiet conditions, some children are unable to cope with auditory distractions in the classroom. They encounter difficulties attending and staying on task which affect academic performance. These children's ability to discriminate conversational speech is adversely affected when there is background noise. Their attending skills may improve with amplification devices, such as FM units, because of favorable speech-to-noise ratios. However, when amplifying these normal hearing children, the potential for damaging the auditory system cannot be disregarded.[28]

Recently, sound field amplification systems have been used in classrooms to create more favorable listening situations. These systems operate similarly to the personal FM units with the teacher wearing a wireless microphone. However, instead of the amplified sound being transmitted to personal receivers, it passes through loudspeakers which are strategically placed throughout the classroom. Advantages of using such a system include the following:
1. Beneficial for children with unidentified hearing impairments of a transient nature;
2. Helpful for children having normal hearing sensitivity but possessing auditory processing problems;
3. Helpful to students with normal hearing when background noise is excessive;
4. Helpful for children with unilateral hearing impairment;
5. Cost effectiveness;

6. Unlikely to be rejected because of cosmetic reasons;
7. High acceptance rate by teachers;
8. Lower repair rates from other amplification devices.[29]

Strides in Audiologic Services in the Schools

While comprehensive audiologic assessments and hearing aid evaluations were done on hearing impaired children in clinics, direct audiologic services were often lacking in schools. For example, *studies have shown that about half of the hearing aids worn by school age children do not work properly when one does not have the services of an audiologist to monitor them.*[30] In addition, even if there are FM systems available, often no one is available to adjust and monitor the units. To relate a horror story, several years ago we evaluated a child who was previously fit with an FM system without any input from an audiologist. While he had a moderate sensorineural hearing loss which required amplification, he possessed a tolerance problem for loud sound. Because maximum output of the FM system was not reduced within his tolerance, he rejected the device after he experienced extreme discomfort. Because of this, it took about six months before he would permit reintroduction of amplification. Further, the excessive amplification could have resulted in additional hearing loss.

Today, Public Law 99-457 (Part H) provides state funding for early intervention services for infants and toddlers (zero through two years of age).[31] While these services are generally provided by a wide array of agencies, some school systems may be providers depending on state mandates and available funding. A number of our local schools are providing services for infants and toddlers with hearing impairment and their families. Public Law 94-142 assures a free, appropriate public education along with any special education services for all handicapped children beginning at age three.[32] These services are to be provided by qualified professionals who have met certification standards which are present in about half of the states. Wisconsin recently adopted certification standards for school-based audiologists with funding being anticipated in the near future.

The American Speech-Language-Hearing Association (ASHA) recognizes the audiologist as being uniquely qualified to provide many of the services needed for the comprehensive management of hearing-impaired children. Some of these services include educating children, parents and teachers about ways to prevent hearing loss; organizing and supervising hearing screening programs; making appropriate referrals for otologic and audiologic assessments; interpreting the audiologic results and holding inservice programs for classroom teachers and other school personnel; acting as a member of an interdisciplinary team giving input about educational placements; making recommendations about the use, monitoring and troubleshooting of hearing aids and FM systems; and analyzing and reducing classroom noise.[33]

Strides in Awareness Of
The Importance Of Audiologic Counseling

Traditionally, audiologists have not had adequate background in counseling hearing-impaired children and their families. The counseling has consisted primarily of information-sharing with little attention devoted to the impact the child's hearing impairment is having on the family.[34] Often, the audiologist is the first to confirm that a youngster has a permanent hearing impairment and has the unpleasant task of communicating this to the parents. This responsibility cannot be taken lightly and requires considerable empathy and compassion. Often the dream of having a normal child has been shattered and the mourning period begins. If the parents' initial reaction is denial, they should be encouraged to have second opinion evaluations. The parents need to be convinced of their child's hearing impairment before they can become effective teachers. Even when there is acceptance, mourning often continues and can last a lifetime. Some become angry and ask "Why me?" Feelings of guilt can persist. Professionals need to realize that mourning is normal and acceptable behavior and that the parents have every right to experience it. Further, professionals need to admit they do not know or understand the mourning the family is undergoing unless they have had a similar experience with a family member.

The public school district, in which the hearing-impaired child resides, is not legally bound to provide services until he/she reaches age three. However, some school systems choose to offer services to these infants and toddlers. Early intervention programs run by counties often provide specialists who are involved with home training programs. Although not all have had formal education and training in working with hearing-impaired children, they most often provide needed help and support for the family. For those in rural areas where no services are available, home training programs such as the John Tracy Clinic Correspondence Course, Beginnings and Parent-Infant Communication can be used.[35,36,37]

Before the parents leave the clinic, a call is placed to a representative from the local parent support group who will offer to visit the parents within a day. These support parents generally have an older child with a similar hearing impairment. Having already experienced much of what the parents whose child has just been diagnosed are going through, their understanding and insights often have a meaningful and positive effect. Further, the support parents can offer coping strategies.

More parent support groups are being formed, some are affiliated with national organizations such as Self Help for the Hard of Hearing People, Inc. (SHHH).[38] These parent groups are becoming more informed of their legal rights and represent a force that is useful in helping meet the educational needs of their children. Further, parent groups serve as a sounding board, enabling parents to vent their frustrations and to share their feelings in an atmosphere of understanding and support.

The roles of the parents in their child's early training are demanding.

While the early intervention specialist might see the hearing impaired youngster several times a week for short sessions, the primary care givers are still the parents and they often become terrific teachers. Much of their child's progress is the result of their efforts. Parents, too often, are not given professional support and encouragement for what they are doing. Too frequently it is assumed that some other professionals are giving them support. Parents need constant reinforcement that what they are doing on behalf of their child is in fact extremely significant and needed.[39] Public Law 99-457 recognizes the family as important contributors in planning and carrying out their child's special education.

Through the years, we have dealt with an increasing number of parents having multi-handicapped hearing-impaired children, some of whom require constant care. Their special children take up most of their time and a need exists for respite services. Concerns should be expressed to the parents about their well-being and the importance of having time to themselves. Referrals are made to agencies that provide these services. The parents need and have the right to know about the specifics of their child's hearing impairment (e.g., cause, type, severity and degree of handicap). They should be given the opportunity to hear how their youngster might hear with and without hearing aids. The audiologist can use prepared recordings or electronic equipment to simulate differing hearing losses. This often helps the parents to make a difficult realization, that their child, even with the help of hearing aids, does not hear normally.

The social penalty paid by the child who displays even a mild degree of hearing impairment is understood best by the child's family. Professionals should never lose sight of that. I was really reminded of this recently with my grandson and the management of his hearing impairment resulting from middle ear infections. I instantly became a concerned grandfather and was no longer an audiologist talking about a routine conductive hearing loss.

More audiologists, particularly those specializing in pediatrics, are realizing the importance of counseling. Some university training programs are addressing the subject in their curricula. Today, the pediatric audiologist generally spends considerable time counseling parents and in arranging for follow-up services regarding management of their child's hearing impairment.

The following scenario could represent a typical sequence of services beginning with the initial detection of the child's hearing impairment. Test results are discussed with the parents using layman's terminology. Intuitively, some judgements are made by the audiologist regarding the parents' immediate reactions. While some parents appear outwardly accepting of the news, having had their suspicions confirmed, others are devastated. Regardless of the parents' reactions, the audiologist responds with concern and compassion and gives them the opportunity to express their feelings. Any questions are answered honestly with an emphasis on accentuating the positive. For example, "You have a normal youngster with a hearing problem who has considerable potential for learning." Still there is no way to soften the blow regardless of how thoughtfully the message has been conveyed. A second opinion evaluation is encouraged if the parents feel the need. Other clinics are suggested where their child can be evaluated. If the cause of the hearing impairment is unknown or a history of hearing loss exists within the family, genetic counseling is encouraged. Also, a contact is made with an Audiologist with the Wisconsin Department of Public Instruction who often assists in the delivery of services.

Some Final Thoughts

It has been a pleasant and somewhat nostalgic experience to reflect over some of the changes that have taken place in Audiology since 1966, my beginnings in the profession. While the primary focus of this discussion has dealt with clinical issues, I will finish with some discussion related to my role as an educator.

The profession of Audiology has become increasingly specialized, and there is considerable support for the professional doctorate to provide the needed comprehensive services to the hearing impaired.[40] Advising students at the entry level, if majors are declared, is desirable. At the undergraduate level, strong academic preparation in mathematics and the natural sciences, in addition to the social sciences, is necessary to provide the necessary background in a profession with immense technological demands.

With a greater interest in management of hearing impairments of infants and toddlers, university programs should address areas of development, family dynamics and counseling with a focus on pediatric audiology.[41]

Graduate level teaching must adapt to meet the needs of Dispensing Audiologists. More courses in hearing aids need to be developed with a greater practicum experience in the hearing aid selection and fitting process. Further, the role of the Dispensing Audiologist as a business person cannot be neglected in academic preparation.

With increased mainstreaming, academic preparation for the Educational Audiologist needs to be coordinated with an extensive clinical experience in the management of hearing impaired children. Because of the many advances in modern technology, instrumentation for behavioral and neurophysiological assessments of hearing demands greater skills for optimal usage. Teaching needs to keep up with these advances in challenging students to make maximal use of their resources to develop ideas and skills for clinical research.

Acknowledgements

I would like to acknowledge Kathryn Beauchaine for her careful review of this chapter and her many helpful editorial comments and also to Kathleen Robl for her assistance in the preparation of the manuscript.

· · · · ·

Bibliography

1. Feldmann, H. (1970). A history of audiology, a comprehensive report and bibliography from the earliest beginnings to the present. *Translations of the Beltone Institute for Hearing Research,* No. 22.

2. Newby, H. and Popelka, G. (1985). The lineage of audiology, in *Audiology,* fifth edition, Englewood Cliffs, New Jersey: Prentice-Hall, Inc.

3. Joint Committee on Infant Hearing, Position statement. (1982). *Pediatrics*, 70, 24-25.

4. Elssmann, S.F., Matkin, N.D. & Sabo, M. (1987). Early identification of congenital sensorineural hearing impairment. *The Hearing Journal*, 40, 13-17.

5. Joint Committee on Infant Hearing. (1991). 1990 position statement. *ASHA* 33 (suppl. 5), 3-6.

6. National Institute of Health Consensus Development Conference Statement. (1993). Early identification of hearing impairment in infants & young children: Consensus development conference statement. Betheseda, MD.

7. American Speech-Language-Hearing Association (1989). Guidelines for audiologic screening of newborn infants who are at risk for hearing impairment. *ASHA*, 31, 89-92.

8. Kemp, D.T., (1978). Stimulated acoustic emission from within the human auditory system. *Journal of the Acoustical Society of America*, 64, 1386-1391.

9. Kemp, D., Bray, P., Alexander, L. and Brown, A., (1986). Acoustic emission cochleography—Practical aspects. *Scandinavian Audiology Supplement,*, 25, 71-82.

10. Bray, P. and Kemp, D. (1987). An advanced cochlear technique suitable for infant screening. *British Journal of Audiology*, 21, 191-204.

11. Kemp, D., Ryan, S. and Bray, P. (1990). A guide to the effective use of otoacoustic emissions. *Ear and Hearing*, 11, 125-131.

12. Thompson, G. and Wilson, W. (1984). Clinical application of visual reinforcement audiometry. *Seminars in Hearing*, 5, 85-99.

13. Kile, J. (1993). Changing demographics related to childhood hearing impairment. *Infant-Toddler Intervention*, 3, 155-164.

14. Epstein, S. and Reilly, J. (1989). Sensorineural hearing loss—Recent advances in pediatric otolaryngology. *Pediatric Clinics of North America,* 36, 6, 1501-1519.

15. United States Department of Health & Human Services. (1990). Healthy

people 2000: National health promotion and disease prevention objective. Washington D.C.: Public Health Service.

16. Kile, J., Kuba, J., Nellis, R. and Becker, T. (1990). Children with Down syndrome: Issues in prevention, assessment and management. Poster Session presented to annual convention of the American Speech-Language-Hearing Association, Seattle.

17. Rossetti, L. (1986). *High-Risk Infants: Identification, Assessment, and Intervention.* San Diego: College-Hill Press.

18. American Speech-Language-Hearing Association (1989). Guidelines for screening for hearing impairment and middle ear disorders. *ASHA*, 31, 71-77.

19. Oyler, R., Oyler, A., and Matkin, N. (1988). Unilateral hearing loss: Demographic and educational impact. *Language, Speech and Hearing Services in Schools*, 19, 201-210.

20. Hecox, K., and Miller, E. (1987). Foundations for the introduction of new hearing instrument technologies. *Hearing Instruments*, 38, 34.

21. Hawkins, D., Morrison, P., Halligan, W., and Cooper, W. (1989). Use of probe tube microphone measurements in hearing aid selection for children: Some initial clinical experiences. *Ear and Hearing*, 10, 281-287.

22. Kile, J. (1977). "Selecting saturation sound pressure levels with a concern for hearing conservation". *Audiology and Education*, 3, 121-135.

23. Seewald, R. (1988). The desired sensation level approach for children: Selection and verification. *Hearing Instruments*, 39, 18-22.

24. Franklin, D. (1984). Tactile aids. *The Hearing Journal*, Feb., 20-23.

25. ASHA report of the ad hoc committee on Cochlear Implants. (1986). *ASHA*, 28, 4, 29-52.

26. Tyler, R.S., Davis, J.M., and Lansing, C.R. (1987). "Cochlear implants in young children", *ASHA*, 29, 41-49.

27. Ling, D. and Ling, A. (1978). *Aural Habilitation: The Foundation of Verbal Learning in Hearing-Impaired Children* Washington D.C.: The Alexander Graham Bell Association for the Deaf, Inc.

28. American Speech-Language-Hearing Association (1991). Amplification as a remediation technique for children with normal peripheral hearing. *ASHA*, 33 (Supp. 3), 22-24.

29. Anderson, K. (1989). Speech perception and the hard of hearing child. *Educational Audiology Monograph* 1:1.

30. Ross, M. (1977). A review of studies on the incidence of hearing aid malfunctions in *The Condition of Hearing Aids Worn by Children in a*

Public School Program, U.S. Department of Health, Education, and Welfare, HEW Publication No. (DE) 77-05002, 3-9.

31. Education of the Handicapped Act Amendments of 1986, Public Law 99-457, 34 CFR Part 303, Part H. *Federal Register*, 54, 119, 26306-26348, June 22, 1989.

32. Public Law 94-142: The Education of All Handicapped Children Act. *Federal Register*, July 1984.

33. American Speech-Language-Hearing Association (1983). Audiology services in the schools position statement. *ASHA*, 25, 53-60.

34. Luterman, D. (1991). *Counseling the Communicatively Disordered and Their Families*, (2nd ed.) Austin, Texas: Pro-Ed.

35. John Tracy Clinic Correspondence Courses—806 West Adams Blvd., Los Angeles, CA. 90007.

36. BEGINNINGS for parents of hearing impaired children—A parent manual (1990). 1316 Broad St., Durham, North Carolina 27705.

37. Parent-Infant Communication—A program of clinical and home training for parents of hearing-impaired infants. 3rd Ed. (1985). Infant Hearing Resource, 3930 S.W. Macadam Ave., Portland, Oregon 92071.

38. Self Help for the Hard of Hearing People, Inc., 7910 Woodmont Ave., Ste. 1200, Bethseda, Maryland 20814

39. Bobholz, Marla, Personal communication, November 22, 1989.

40. Goldstein, D. (1989). Au.D. degree: The doctoring degree in audiology, *ASHA*, 31, 33-35.

41. Matkin, N. and Oyler, R. (1987). National survey of educational preparation in pediatric audiology, *ASHA*, 27, 27-33.

So Your Child Has Been Tested
What is an Audiogram?

Parents are given a copy of their child's audiogram. As carefully as the audiologist tries to explain that it charts what their child can or cannot hear, the parents do not understand the audiogram.

There are so many variables, and the terms are so technical. What does it mean when applied to an infant or young child?

The test is given in a sound treated room, or for newborns the ABR (Auditory Brainsteam Response) test can be administered while the infant is asleep. The ABR test is used not only to test small infants but also children with other disabilities. For older children behavioral techniques can be employed.

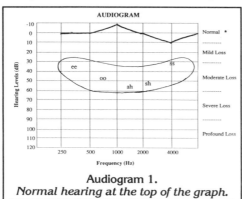

Audiogram 1.
Normal hearing at the top of the graph.

The audiogram is to show how loud a sound must be for a child to hear it. Normal hearing for everyone is at the top of the chart showing -10 to 10 dB. (dB means decibels. This is the term used to measure hearing.) [Audiogram 1]

The volume of normal conversational speech is in the enclosed area which means it is in the range of 60 dBs. It is Daniel Ling's *Five-Sound Test* (Ling 1988)[1]. These five sounds represent the Acoustic Range of speech sounds.

Mild Hearing Loss

Now what if the child has a mild hearing loss? [Audiogram 2] If the graph falls as low as 30 dBs, the child may hear in a quiet room when spoken to directly. However, such a mild loss can result in an educational disability, showing speech and language delays. Here he will miss some consonants and therefore not develop normal vocabulary nor easily grasp new concepts.

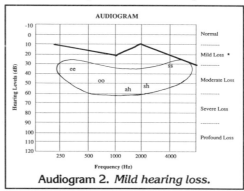

Audiogram 2. *Mild hearing loss.*

Moderate Hearing Loss

A moderate loss—30 to 60 dB range—will mean this cuts

114

across normal conversational speech. [Audiogram 3] Hearing aids are required. But depending upon the malfunction of the hearing mechanism, there may be some distortion of what the child hears. He will benefit from the services of a speech therapist as his speech may show imprecise high frequency sounds. He may also be depending upon lipreading even though he may not be aware that he does. He will be most comfortable if he can see the speaker. The classroom teacher should ask the child answering the questions to hold up his hand before speaking so the hearing impaired child can locate him.

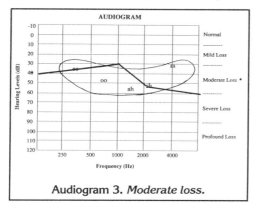

Audiogram 3. *Moderate loss.*

This child with a moderate loss may miss directions and therefore fall behind in classroom assignments. The regular classroom teachers must understand his behavior: he is not paying attention because he is missing so much that he gets lost and seems to give up. This behavior should indicate he needs additional help in building vocabulary and concepts. A well functioning FM system can prevent these problems.

Severe Hearing Loss

Severe hearing losses [Audiogram 4] fall in the 60 to 90 dB range. These children cannot hear speech at all without a hearing aid. They need continued help from the Speech Therapist. And careful attention must be given to develop language. These children are most frequently in day classes for the hearing impaired. Their teachers use Total Communication methods which means speech and manually coded English.

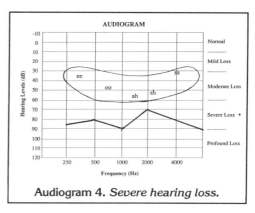

Audiogram 4. *Severe hearing loss.*

If the children with severe hearing losses are mainstreamed, they will still need the support of trained teachers of the hearing impaired to reinforce what is taught in the mainstreamed classes. FM systems are the most helpful in both self contained classes and in mainstreamed classes. And speech therapy is essential.

Mainstreamed classes may have interpreters who will use manually coded English. The purpose of the services of itinerant or resource teachers is to help in reading comprehension, develop vocabulary, and reinforce topics taught in the reguar class.

Profound Hearing Loss

Six percent of children with hearing impairment have profound losses. [Audiogram 5] Remarkably, with early intervention with hearing aids and family support, many of these

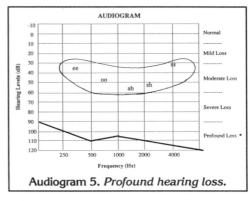

Audiogram 5. Profound hearing loss.

children can and do develop intelligent speech. It does take continuous speech therapy and tutoring in academics to be successful in mainstreamed classes. Usually these children are accompanied by interpreters.

However, these children with profound hearing loss and in many cases, severe hearing loss are usually the ones attending public day schools or classes and public residential schools. In 1986 the Directory of Services for the Deaf, *American Annals of the Deaf* reported that 25.7 percent of the enrollment took place in public residential schools, and 6.9 percent in public day schools. Day schools mentioned in this study reports on separate schools for the hearing impaired in large cities, not day classes found in regular public schools.

As mainstreaming becomes accepted in communities, the enrollments in all special facilities for the hearing impaired lessens. Residential schools, day schools and day classes are finding they have many children with added problems. Their Adaptive Education Departments have grown. Even though local schools try to accept all children, they soon learn that the multiple handicapped deaf children require services beyond their staffing.

Today one of the factors contributing to the presence of a hearing loss in infants is low birthweight. And, unfortunately, other handicapping conditions may also be present. All these added problems must be considered when relying on the audiogram to predict school success.

Illness during the first few months may result in a hearing loss. As many as seven out of ten children have middle ear infections such as otitis media.[1] If this condition is not treated with antibiotic drugs or having tympanostomy (tubes placed in the ear drums to allow drainage), it can become chronic. Middle ear infections are most common in cold, rainy weather. From this condition, a child can develop persistent middle ear fluid. These children can have enough of a hearing impairment during episodes that they fall behind in acquiring speech and language at age level. Some develop articulation problems that persist even after the infections have cleared. This is why such children require regular audiometric testing to be sure the condition does not become chronic.

Audiologists must rely on parents as they tell how and when the child seems to be inattentive, or not aware of sounds in the environment, or when spoken to from a distance or another room. Schools regularly test children in kindergarten and third grade. But otitis media most frequently develops in the first years, long before the child is old enough for nursery school or kindergarten. Children in day care centers are exposed to infectious diseases and must be watched for signs of ear problems.

References

1. The Five-Sound Test by Daniel Ling, Ph. D. *Foundations of Spoken Language for Hearing-Impaired Children.* Drawings by James Davel. Alexander Graham Bell Association for the Deaf. page 67
2. G. Scott Giebink, M.D. Medical Issues in Hearing Impairment: *The Otitis Media Spectrum. Our Forgotten Children: Hard-of-Hearing Pupils in the Schools,* editor, Julia Davis. Self Help for Hard of Hearing People, Inc.
3. Audiograms made by James Davel.

· · · · ·

Speech

Speech can only develop within the confines of a language. The goal of speech is to convey meaning. Spoken language implies meaningful speech.

The Normal Hearing Child

Early babbling is the beginning of spoken language. We parents and caregivers constantly talk to the infant. The infant babbles all the more with this attention. And the baby begins to mimic the speech sounds he hears. All this is a pleasurable experience. The infant enjoys this activity even if no other person is around. He experiments with many sounds—many that are not even in our native tongue. Eventually the infant is able to match the sounds we make and we encourage him to repeat them. And all this while we are talking to him about all that is going on around him. We know perfectly well that he does not really understand the actual words, but the pleasant tone of our voices gives him a feeling of well being. In addition he is becoming accustomed to the pattern or sound of our speech. He is being imprinted by the intonation and rhythm of his mother tongue.

This hearing baby, within the first year, recognizes groups of sounds— words. Simple words frequently used begin to have meaning. He can mimic a dozen or more words that first year such as: "Mama. More. No. Bear. Bye-bye. Up." And every day his understanding grows. He responds to his name. He recognizes familiar faces and voices. He is well on his way to become a fluent speaker of his "mother tongue".

Speech implies oral expression. To be understood it must be expressed in the community accepted form—language.

Mild to Moderate Hearing Loss

The hard of hearing infant is difficult to identify. Mother and the care-givers hold him, bend over him while changing and dressing him, when feeding him, putting him in his high chair, in bed, and play pen. He does hear much of what is said to him at such a close range. He is the child who is not identified as having a hearing loss until he enters school. Parents try to disregard their concerns by telling themselves that he is too interested in play to pay attention. Or they rationalize that he is a dreamer and lost in his own world. He is quiet and a good baby. Certainly nothing is wrong.

While most states do audiometric testing on newborns at-risk, only 18 states require it for all newborns. Hopefully our new health standards will mandate this immediate testing.

However, infants may not be born with a hearing loss, but develop one at an early age due to illness or infections. These are the children for whom the doctors must take a mother's concerns seriously and arrange for audiometric testing immediately. No child is too young to be tested. Read Dr. Jack Kile's article on audiometric testing of infants. (pages 94-110.)

Severe and Profound Hearing Loss

Our hearing impaired baby begins to babble. He responds to facial expressions. He smiles, but gradually his babbling tapers off as he gets no sound reinforcement. He does not hear his own babbling. I have seen a video tape of an infant who is moving his arms and legs, but making only a few babbling sounds. The father put the hearing aid on the infant and immediately the baby began to babble in a very normal manner. When the father spoke to him, he moved his arms and legs even more and babbled back. The hearing aid was removed and the child became quiet as he did not hear his father or his own voice.

Parents, if not guided to encourage the infant to babble, stop talking and singing to the child. Even if the child has a severe loss, he is aware of some sounds when the parent is holding him. The child feels the body vibration. Also the infant is responding to a pleasant facial expression and the physical enjoyment of being held and loved.

A child who does not hear but is exposed to consistantly presented signs, responds appropriately. He begins to understand the signs and mimics. Many deaf parents report that their infant can sign many familiar words and requests as early as seven months of age.

This hearing impaired child is learning to communicate, *but he is not automatically learning to talk.*

To quote E. Ross Stuckless, a professor at the National Technical Institute for the Deaf at the Rochester Institute of Technology in New York: "Acknowledging that most deaf children have a greater propensity for learning ASL (American Sign Language) at any age than for learning English, it is unwise to delay the child's introduction to English beyond the period of optimum language development."

And it bears repeating time and time again—All children are biologically programmed to speak during the first three years. Eric H. Lenneberg stated as early as 1970 that language is indirectly connected to the action of the genes. This genetic control accounts for the fact that normal children all over the world go through the same sequence of developmental stages as they learn to talk, even though they may be acquiring very different languages.

Sign language without the development of speech is not in the child's best interest. To move into the real world he would be better served if he has speech. It is unrealistic to think that the man on the street, the foreman, the clerk, the doctor, the insurance agent, the garage attendant, the neighbors are all going to be fluent in sign language—what ever method. Nor do we dare let our hearing impaired child think that an interpreter will be at his elbow for all every day situations.

Amplification

Only ten percent of all hearing impaired children are totally deaf. That means that 90 percent of the children have some residual hearing that can be amplified.

Properly fitted and maintained hearing aids give the hearing impaired child maximum exposure to talking. When the child is preschool age the the child's own hearing aid is best utilized. The heavy, bulky FM systems are not appropriate for the activities of a toddler. However, by the age of four or five, the best way to overcome background noise is for the child to wear an FM system. The teacher's speech is always at the optimum distance—six inches from the mike. The systems used in schools are sophisticated enough to also pick up the voices of the other students as they answer questions.

Speech Therapy

I began this essay on speech, so back to the theme. I almost hesitate to tell the truth about learning to talk. It is the most difficult, the most demanding of minute muscle control known to man—and yet toddlers can do it.

English speech is made up of 46 sounds. (Phonetic sound of the letter, not the letter name.) But not in isolation except for the sound /a/ as in *a dog*. There are 30 consonant sounds. In some instances, two letters form one sound such as /sh/ and /th/ and /ng/. Some are not voiced which means the air stream comes up over the relaxed vocal chords, while others require the vibration of the vocal chords. In addition to this difference there are nasal sounds /m/n/ng/; some are fricatives made by forcing the breath through a narrow opening between the teeth /s/, or teeth and lip /f/, or tongue and teeth /th/. The /th/ sound may be either voiced as in *th*at, or non-voiced as in *th*ink. The voiced partner for /s/ is /z/ and for /f/ it is /v/. Plosives are sounds with a stop motion as /p/t/k/ which are breath stops and /b/d/g/ are voiced stops. And all these consonants can be blended as in *bl*ue, *dr*um, *sp*ot. And even this is not the whole story as consonants have variations if starting a word, or in the median position or a final sound—and that too depends upon how the next word starts.

There are 16 vowels and diphthongs. While diphthongs are blends of vowels, there is a glide that produces a sound different from the two vowels.

A syllable is the smallest sound "byte" that should be drilled. A syllable includes a vowel and a consonant. The drill should immediately put the syllable into a word or phrase. All this exacting drill is only for developing sounds the hearing impaired child has not acquired in a more natural situation. There is a "melody" to every language. Even if we are not close enough to understand a speaker, we can tell if it is a statement or a question. We do not speak in separate words, but in phrases: *the jolly old man, the little brown dog,* we went *to the store*, we watched *the football game*, its time *for lunch*.

There is more to speaking than articulation. There is intonation, stress, and rhythm. And as mentioned before, phrasing. Not only are the mouth cavity, the tongue (which has eight muscles), and vocal chords required to make minute adjustments, also the diaphragm which controls the breath is involved.

Enough said. Speaking is the most remarkable feat humans master. If a child is not hearing the complete roster of speech sounds, he needs help from a speech therapist. The regular teacher in a mainstreamed class has neither the knowledge nor the time to coach and drill an individual student.

The advantage of mainstreaming is that the child lives in a normal speech environment. If, however, interpreters act as mediators for the child who is apt to give the answer in sign, then the "normal speech environment" is thwarted.

On the other hand, in classes for the hearing impaired there is not that "normal speech environment". Teachers must draw the fine line between using signs and encouraging speech. Observation shows that teachers who have a speech background intuitively put the emphasis on an oral response.

This becomes more difficult in the advanced grades as subject content must be stressed. The collaborative work of the teacher of the hearing impaired, the speech therapist, and the regular classroom teacher is so important. The teacher in the regular class needs to encourage the hearing impaired student to speak for himself.

Jenny Van Straten Dillard, who successfully integrated into the regular high school in her home town with an interpreter says,

"Every time I speak, I practice. With practice, I improve."

References

Lenneberg, Eric H. "What is Meant by a Biological Approach to Language", *American Annals of the Deaf*, 115, (March 1970).

Ling, Daniel (1988). *Foundations of Spoken Language for Hearing-Impaired Children*, Alexander Graham Bell Association for the Deaf, Inc.

Ross, Mark (1990). *Our Forgotten Children: Hard-of-Hearing Pupils in the Schools*, Editor, Julia Davis. Self Help for Hard of Hearing People, Inc.

* * * * *

The English Language

The English language is a conglomerate of many languages. Yet it does have its own rules. Word order is an all important requirement.

"Mary dress blue party."

This tells us what she wore and where, but you would get strange looks if you spoke this way.

"Mary wore her blue dress to the party." would be acceptable.

To illustrate this "language problem" may I quote from a study I did in 1974.[1] It included the post rubella students who were 9 to 10 years old, and those students with other etiologies, but the same age, a total of 33 children. There were 26 pictures in the study. However, one will suffice to illustrate the problem. The study an-

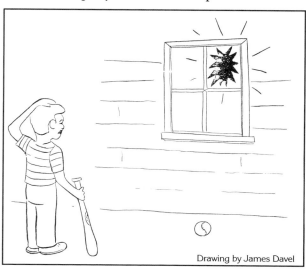

Drawing by James Davel

alyzed all the language constructions, but for brevity, just a few sample sentences are given here without rating the grammar. All the students in this sample have average non-verbal I.Q.s.

1. Ferris, Margaret H. *Linguistic Analysis of the Language of Post-Rubella Hearing Impaired Children.* (1974)

The teachers tested the students individually. The teacher could ask, "What happened?" The vocabulary was kept simple so that was not a problem. The children either spoke or signed. The teacher gave them several chances to give the best answers.

The boy broke the window.
The boy is a ball on window. Broke window.
*The boy played ball and broked the window.
Boy hit window broke.
The boy broken the window.
The boy hit ball window.
*The boy has bat and break the window.
*The boy is broken window. Ball hitting window.
The window broke.
The window is broken.
The boy is broke the window.
The boy throw ball window.
The boy broke window.
*The boy is hit. Window broke.
The boy is broke the window.
*The boy is house crash. Bat the ball.
The boy broken the window.

Other etiologies:
The boy window broke.
*The hit the window, baseball. They broke it.
*The boy put the ball in the house. The glass cracked.
The boy is throw the ball.
The boy is broke window.
*Boy hit ball. Broke window. Naughty.
The boy break the window ball.
The window is broken. The boy is throwing the window.
The boy broke the window.
The boy has broken window. The boy said, "Forgot."

Hearing students, same age, from regular class.
The boy broke the window. (6 same reply)
The little boy broke a window.
*A boy broke a window while he was playing baseball.
*The boy broke a window playing baseball.

This picture involves two actions.* We see only the result. The boy hit the ball and it broke the window. Not many of the children attempted to include both actions—even the hearing students.

By the age of nine our hearing children have mastered all the constructions of the English language. Our hearing impaired children still have a long way to go. Notice that the other studies reported in the book make the point that even a small amount of hearing improves the language ability of the child. This is certainly a strong argument for early diagnosis and wearing a hearing aid.

One other problem is that the most common verbs are the irregular ones: to be, to have. And you recall the saying we learned about the auxiliary verbs: "am, is, are, was, were, been, be". With regular verbs, there are only these forms: "to walk: walks, walked, and walking". Try "to go, went, going, gone". None of these variations is easily lip read. One must depend upon the context of the sentence.

We not only have the grammar of the sentence to consider, but also the meaning of the words as they fit the topic. For instance, the director of a program died, and the next day the teacher tried to reassure the students that they should not be sad as he had gone to Heaven. One nine-year-old objected, "No, mother read in paper. He was out . . . standing in his field."

I recall analyzing a primary reader. When the mother did not hear a *sound*, she went to look for the toddler. She found him *safe and sound* behind the couch where he was *sound asleep*. Three meanings for the word *sound*. I would not attempt to list all the meanings for the verb *to run*.

Here we have dealt with verbs. Language is also subjects, objects and adjectives, adverbs, and prepositional phrases. The complication of clauses, add conjunctions, to say nothing about idioms, expressions and slang which add to gaining command of the language. Passive voice is difficult to master. There is direct and indirect discourse.

It is obvious that our language has a rigid code and that there is little leeway in spelling. Even a child with a mild hearing loss is missing much that gives him the normal listening experiences needed to become competent in the understanding and use of language.

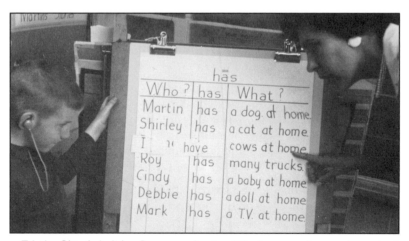

Edythe Sitte is helping Duane understand the language lesson. The chart helps children use the irregular verb: to have.

For regular verbs one adds an -s, -ed, or -ing. But irregular verbs, which are the more common, the whole form changes.

123

Developing An Academic High School Program
1970s

Looking Beyond High School

Originally the whole Oshkosh program for deaf and hard of hearing children was held in one building. In the 60s the children were placed in the buildings where they would be with hearing peers. The older students moved to a high school, but the program continued to be self-contained. They did attend non-academic classes such as gym, art, and shop and home economics classes. A few did go to high school math classes. David Thomas, the high school instructor, also developed a work study program. He accompanied the students to work sites and acted as mediator between the place of business and the student.

At this same time Wisconsin introduced Signed English. The oral staff had to learn sign language and then teach the students. The elementary program hired a deaf teacher so the mastery of sign language moved swiftly at this level. And the staff took courses in sign language.

It was at this juncture that parents of the children still in the elementary program became concerned that their children were capable of more than merely work study programs. These parents worked with the teachers and convinced the administration that a more comprehensive program was necessary. These were the parents of the post rubella children. Many had older children and knew what general education was and how necessary it was for their hearing impaired children.

By the time this large class of students was in high school, there was a staff of six teachers and four interpreters. These students could then attend classes in the regular high school program. Scheduling was difficult as several students had to take a class at the same time to get the benefit of an interpreter. In one case a teacher of the hearing impaired team taught a science class.

These students did go on to technical colleges and universities. As clients of the Department of Vocational Rehabilitation—DVR—they qualified for financial assistance and could request the services of note takers and interpreters. The work study program had also continued and Mr. Thomas assisted these graduates in finding employment. Then, as now, the students had been guided in classes and activities of their strengths.

So it was the parents of the post rubella students that encouraged the development of an academic high school program.

．．．．．

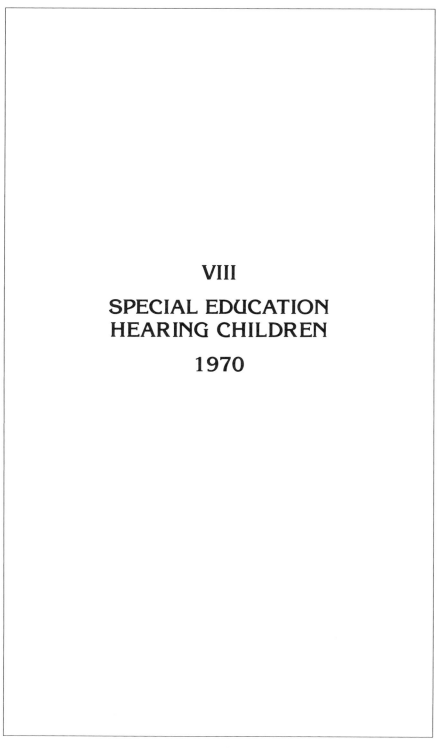

VIII

SPECIAL EDUCATION
HEARING CHILDREN

1970

Robust, Happy Children

My class of nine primary educable mentally retarded—EMR—children were at another school. There were several classes of special education students and the regular classes.

I was able to bring some equipment to start the class, and through the years I had purchased many extras. I did have my collection of Little Golden Books and many toys, but largely the room was regulation—a couple tables and little chairs. After a few days, the clatter of the activities on the hard wood floor sent me to the carpet shop to buy, on sale, some rugs. What a difference that made.

It was a different world, these children could hear. But, surprise of surprises, they did not understand very much. In no time I took out my bag of tricks that were stand-bys for teaching the hearing impaired. They needed help with saying simple sentences, not fragments of sentences. These children had established these sentence patterns since early childhood and were very difficult to correct. One little girl, Jane, told me about her mother, "Her baked cookies." Try as I would to give her the correct form, she only repeated her sentence.

It took carefully planned, step-by-step lessons to develop correct patterns. All the students needed speech therapy. This became part of every lesson. I gave them the model and through games, got them to practice correct sounds and words, phrases and simple sentences and questions. Stars worked wonders.

Chart stories, a stand-by for teachers of the deaf, worked equally well for this class. We all rushed home after school to watch "Flipper". We developed stories about the dolphin. The fish was easy to draw and they soon were able to give a sentence or two about Flipper. They could manage stick figures, cars and trucks, Christmas trees and houses.

Playground activity was a problem. One day they wanted the jump ropes. I had to take one end as turning the rope was not that easy or even just to swing it back and forth to jump over it. But alas, what they really wanted to do was to swing the rope like cowboys—rather dangerous on the playground. But we did manage to play some simple games and two of the boys got really good at making baskets.

One of the most pleasing developments in this class was their learning to enjoy stories. In the beginning we would have a period to look at books—because I insisted. But they flipped through them, many times upside down, and cared nothing about looking at the pictures. Gradually they began to enjoy my reading and telling the stories. And as time went on, they could help in the telling, and acting out the stories. Eventually they each had a favorite book. One girl, on her own, lined up several chairs, and read her story to "her class".

One husky lad would get restless and before he could get into trouble or disturb the other children, I would say, "Donny, let's move the play furniture. I think we would like the stove over here." He used up his energy and then was anxious to play in the new setting.

All one wall was a blackboard. The children did numbers and beginning printing on the board. And, of course, they all had papers to take home to show mother.

The goal for that school year was to have close contact with the parents. At this, I was an old hand, and fortunately so.

I visited Tommy's family before he entered my class. In addition to talking about the general level of his activity, and the feelings the parents and siblings had, his father gave me the exacting information about his medication. Fortunately I had this as on the second day he was in school, the principal, who was to give the child the medicine, was gone. Fearing that skipping the medication would be dangerous, I knew what he needed.

The father wanted to know if anyone at school could give mouth to mouth resuscitation. The school nurse stopped at our school several times a week, but was not there all the time. The father told me what emergency steps to take.

One morning I had the name of a new girl who was assigned to my class. At noon I phoned the family to make an appointment to visit them.

I learned that Mattie was the same age as Tommy and was glad they could be together afternoons. I explained that the other children were beginning reading and printing and that the morning was best for those activities. The afternoons were less structured and would be better for the younger children.

My year in this program showed me what the mentally retarded child needs without the added problem of a hearing loss. However, the needs of a mentally retarded, hearing impaired child are more complicated. This I was to find out in my next assignment.

* * * * *

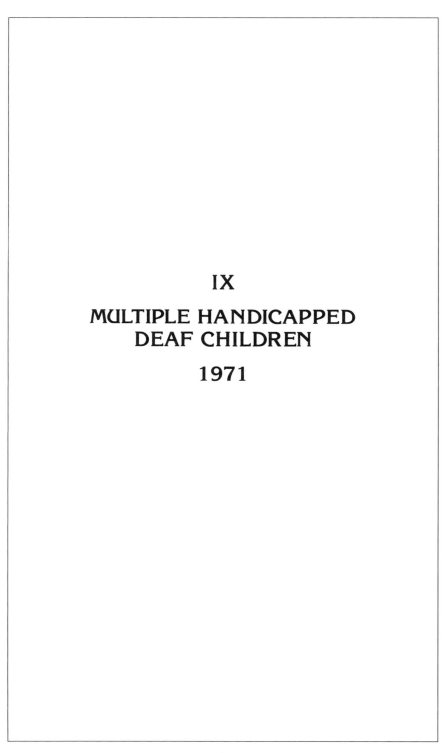

IX

MULTIPLE HANDICAPPED
DEAF CHILDREN

1971

Sign Me In

After a year of teaching a class of primary educable mentally retarded students, all with normal hearing, I was offered, as promised, an opening in the Hearing Impaired Department at a junior high school to start September 1971.

The teacher who had the class had retired. I got her room, but not her class. The elementary multiple handicapped, hearing impaired class was now ready for junior high, age wise. There were six students: Shirley, a large child with birth injuries; frail little Debra with multiple handicaps; Cindy was active and academically low; Steve lived at the Winnebago Mental Health Center. And then there was Dean, slight of build, well coordinated and with normal non-verbal intelligence, but with no interest in anything that did not have moving parts. His scholastic achievement was inexplicably low. Before the end of the year, the sixth student, Mavourneen, moved out of state. And the class settled down to the five students.

The summer before taking this class the Wisconsin Division for Handicapped Children, Hearing Impaired Program sponsored a week's training in sign language. Wisconsin was moving into Total Communications for most day classes. The training was held in a posh resort in the north, but we were kept so continuously busy all day and evenings that it could have been held in a basement in town. However, the meals were sumptuous. Perhaps to make the change more palatable. I was then directed to conduct my class in the manual mode, as speech training for this class had been a dismal failure.

The wing had been added to the junior high school to accommodate the classes for the hearing impaired. In the beginning it housed all ages of hearing impaired students from the ten surrounding counties. However, there had been no integration within the school, other than perhaps physical education for the junior high students.

There was also an art class for our older children, but not with the hearing students. And our children went to lunch a half hour early, so even eating with the regular students was denied. The reason given was that the lunch area—tables let down in the hall near the kitchen—did not afford room for these additional children. Also the little ones might be pushed by older, active regular junior high students.

By the time I joined the staff at the junior high, there were just the two of us teachers for the hearing impaired. The younger children had been moved to a regular elementary school so they could be with peers and have normal contact. And the high school age students moved on to North High School.

The other teacher, Marlene Tucker, was able to integrate students through close cooperation with the regular staff. She carefully followed the students' progress, over-saw their assignments, assisting where they needed help.

I tried some integrating. I choose a placement where each child showed some promise. Steve had a Grandma Moses art talent. The art teacher tolerated his hyperactivity and disruptive behavior for one quarter. Shirley started sewing class, but after a few lessons, the home economics teacher gave my class a sewing machine. The boys did well in woodworking class. The teacher was accepting. Dean was exceptionally good.

All these classes met at different times, so I was unable to leave my classroom to go with the student needing help.

It was during this junior high experience that I recognized Dean's talent for fixing things. He fixed clocks, radios, the movie projector, the sewing machine, and put together a Wankel rotary engine. The boys made a train table in shop. Steve built the city from small blocks from preschool days. Dean kept the switches, the engine, and lights operating. We drilled holes in the train table and strung tiny Christmas lights up into each house and building. Our village looked most real. We went to visit a train buff and got many ideas to incorporate in our train set-up.

However, we shared very few activities or resources with the regular junior high students. Even the library was beyond my students' reading level. There were some books about travel that we could enjoy. But one incident showed what our limitations were. Steve found a book about his hobby— trains. I watched him page through the book, and then disappointment grew on his face. He looked back at the title, and again went through the book, but could not find one picture about trains in *Training for Track*.

After that we went to the Public Library to the Children's Department once a week.

On one of our walks through the park near school we found a plastic container about the size of a salt shaker filled with old coins. We wrote a newspaper ad in Lost and Found and patiently waited for an answer. One never came. After several weeks the principal said the coins were ours. One of the teachers brought us a book on old and rare coins for us to study. The coins were worth over four dollars, only 83¢ in face value.

Several weeks later the boys found a pair of flippers for swimming in, of all places, the shrubs near school. Steve and Dean were anxious to take them to the principal's office. And they waited. Only a week, in this instance, for the next time we went to the YMCA for our weekly swim the life guard said, "Your boys walked off with a set of our flippers last week."

Too bad the flippers didn't become theirs!

For one six week period we were fortunate as a practice teacher in the art department took our whole class. She helped the students make a huge paper mache fish five feet long just like the one in the Jacques-Yves Cousteau story we read. Because our classroom was small, it was suspended from the ceiling.

The reading level of my class in regular texts dealt with little children and was not emotionally or socially satisfying. We particularly liked the *Reader's Digest* stories adapted to lower reading levels. These stories were about adult interests. The Cousteau story was one such tale. Our huge fish made it all the more real.

There are excellent reading series for children and young people with reading problems. The vocabulary is carefully controlled, but no particular attention is given to language construction. The hearing child at the third grade level, age 8 to 9, has mastered all language constructions. Not so the deaf. They have much deeper and more profound language problems. In the Cousteau story the divers named the huge, ugly fish—Pretty Boy. It went on to say, "He followed them." My students easily and quickly signed those three words, but they could not tell to what or to whom the pronouns referred. They could not supply either, "The fish followed the men." or "Pretty Boy followed the divers." (At that time I did not know about placement in space to indicate the people or objects in sign language.)

Another story about Red Adair, who fights oil rig fires, needed further explanation. The refined oil in the little "3 in One" can was not sufficient to bring the understanding of an oil well "burning out of control". So off we went to a service station where the attendant showed us heavy lubricating oil, let us smell gasoline, and showed us the sign—NO SMOKING. He explained about fire and explosions. I interpreted in sign language.

We did have permission from the parents to make field trips and these spur of the moment excursions. All were for enlarging the understanding of the community and bringing meaning to the language and reading lessons.

Among the pamphlets left in the classroom was a listing of all the names and addresses of the home offices for all the railroads in the United States. Steve had written on his own to each and the PR people sent him brochures and other interesting information.

One of our trips was for Steve's pure enjoyment. The SOO Railroad Line staged a derailment outside of town. We watched a huge crane lift the boxcars back on the track.

At the airport we were bused out to the control tower, and it was Dean who watched through the binoculars as a large plane landed and a smaller one took off. We got to sit in a plane that had just returned from Alaska. It was back to class to study the map.

Routine trips to the hobby shop, the fabric store, and most frequently to the grocery store helped the students learn to make purchases and handle money. While we all went to the store, eventually only one student would go in with the list to select the items and make the purchase. Our arithmetic problems were real.

We cooked in our classroom as the home economics classes were fully scheduled. We had our own small budget for food. We constantly blew fuses as our classroom was not wired to have an electric frying pan, a toaster, and a hot plate connected all at once.

We took pictures and more pictures of every activity in school and in the community on our trips. It is said that we learn 85 percent through vision. However, what we see would be only a series of meaningless activities if not accompanied by language. In addition to the students learning sign language—I was continuing learning too, taking evening classes—I did not neglect lipreading and speech drills. Only Cindy and Steve had usable residual hearing. However, in the store they had to be able to lipread and ask simple questions. All wore hearing aids as it is my contention that environmental sounds are essential for one's safety and for orientation. This even when speech discrimination is not possible. The awareness of sound, its duration, and inflection assist in lipreading. With their desks in a semi-circle and my chair on wheels, I could easily move to within the optimum distance for the best function of their hearing aids.

In the fall the parents told me that the girls had matured during the summer, so we continued the health lessons. They signed "finished, finished", and were not interested. In a matter of a few weeks the unpleasant truth had to be accepted.

Gradually our signing improved. We did have the help of one other staff member, Carol Fredrickson, who came weekly to give us added experience. All the students came from hearing homes, nor were any of their parents or foster parents taking signing classes. Therefore the students only experience was in school. My students found little companionship with the other junior high hearing impaired students who were very busy integrating into the regular classes. However, many of the regular students became interested in learning some signing and came in at noon once a week for lessons. And the boys in the school were most interested in our train set up. So the regular students made every effort to greet my students in the hall. And by this time we did share the lunch hour.

We did have behavior problems, attention spans were short. The junior high no longer had recess, but we found it necessary to take a few minutes break. Normally the regular children had a few minutes as they moved from class to class, but our students remained in the same room. In psychology there is a term called "time out". My students had the technique worked out. When we all felt frazzled, they would suggest I go get a cup of coffee! The teachers' room was a few steps away from our classroom. I came back refreshed and they were willing to resume class. One morning we all decided to go outside for a few minutes. They rushed to their lockers and before I got into the hall, a fire drill sounded. Usually teachers were told of such a drill, so I said, "Who did that?" And my students turned to one who had pulled the alarm near the door. Everyone in the school went out. Needless to say the students undressing for gym were not happy. In no time the principal was in our room. He stood beside the miscreant and told me how serious this conduct had been. He expected me to sign this warning, which I did. However, his lecture would have been more effective if he had faced the culprit. His body language and facial expression would have carried his message. What he did not know was that the girl had no idea what the fire alarm box would actuate. She had pulled the alarm as you might flick a light switch. It was time for a lesson on fire alarms and safety and when it was permissible to sound the alarm and who was to do it.

Our goal was to acquire more mature behavior in relationships, to finish our assignments, and be responsible for our actions. And all things considered, our two years in the junior high school did accomplish these goals. And we looked forward to moving on to the North High School.

· · · · ·

On To High School

In early spring of our second year at the junior high school, arrangements got underway for our move to high school. There was one teacher at North High, and I naturally thought my class would move there. At the meeting to make plans, I was surprised that the general feeling was that my class would move to the West High School.

"Your class would fit in with educable retarded program. We have trouble integrating our normal hearing impaired students as it is."

Shortly after this meeting I met with the assistant principal at West High School. He showed me a small conference room located in the middle of the building.

"This should be adequate for only five students," he said. He was sure it would be acceptable.

How was I to point out it would never do? How to sound firm and yet not ungrateful?

I began, "My students will be with me all day. We have our own over-head projector, and there is no screen."

"One can be put up."

"And no chalk board."

"That too can be added."

Now came the touchy part, "We also have our own sewing machine and we need a large table for projects and crafts."

"I thought you were to join some classes for the special education students," he said.

"My students were not integrated with the special education students in the junior high. I use sign language with my students."

A shadow crossed his face.

I hurried on, "My students are very shy, and would be uncomfortable with this wall of windows toward this busy hall."

"I'm sorry, but all our regular classrooms are in use." But he did not sound sorry.

"But," I persisted, "six to eight deaf children constitute a class. And their needs are unique."

"I will see what can be arranged. It will mean moving several classes around." He implied it would offend the regular staff.

At whose intervention I never knew, but several weeks later I was assured a room at the south east corner of the high school would be available. It was in the English wing, and right down the corridor from the special education classroom and kitchen-shop room. It had two large windows to the south, a chalk board along the front wall, a built-in cupboard and movable bookcase, a large table, the five desks, and plenty of room for our sewing machine and over-head projector on a cart. And, of course, racks for our screen and maps. I had only to bring my carpet to make the room acoustically ideal.

And my students were to have their lockers right outside our room—even though this hall was used by seniors.

And the assistant principal said, "Buses stop at this corner."

The several days of orientation for teachers before the students arrived in the fall were filled with meetings: general meetings, special education meetings, deaf department meetings, and meetings for the new staff at the high school. My walking the new halls—there was by actual count one mile of hallways—to become acquainted with the cafeteria, the nurse's station, and the offices was limited as I had only recently had the cast removed from my broken ankle. By the end of each day my leg was swollen and painful.

This accident happened several weeks before school recessed in June. My absence the last days meant that the substitute had to pack for the move. In the last years as classes in the deaf department left our wing at Webster Stanley, old texts, workbooks, and supplies had accumulated in my cupboard. All this arrived at high school in room E-22.

Any time spent in my room was a treasure hunt. Most valuable were the boxes which contained my file of pictures collected and cataloged throughout many years. Once these pictures were placed in my new filing cabinet near my desk, and I found chalk, I was ready for class. The other packing boxes were pushed to the back of the room.

Day One

At junior high the buses, vans, and cars for the students pulled up in the driveway adjacent to our wing, so I was lulled into thinking transportation would move smoothly here at high school. Did not the buses stop right outside our door—at our very corner?

However, all my students wore or carried identification. Not only my students, but all the freshmen would need some help in locating classes. Shirley and Debra rode rural buses, and they had the bus numbers. Debra had two sisters at high school who came in to see me during the week of orientation and assured me they would help Shirley and Debra. It was not until they arrived the first morning that I discovered that the rural bus pick-up was not at our corner, but at the far north west side of the school a quarter of a mile from our room. It was near the student parking lot, the civic auditorium, and gym.

"Not to worry," Debra's sisters told me. "We will come for the girls at lunch time and after school."

Cindy and Dean lived in boarding homes in Oshkosh and had been riding city buses for two years. Their social workers and boarding mothers had ridden with them before school started to familiarize them with the new route.

Steve, who had lived at the Winnebago Mental Health Center in the Children's Unit for many years, was transported by a van from the Center. (There was a school at the Center, but his hearing loss was the primary educational handicap.)

The first morning all arrived on time. We brought the locks from the lockers into our room to practice the combinations. I copied down the combinations knowing they would need much more practice. We arranged our room, and I had prepared a mountain of seatwork. All had been mailed the lunch tickets for the first week. It was an all together pleasant day.

At the close of the day Debra's sisters arrived and took the girls. Cindy and Dean waited at our corner and I watched them get on the city bus. I waited with Steve as there were many private cars and vans. His ride never came, so we returned to the room. He helped me put things in order, and I drove him to the Center which was more or less on my way home.

Finally at home I rested my swollen leg for a few minutes before getting dinner. No sooner was I settled when the phone rang. It was Shirley's foster mother.

"Shirley missed her bus. The principal phoned to say she would be waiting in front of the school near the flag pole. I have driven around and around the school and can't find Shirley. And all the doors are locked."

"Oh, my. All you can do is call the police. No way would she know which way to walk."

"It's five miles. Where can she be?"

"Call the police is all I can suggest."

Later, much later, Shirley's foster mother called to say she had been found in town at the shopping mall near the transfer point for city buses.

As we pieced together the story, Debra's bus arrived first and Shirley, even with her bus number, was faced with over a half dozen buses that shot in, expected the students to be lined up, and then roared off leaving her alone. She began circling the school, crying and rapping on windows until she came to the principal's office. With her identification Dr. Traeger was able to phone her home. He wrote a note for Shirley that said she was to wait at the flag pole where he took her. Alas, his hand writing at best was none too easy to read, and Shirley had a limited reading ability. Nor, of course, could the principal sign. Shirley, not understanding the direction that she was to wait, boarded a city bus and at the transfer corner wandered about.

I spent the second day at West High School arranging transportation.

· · · · ·

The High School Experience

Can one be accepted and rejected in the same situation? Being part of the West High School staff was the most rewarding experience I had of the seven schools in which I taught in Oshkosh, Wisconsin. My room was in the English wing. Teaching hearing impaired students is one of communication, so I felt comfortable and welcome.

Yet it was the worst possible placement for the lads in my class. Educators and parents talk about mainstreaming of handicapped children, but my multiple handicapped hearing impaired students were not welcome in the same building with the regular hearing impaired classes. It was thought my students' behavior would have an adverse effect on the acceptance of the other deaf students, therefore we were the only hearing impaired class at West High School.

Who were my students going to find as friends? Who would be able to communicate with them in sign language? At no time is one more alone than in a crowd, in this instance, with 1,200 regular students.

The girls fared better. One had two sisters in high school. Another had sufficient residual hearing that she could easily communicate with the girls in special education. And the third one, although she was profoundly deaf, was comfortable with her classmates and their friends.

Not all was as bleak as I anticipated. The first week of school a sophomore lad, Tom Harris, came to our door and asked, "Can I help with your students?"

Tom was medium height and had blond hair that fell about his ears as was the style in 1974. He came to our room one period each day, learned sign language, and befriended my students, not only in our room, but also sat with them at lunch time.

Peer tutoring was Tom's gift. He patiently encouraged them to do their lessons, helping only enough to show them how. He also did his homework which set a good example. He was so much a part of our activities that he appeared in many of our classroom pictures. My favorite was one where he

136

was in earnest conversation—no—in consultation with our social worker of many years. Tom spent time with us all his years at high school. In the spring of his senior year he got his GED (graduation equivalency diploma) and joined the Marines. The next year he paid us a visit—tall, straight, in dress uniform. Our girls melted.

Freshman English classes study "The Miracle Worker". The teachers asked if their classes could visit our room. My students enjoyed this attention and gave a demonstration in sign language and fingerspelling. Then I would show them the added problem of the deaf-blind who must read fingerspelling under the palm of the hand. Following these demonstrations many of the regular students came to help my students and to learn more sign language.

Two students continued to come regularly for a period a day. Chris Williams and Sue Campbell not only learned Signed English in our classroom, but went with the entire staff of teachers for the hearing impaired for an advanced course given by the University of Wisconsin-Milwaukee in Fond du Lac.

Sue Campbell received her degree in Elementary Education, but took most of the course work for teaching hearing impaired children. And she did teach a preschool class in Lincoln, Nebraska, putting emphasis on parent education. Presently she teaches a regular fifth grade in Fairbanks, Alaska.

Chris acted as an aide and interpreter with one of my students who took regular typing. She too kept a watchful eye on the girls.

The original intent of moving to West High School was that my students would join some EMR classes. So off the boys went, not to the special education shop, but into beginning Woodworking instructed by a teacher who had experience with handicapped students. However, after several weeks when we discussed the behavior of my students, their limited ability to follow directions and the safety factor, the set of his jaw told me this would not work out for Steve.

The set-up for a shop project for the EMR students did not seem promising at that time. Their activity took place in an all-purpose room mornings where they had an assembly line project making tip-ups for ice fishing. My students could not spend the entire morning in such an activity.

My three girls and I joined the afternoon cooking class in this all-purpose room. All was fine if you did not object to sawdust in your pudding. With two teachers and an aide and two classes, there was limited room to cook—with only one stove.

And the instruction was on two levels. The EMR students, older girls, were ready to prepare recipes, while my students were still learning the names of the kitchen utensils: sauce pan, mixing spoon, measuring cup. And the math necessary for measuring: teaspoon, tablespoon, ¼ cup, ½ cup, pint, quart; and directions: mix, stir, add, boil, simmer. All these were terms that we still had to drill. Added to this there was subtle teasing that we teachers could not identify the source. So back to our room for basics.

I am pleased to report that the all-purpose room gave way to the kitchen, and the shop moved next door to a room now equipped with a power saw, hand tools, and cupboards for paint and supplies. Here my students were accommodated. I worked with the shop teacher and all my pupils participated. This, however, did not happen until several years later. We were able to work alone in the kitchen, and one year were joined by a small class of younger EMR students. By this time they also were in my class for a period of job readiness.

This group was delightful. Each day during the period one student could take a turn being the teacher. I prepared the lesson, seatwork and answer sheet, then sat in the back of the room. By this time the EMR students had a rudimentary signing ability. As you might expect the most recalcitrant student became the most demanding instructor.

Sewing went much better as our class had a sewing machine given to us at junior high school. In addition we were supplied with a new portable machine. So now on our large table we could lay out patterns and work on crafts. From the many scraps from our sewing projects each girl made a crib size crazy quilt as each had infant nieces and nephews.

Cooking and sewing with limited shop work was not what the boys needed. I began talks with their parents and the director of our program to consider their transfer to the Wisconsin School for the Deaf at Delavan. At this residential school the boys would have role models as many of the men instructors were deaf. They would have friends, and most important there were all sorts of after school activities.

Dean, a farm lad, had been driving farm equipment for years, but there was no way he could take drivers education in our building. He could at Delavan. And Steve — let me tell you about Steve.

The Railroad Buff—Steve

If Steve had no handicaps and could develop his talents, age 25 would find him buried behind a mountain of books seeking minute information for his doctoral thesis. He studied even the phone book with intensity.

He was a delight for librarians. No student used the library so thoroughly— the files, the maps, the over-sized books, the flat pull-out drawers. He could use the card catalog and retrieve any information. But then the sad truth surfaced—he could not read. He read words here and there, but not the text. He brought a book back to our room titled *The Block*. It had endless pictures of the ghetto and not one about the manufacturing of cement blocks which his father used to do.

A less kind, but more realistic picture of Steve was that he was a pack-rat, a scavenger. This trait, his social worker said, was typical behavior for a institutionalized child. Steve had lived at the Winnebago Mental Health Center for nearly six years. He was not a disturbed child. Hyperactive, yes, but very much interested in the community and all that happened. He loved the SOO LINE RAILROAD which obliged him by having endless derailments in our area. He had written to every railroad corporate headquarters in this country—many times. The PR men sent him pamphlets and brochures and articles which he had carefully organized in drawers and boxes in his room at the mental health center.

Steve was a loner. The residents in the Childrens Unit are there for a relatively short time. It had few activities and no sports. Considering that Steve had motor problems, his coordination was that of a wet noodle, so he did not enjoy sports. The Center did have a farm. They raised cattle, crops, a vegetable garden and chickens. All this Steve enjoyed.

Through the years there were hopes that he could be placed in a foster home, but nothing worked out. His social worker and wife took him home with them two nights a week and often on a weekend. On the days that he was to visit them he began packing at noon for the 3:15 dismissal.

When we drilled a language principle, he did well. However, it did not carry over into his writing, talking or signing. His spelling was good. His audiogram showed peaks and valleys. Add to this his spastic involvement meant that his articultion was affected. This would have been so even if he had no hearing loss. His signing was over-blown and filled with added gestures. He printed due to his difficulty with motor control.

He was on medication—Ritalin. Generally his behavior was acceptable. The very first week we started at the high school I expected he would have trouble adjusting. And his behavior was "off the wall". I immediately called his social worker who was on vacation and so I asked to speak to a psychiatrist.

The doctor said, "Every six months all medication is stopped and the patient's condition re-evaluated. This week was Steve's time for discontinuing his medication."

That first week the administrator at high school who handled behavior problems was in our room repeatedly. Our first impression was not good.

For all of Steve's love of books, he rejected reading lessons. The attention and drill necessary to comprehend the language was too demanding. He was perfectly satisfied with words. However, I was not, so we struggled, but with very little success.

He had a Grandmother Moses art talent with an eye for detail. All of which was most surprising with his poor coordination. There seemed to be no way to schedule him for a regular art class. His general behavior precluded an attempt to intergrate him.

Because he lived in an institution and missed family life, he enjoyed home tasks—cooking (he made a toque), and washing dishes. He also did this at camp. At school when the whole Special Education Department prepared a Christmas dinner for 45 guests, Steve washed all the dishes and pans— enjoying every minute of it. He enjoyed making a tote bag on the sewing machine, sewing on buttons, and ironing. (I kept a few family items for practice.) He vacuumed so vigorously that he raised cement dust from under the tiles right through the rug.

He did everything with gusto. I mentioned he was a scavenger. He had a collection of empty beer cans in this locker. The school administrator, who was our constant friend, and I did not know that collecting beer cans was a legitimate activity. We made him throw out the stinky things.

Steve was beginning to notice girls and became flustered with the young practice teachers. The more they tried to help him and give him added attention, the more uncomfortable he became. Certainly at Delavan he would have a more natural contact with girls in many activities—ones he could communicate with and share activities.

Steve was a "group" of contradicitons: awkward, yet had art talent; had understandable speech, but jumbled language word order and limited vocabulary.

Steve was accepted at the Wisconsin School for the Deaf where he would be better served.

Author's Comment
Today Steve lives with a brother who is his legal guardian. He works in the kitchen of a country club. Recently I was doing some work in the Oshkosh Library when I became aware of two young men who were talking about trains—and there was Steve.

· · · · ·

Fixing Things — Dean S.

Dean S. had one love—fixing things.

All academic work he swallowed whole avoiding any taste or trying to understand it. He did his seatwork rapidly with no thought.

He wanted to do what he wanted, when he wanted and usually couldn't be bothered with academic work. This behavior was evident in shop class and in physical education. The accident outside the janitors' area (with whom he spent his lunch hours) was a result of his going ahead on his own and not following instructions.

He liked to help shovel snow. When it was possible, I said the boys could go the last hour of the morning. He sulked. Another time I excused them immediately with a pass for an hour. I never saw them again all morning and when they returned they were not cold, but were munching candy. When I said they may not go, Dean sulked the entire morning.

The assistant principal in charge of discipline came in to straighten out the misunderstanding. The next occasion the same argument occured.

Dean did not have a learning disorder. A student who can follow a complicated diagram for the repair of a sewing machine or construct a model Wankel rotary engine or fix a small gas engine is not multi-handicapped. He manipulated teachers all of his school years. He needed to have immediately a staff of teachers who were on to the ways of deaf students—with mostly men for instructors.

Some weeks after school started the gym teacher reported that Dean did not yet have his gym clothes. He did. They were in his locker near our classroom. A deaf child can outsmart a regular instructor every time!

Dean claimed that the other students laughed at him when he wore his hearing aid so he took to hiding it in the room before going to other classes. Other students molested him on the bus and in the lunch room. His money was taken out of his wallet, and his food from his tray. They knew he could not name them.

The instructor of small gas engines was a friend of the boarding family where Dean lived. The instructor had occasion to visit at their home and took Dean to the school shop some evenings. Dean did wear his hearing aid and the instructor learned that even then he did not understand speech through his aid. The instructor then realized what a handicap Dean had.

In the regular small gas engines class he could do the work when shown how, but could not read the text nor participate in the question and answer periods. All of this must be taught in conjunction with the language needed.

Because Dean was so talented in manual work, he needed to have the best training.

He appeared embarrassed to do the drill for better speech, and on the other hand, he did not want to bother with signs. Lipreading was fair. However, his academic work was very low. Yet he had better than average non-verbal intelligence. He was well coordinated, wiry, and should do well in sports. However, he needed the rules for games. He played baseball with his brothers.

Dean reached the age when he was very sensitive about his hearing loss. He would not wear his aid out of the room for so much as getting a drink of water. He constantly closed the window shades as there were students around the building who might look in. He kept a panel over the small window in our hall door for that same reason. Nor would he walk down the hall with his classmates who were signing to each other. When the assistant principal attempted to urge him to wear his aid to other classes, he dissolved into tears.

141

He was much happier with adults and was a real friend and helper to the janitors with whom he ate his lunch. But Dean needed friends his own age. He was happy at home with his many brothers. The boys had a workshop where they repaired bikes. The father repaired farm machinery so the boys had good instruction. Dean used speech at home and did lipread. None of these emotional problems showed up at home.

Recommendation: Immediate placement at the Wisconsin School for the Deaf where all the students and many of the teachers have profound hearing losses. He would be able to relax, learn and accept signing, and apply himself to academics as well as participate in all the social activities.

Author's Comment

Dean did transfer. He soon got his driver's license. He had been driving the farm equipment since age twelve.

At Delavan he was on the ski team and the swim team, and also wrestled. And the following year when my class visited Delavan we met him in the library withdrawing a book.

Since graduating from Delavan at age 18, Dean has worked at a tool company. Recently he purchased a house and is doing the renovating himself. A brother says he manages his own affairs and gets along fine at work. His friends understand his speech.

He has had many trucks and cars, and also a small tractor with a backhoe and does contracting.

Dean's many talents make his life full and rewarding.

· · · · ·

Socializing

My multiplex hearing impaired students at Webster Stanley Junior High School were sent to the West High School because they were high school age and tall. In no way could we be part of the high school program. The reading level was second grade. Integration was to be with the mildly retarded students. And that was not always possible.

Integration is supposed to benefit the student in as much as they will observe and emulate peer behavior. *This is a doubtful premise for multiple handicapped children. And for the general population of deaf students, acceptable behavior must be taught—both at home and at school.* This is a concern for all parents and teachers.

For instance, my class of multiple handicapped students was given front row seats for auditorium peformances. At the Christmas program we sat practically under the baton of the choir director. Some 200 students were singing "Joy to the World" when one of my lads indicated his watch. I was not sitting next to him, so he stood up and again pointed to his watch and signed that it was lunch time. There were 1200 students in the auditorium who knew it was a few minutes after the bell, but sat quietly until the program was finished.

While the student could not hear more than the drums, still by this time he should know the accepted behavior at a program. When we went to a play we learned the story ahead of time and our friend Sue Campbell was often in the play. The other students in my class thoroughly enjoyed the plays. They enjoyed being part of the student body.

One other situation illustrates the immature behavior. In our joint cooking class with the younger EMR students we prepared a dinner and invited several special education teachers. It was a dinner, not a lunch, and all ate heartily. And they cleaned up swiftly and then ran down the hall to the cafeteria—they did not want to miss lunch. That might be because teenagers have tremendous appetites. No, they could not break the routine.

Routine

All of my students, whatever age, are most comfortable with routine. One of the mothers of the preschooler sent me a note saying the school was not to have anymore two day holidays. Her son hung on his coat in the closet and then pummeled her and pulled at her apron. She was keeping him from school. It was the two day teacher's convention. The other children in the family attended a parochial school which did not have days off at this time.

Understandable for preschoolers, but the high school lad that was not interested in "Joy to the World" because it was breaking up his routine was immature. He had been patient long enough. He paid no attention to the auditorium filled with students sitting quietly.

This same December it was time to schedule for the next year. We went to the library where scheduling was taking place when it was our turn even though there was nothing to debate about—I taught, or the special education woodworking teachers taught, the students. But we joined the throngs—when in Rome . . .

That was the winter that our wing was being painted. We were told that when the painters arrived we would have to find another room—wherever one was vacant for an hour. When our time approached—the painters were in our hall, one of my lads pushed all the equipment and furniture to the center of the room. (During the summer our moveable bookcase needed to be emptied so the rooms could be cleaned and nothing heavy left in the cupboards.) Well, my lad, slight of build, moved that full bookcase. We had lots of boxes and materials and equipment in our room—now jammed in the middle—most on top of the desks. For whatever perverse reason, the painters did not come on our schedule. So for a week we lived in the mess. We barely survived the disruption when the painters did our room.

Soon after that I wrote a note to our principal, Dr. Traeger, saying that I was quitting. We had enough problems and now he had scheduled Christmas.

That morning Dr. Traeger came into my room actually worried. He did not see the humor in it. I had to explain it. Explaining a joke or "smart" saying does not make it funny. Actually Dr. Traeger was always very understanding and compassionate. Perhaps too much disruption of routine had gotten to him too.

The assistant principal in charge of scheduling sent me a notice that one of my students could not graduate as she had no physical education credits. This was the girl with many major handicaps, among them was a heart condition. I asked him if he was planning to give her the diploma post-humously. We had been in that building for five years and he did not really know my students. That was not my only problem.

Don't Bend, Fold, Or Spindle

Grades at the high school were made out on computer cards. The class and subject were stamped on the card and any number of holes. I complained that the subjects my students studied did not match the high school English course. The parents would want to know how the student was progressing in signing, lipreading, speech, written language and reading. I needed more cards to indicate this. Seems this was impossible. So I took a sharp scissors and cut out the subject. When I turned in the cards the office girl blanched. I thought she would faint. And here we go again. In no time the assistant principal came into my room. He said, "I don't need this."

This seems to have been reported to our deaf department supervisor— wasn't everything. And he said to go with the crowd and then send home written reports.

I report these things so that parents understand that trying to get the best education for hearing impaired students has pitfalls.

One other situation. One lad was uninterested in math. I wrote a letter to one of the math teachers who had advanced classes. (We had a total high school staff of 75 teachers, and the math department was somewhere in the heart of the building.) I asked if my student could attend his class. I would furnish the work sheets, but hoped that my student would see how the regular kids worked and want to emulate them. A copy went to the principal. Eventually I had his answer. "No, I will not accept your student. I will find a lad to tutor your student."

And so he did. A tall, charming young fellow. My student would have nothing to do with him, but my girls developed an interest in math. Pictures show them so pleased and laughing and happy at the attention. So I was left with working with a less than enthusiastic math hater.

Off To Delavan

One by one I recommended Delavan for my lads. They had been happy at

144

the junior high, but this was another situation and there was teasing. Dean S., my talented lad, was able to take regular Woodworking and Small Gas Engines—he had helped his father and brothers repair farm machinery. All hands-on he could do, but not read the text. He was riding with me and the class one day and indicated that the engine was not performing correctly. He could feel it. When I took it to the garage, he was right.

He always worked the projector and sat in the back of the room waiting for us to pull the shades, lower the screen. I happened to glance at him and he was trying to pry the top off of an old aerosol can. Screaming at him would do no good. I frantically waved my arms and he did look up.

I marched the class across the hall to a journalism class and asked the teacher to tell my students how dangerous this could be. I thought it would have more impact than if I told the students.

It so happened that a friend of the teacher had a nine-year-old son who was alone in the basement while the parents were shopping. He had put the aerosol can in the vise. It exploded and they found their son dead on the stairs where he bled to death. I put all my skill into signing this horror story and hoped my students all realized how dangerous this "empty can" could be.

So many things our hearing children learn—"over hear" as Leslie Halvorsen stresses. All these things we must consciously teach the hearing impaired child. This means the hard of hearing child as well as he does not pick up this information freely.

When one of my students transferred to the state residential school, he was put in the dorm with his age peers. Within the week he was transferred to a younger setting. To think that for two years he had been in a high school setting in a regular school when his coping skills were not at that level—even in the all deaf school. This had nothing to do with his academic level, but with his socializing.

Mainstreaming and inclusion must take into consideration the maturation of the child. Is he or she ready to cope with the peer age group?

Parents of infants and toddlers often remarked that their children had no fear. Normally a parent can caution a child and even one as young as 18 months or a toddler hears the fear in the parent's voice. Not so our hearing impaired children. So we must be ever vigilant. It is no wonder that we all tend to over protect our hearing impaired children.

Adult Behavior In The Work Place

A recent study says that, "Eighty percent of the people who fail at work do so for one reason: they do not relate well to other people" (Bolton, 1979). If this is true of the general population, how much more so it is for deaf employees.

They do not seem to understand the work ethic in such a simple matter as being on time or getting word to the job site that they are ill.

They tend to blame co-workers for mistakes.

Because our hearing impaired workers do not over-hear conversations at work or in the lunch room, they do not have the opportunity to acquire socializing strategies that the general population absorbs naturally.

Today's highly skilled jobs *require that deaf workers pursue advanced training* and especially to *improve their command of English.* Our young people are being trained for technical jobs. And what a shame if they fail because of inappropriate behavior.

Parents and teachers must be cognizant of the need to teach the children accepted behaviors. It must start with toddlers and be continuous there after. *For life experiences to pass before the deaf or hard of hearing child will not benefit him. We, the parents and teachers, must develop the means to have our hearing impaired children fully understand and practice accepted behaviors.*

References

Bolton, R. (1979) *People Skills.* New York: Simon & Schuster.

. . . . .

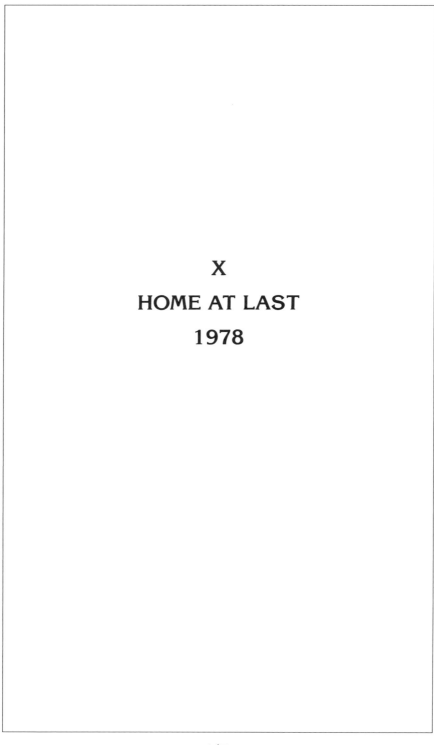

X

HOME AT LAST

1978

Home At Last

I moved to Lincoln, an elementary school, to teach the multiplex class—multiple handicapped deaf class. Asking for a regular hearing impaired class fell on deaf ears—did I not have a Masters Degree in Special Education and was the one qualified to teach this class.

However, particularly pleasing was that I would be with the staff of teachers of the deaf. I would have lunch with them everyday, be part of the give and take that makes for staff cohesion.

The rooms were large, mirrors and boards were a plenty and of course, I had my flying carpet—the third flight for it. And the teacher in the Deaf/Blind class offered a work bench.

My students were eager children, two with crutches, and the others with various problems. The only difficulty was that the lunch room, also used as the art and music room, was in the basement. But we took it slowly.

Art teachers are a flamboyant crew. Their projects are large, colorful and fun. And elementary schools are always bright with art work displayed in the halls. I welcomed the creativity for my students.

My students had physical therapy that took place in the gym. And I had an aide, Mrs. Johnson, who so frequently came to my assistance in the beginning days.

Nancy Spalding taught Adaptive Physical Education. She had one glaring fault—she did not notice that my students had physical disabilities. The period with her was a joy. There was not an activity that she could not adapt for my kids.

Our room had a little sink and better wiring than the older schools. We cooked up a storm and always had another class to invite.

Having had several years under the tutelage of a knowledgeable carpenter, I felt able to continue woodworking. And the children made several projects—wall shelves, bird houses, hanging baskets for flower pots. We practiced pounding nails—straight. We sanded and stained. We made presents for mothers.

We still had our sewing machine, and ironing board and were always busy with projects. Seems we must have taken time for arithmetic and reading—am sure we did. The library had books we could enjoy at our reading level.

We spent only one year in the elementary building and then flew up to Merrill Middle School.

· · · · ·

148

Dé Jà Vu
1959 and 1979

It was an evening in early June 1979 when I received a phone call from the Director of the Atlantic Provinces Resource Centre for Hearing Handicapped.

Dr. Peter Owsley asked, "Will you teach the Introduction to Phonetics in my teacher training program this summer?"

My first reaction was that he was visiting in Wisconsin, but no, he said he was calling from home in Nova Scotia, Canada.

"My speech teacher has become ill and I thought you would enjoy the experience. And you and Garwood can spend the weekends visiting in his home state of Maine."

I thought of my many years teaching classes of multiple handicapped deaf students where the emphasis had not been on speech. I hesitated. "It has been years since I did phonetic transcription."

"You can do it. We have other teachers on the staff to help and the curriculum is mapped out. I will send it to you."

I talked it over with my husband and we both thought it was an interesting prospect.

Dr. Owsley sent me the air fare, but the description of the course was one paragraph. But I was committed. I made a hurried trip to Milwaukee to confer with my college instructor, Professor Alice Streng. I asked, "What if Ling is the method?" Then you have nothing to worry about, "Ling is Streng, Streng is Ling." So basically I did have the background.

I arrived in Montreal and was questioned by immigration. "Are you planning to stay a few days or a week?"

"Oh, no, I am to teach for a six-week period."

"And may I see your work permit?"

Luckily I was admitted as the "paper work" took several weeks. The officer I finally met to get the permit said, "If you had come through Halifax, I would not have let you enter."

I was accustomed to giving talks about teaching hearing impaired children—general talks of say a half an hour. These classes lasted an hour and fifteen minutes every day for the entire six weeks. The class consisted of a dozen teachers from many other fields who were now specializing in deaf education. That first morning I discovered they did not know the meaning of "phonetics"—the study of how speech sounds are made, so I had a small edge. The school had a remarkable professional library so assignments were easy to develop.

149

The class was a delight. The students were eager to learn and any written assignments came in beautifully typed without my having to use "behavior modification". We developed many projects and all learned to be tuned to every speech sound and how it was made.

Two members of the class were fluent in French. This allowed us to study accents. And to develope an interesting project. We connected a head set to a small T.V. and turned it so only white noise came through. The "student" wore the head set. The instructor, one of the French speaking students, attempted to teach come simple French syllables, words, and phrases. The "student" could not hear him, but only watch him in the mirror.

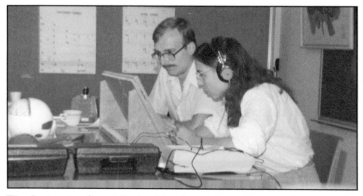

The instructor found he had to show where the sound was made, whether a nasal sound or a plosive one.

We the class could see what an effort it took to learn the French pronounciation and how much repetition it took to establish the correct pattern. It was very revealing. How do we show our deaf students how to speak? And what does it mean when there is no residual hearing to amplify?

My introductory class used *Speech and Deafness, A Text for Learning and Teaching,* by Donald R. Calvert Director, Central Institute for the Deaf, and Associate Professor of Audiology, Washington University, St. Louis, Missouri and S. Richard Silverman, Director Emeritus, Central Institute for the Deaf, Professor of Audiology, Washington University in St. Louis, Missouri (1975). This was an Alexander Graham Bell Association for the Deaf publication.

The second semester the students would have Dr. Daniel Ling's text books and learn his methods.

I did not make it to Maine, but I returned invigorated and anxious to work with my class that flew up from the elementary school. I did encourage more speech and spent a session working on speech improvement with several lads from the other hearing impaired class.

· · · · ·

150

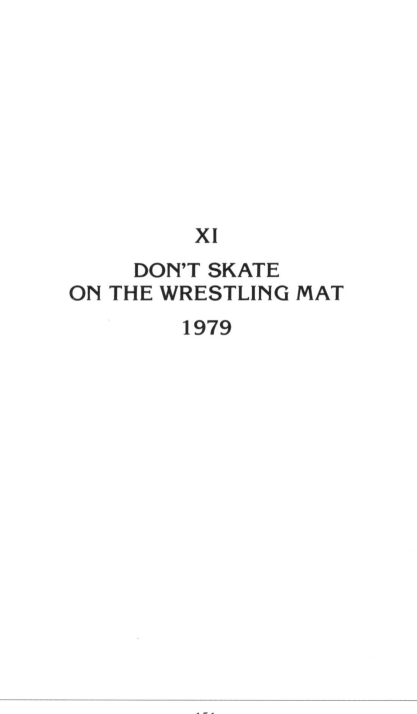

XI

DON'T SKATE
ON THE WRESTLING MAT

1979

Don't Skate On The Wrestling Mat

Merrill Middle School meant a great change. Regular students in 6th through 8th grades are lively, fast moving and here we were on the first floor near one of the doors. One happy surprise was that the room was carpeted for us!

Nancy Spalding came to continue our physical education. Here she had to improvise as the gym was never free for us—we had exercises in our room

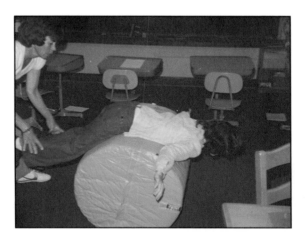

Nancy Spalding, Phy Ed teacher, with Teri on the roll.

as she secured all kinds of equipment for us and put us all (teacher too) through the paces. She had the children skiing on the gentle terrace outside our room using their crutches as ski poles. Let me tell you about tennis—my students were seated in a good center position and I ran for the balls (I was included in the exercise), some fun. We flew kites, we fished, we rode horses. When Teri discovered she could guide the horse with the reins and he would go where she wanted him too, she was thrilled. Swimming at the YMCA was probably the most remarkable experience for my students. These children, who could not walk without their crutches, could walk in the water.

It was a year before Teri would move away from the edge of the pool. Finally she grew brave enough to swim across the pool. That was so much fun she struck out down the middle of the pool toward the deep end. I swam beside her fearing she might tire and panic, but she made it. She was willing to swim back near the side, much to my relief.

There was a second new pool that was only three feet deep throughout, and several degrees warmer. Here we played games with other special education students.

Then that Nancy Spalding brought a canoe to the pool. That day we went to the high school pool. But what really got us into trouble was roller skating. We did get to skate in the gym and how fortunate, there was a large mat on the floor. Just the thing, should our students fall. They moved slowly like little children trying out skates for the first time—after all their parents had not thought to get them skates to roll down the sidewalks at home. All was going well when the teacher, the coach for wrestling, came in. I will leave it to your knowledge of men to imagine what then transpired.

We skated on the floor to the side of the mat and in came several girls with pails and mops to clean the mat in preparation for the meet. I could not resist the opportunity to say, "Why are girls doing this housekeeping? They don't wrestle. Seems that should not be women's work."

It is fair to say I never did get along with that gym teacher. Even my apology was refused.

Never mind, we continued to have many experiences because Nancy Spalding refused to see my class as handicapped.

Lunch time did require adaptive procedure. The regular students got their lunches from tables set up in the hall and moved onto the bleachers in the gym to eat, balancing their trays on their laps. No way could my students carry trays when they had to use both hands for their crutches. So we ate in our room. Every day was a party. Both the aide, Peg Kinderman, and the interpreter, Phyllis Clarke ate with us and often other students with a broken leg or a behavior problem joined us.

We did join the regular cooking class. The teacher put the items we would need for the day's cooking lesson on a center table and each cooking station—there were six or more stoves, sinks and tables—sent a student to get the items, but even that required that I carry the items. By then my students were old hands at measuring, stirring, cooking and baking.

One time we all made peanut butter cookies and they were for a teachers' meeting. The following day the class again made peanut butter cookies for themselves. The teacher suggested we press sugar on top of each cookie as we marked it with a fork. Chris was able to get a great deal of sugar on his cookies. We all did. They baked just right and we could take our batch to our room. However, some wag had put salt in the sugar canister! Not one of the cookies could be eaten. Back to doing our own cooking in our room. I brought a small roasting oven and we mixed and baked. Soon we used the grill and got good at making pancakes.

We were not always successful as the day we beat and beat the pudding but it did not thicken. We checked the box and it was not Instant Pudding, but required cooking to a boil! We learned it was important to read the directions.

We joined the woodworking class. And did well, but many of the tools required holding them—actually all required holding them. After one semester I requested that we return for the special education shop at the high school. So several afternoons a week we were bused to the high school

Pancakes Anyone!

Adaptive Cooking

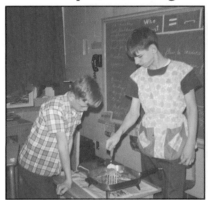

⇧ Dean and Steve at
Webster Stanley Junior High School

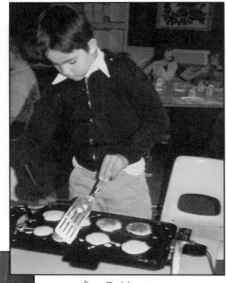

⇧ Bobby at
Lincoln Elementary School

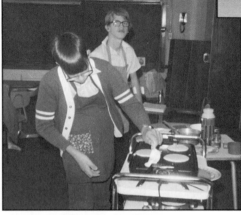

⇦
Tom and Chris at
Merrill Middle School

West
High
School
Cooking
Class

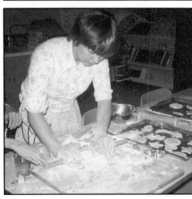

⇧ Cindy baking cookies for the
Children's Christmas Party for the
entire Department for the Hearing Impaired

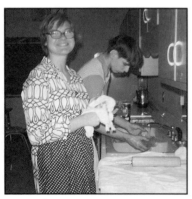

⇧ Clean Up Crew
Shirley and Steve

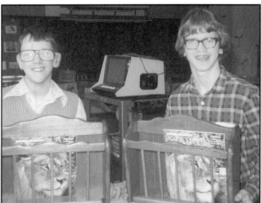

⇨
Tom and Chris with magazine racks made in regular Woodworking, Merrill Middle School.

Teri with lap tray made in
⇩ adaptive woodworking.

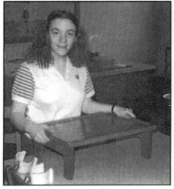

Teri's father made
this workbench. ⇨
Tom, Chris, and Teri are sanding the workbench.

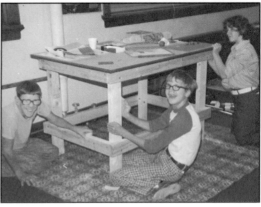

and could work at our own pace. We joined several other handicapped students and shared the instruction with their teacher. We had the choice of going to the shop room in the middle school during the lunch hour where we could work alone, but we opted for sharing a class.

The school was almost directly across the street from a fire department. We were not only interested in the fire trucks, but in the fire fighters' living quarters. And that meant climbing a great flight of stairs. We did and then a fire fighter carried Chris down, showing the special hold.

We had an interesting reading program. The students were followers of Little House on the Prairie and Ben and the Bear (you recall that Bear was really a monkey that accompanied Ben who drove a truck). We created stories for Ben and the Bear. This gave us the idea of creating a moving van company. We drew and painted a huge van on huge sheets of paper which we put up on one board, and created our own company. We then got jobs—moved T.V. sets from a store in the towns where the students lived. Had to get the accounts and checks. Had to look up addresses.

I did have to guess how one of the continued stories on the Little House on the Prairie would come out. A girl had been sexually attacked and I had to

155

explain what happened. I did not anticipate that she would fall and be killed. The children were not sure but that she really died. Luckily we found a T.V. magazine that told about her career.

While we were at Merrill, Chris had more surgery on his legs and his new braces allowed him to stand tall. He was so pleased. We visited him in the hospital.

Our middle school days drew to an end and this class looked forward to moving to North High School.

Finally the special class would be part of the North High School program for the hearing impaired. Some of the shops and rooms were on the second floor and Teri got to wear the key to the elevator. The students had a special program to meet their needs. They also went out to the Work Adjustment Center with Mr. Thomas, one of the high school teachers in the Hearing Impaired Department. They learned work skills.

One lad, Tom, transferred to the Wisconsin School for the Deaf at Delavan where I hoped he would have many friends. However, his mother reported that in the dorm and free time he was teased. (Deaf children, like all children, tease the children with additional problems.) One Sunday he hung back from the group crossing the street to church and was struck by a car and seriously injured. However, he eventually did learn many useful skills.

Recent conversations with his family are showing Tom to be leading a busy happy life. Although he did not pass his driver's test while still at Delavan, he did so at home. This gives him freedom to drive to the Fox River Industries where he works. Here it was suggested he have a lap top computer. DVR could not believe how successful he was able to use it at work and shopping. His speech is minimal and there is not an interpreter to be with him at work or shopping in the small town of Berlin.

He enjoys going to all the sporting events at the high school, and watching sporting events on T.V. He drives his grandmother around. He still lives at home, and if his mother is at work, he can cook. His health is stable and he is busy and happy.

Teri works in the Brooke Industries in her hometown now. On Friday afternoon she goes to the Advocap office to work. She has a motorized wheel chair that she uses to go shopping and around town. However, at work she manages fine with her crutches. She too has become a good cook at home.

Chris is still with the foster family that now are his legal guardians. He too works at a sheltered workshop, Ripon Area Service Center. Chris works in the packaging department. This center, as the others, do contracting for jobs from local industries.

. . . . .

156

XII

SIGN LANGUAGE

Pragmatic Issues and Anecdotes Regarding the Real World of Deafness, Communication and Sign Language

By Leslie K. Halvorsen

I've heard a lot of things in my life, including "I just can't keep my eyes open anymore, I'm going to bed." Never, however, have I heard anyone say, "I simply *must* go to bed, I just can't keep my ears open anymore!"

American Sign Language is structured in a succinct visual manner for a reason . . . a sense-able reason. And what is that? The fact that the eye is prone to fatigue. The ear is not. The ear never closes. Students with normal hearing can lay their head on a classroom desk and still hear what is going on. They can even close their eyes while taking a brief "snooze" and still be capable of jumping in response when their teacher says, "And what do YOU think about that, Johnny?!" Deaf students cannot. Deaf students must keep their eyes open every second of every waking day in order to keep abreast of things in an astute manner . . . in order to keep pace with society in general. Infants with normal hearing can appear to be half-asleep in their buggies and cribs but still they are ingesting the sounds of their environment (and they are learning the meaning of those sounds). Dying folks generally maintain an acute ability to hear and understand what is going on until their last breath is gone even though they may not be able to keep their eyes open. Deaf infants and adults are substantially cut off from the world the minute their eyes are closed.

Deaf people hear visually and kinesthetically . . . they hear through their eyes and they are drawn to sound through the sense of vibration. They *think visually* as opposed to auditorially.

It is important to realize that there is a very unique difference between American Sign Language (ASL) and signed English. ASL is designed for the eye. English is designed for the ear. It matters little if English is spoken or signed, both modes of the language can be rough on the eyes. ASL, however, doesn't require near as much eye strain.

The ramifications of deafness and severe/profound hearing loss can be far more complex than we, as hearing people, might suspect at first thought. It would be unfair to say that deaf individuals are born with superhuman extra-sensory systems. What does seem to occur, however, is that they generally utilize every aspect of the sense-able system they have, *but can only use it when given the opportunity to do so*. In other words, since their "ears" do not hear, they must be allowed to use their eyes to receive information, and their hands to impart information to the world around them.

How vividly I recall the first day that I, as a speech pathologist, ran into

158

deafness about 20 years ago. "Ran into" is an apt phrase. Why? because I was left feeling stunned, to say the least. Nothing in terms of diagnostic procedures and tools that I had used successfully during the previous years with children or adults who had mild, moderate or even severe hearing losses seemed to be appropriate. I even doubted this person was deaf! Hard of hearing, possibly, but deaf? It sure didn't seem so in spite of the fact that a referral source provided documentation indicating so.

Prior to actually meeting this profoundly deaf young woman, I spent considerable time wondering how I would communicate with her . . . how I would give instructions related to evaluating hearing, language and speech. I finally decided that the best approach was to prepare a "written backup" of what I wanted to say just in case she could not read lips. Why did I feel it necessary to worry?! After all, my professional training had led me to believe that deaf people were born with an innate ability to read lips. But worry I did. (Thank heavens for common sense!)

Experience has since taught me that speechreading (lipreading) "Hvordan star det til", "O-ai-dekite ureshii", "Danke schone" or any phrase from a language a person has never heard is virtually impossible. Why, then, does society presume that young deaf children should be able to do it? (By the way, speechreading a *sentence*, from a language one is familiar with, is much easier than speechreading a single *word*. If your child is not understanding something, *add more information*, not less. Additionally, rephrase the sentence if necessary. Simply repeating the word or sentence will do little good. Example, if you have said "Hurry" and your child is not responding, say, "Where is your jacket? Come—now. We must hurry. Grandma is waiting for us." But, back to the story about my first experience with deafness . . .)

On the night preceding that first encounter, I wrote a two page greeting in my best penmanship which, in essence said, "Good morning . . . my name is Leslie Halvorsen. I'm happy to meet you." Eventually I got around to saying, "It is my responsibility to test your hearing, language and speech and I would like to start with . . ."

In a way, I felt no qualms about my ability to test her hearing. It would be a simple task (if testing hearing can ever be considered simple . . . and it can't be). In other words, if she didn't raise her hand when I subjected her to audiometric pure tones, then she was profoundly deaf. However, testing her language and speech might be quite another matter . . . and I sensed it. I felt alien to the task.

What did "deaf" really mean, I asked myself. After she left my office, I jotted the following notes:

"I met the deaf girl today. She looked skeptical, but she smiled. She was very congenial after a few minutes and seemed to be a very good lip-reader. She didn't utter a sound nor did she move her lips one iota. (I talked with voice, she responded to me by facial expression and writing.) We had a productive meeting . . . until I stopped *telling* her things and started *asking* more specific questions. Then she hesitated. I sensed her frustration . . . and felt my own. I pulled out my "best penmanship". In quick fashion, we were communicating well. After a while, when my hand tired of writing, I said to her, 'Would you please move your lips. I can speechread.' She complied. That worked much better for me. I felt more at ease."

(Umm . . . wasn't it supposed to be the other way around?? Wasn't I, the hearing professional, supposed to be putting her at ease? But instead, she was putting me at ease!)

I felt at ease about everything except for the possibility that she wasn't deaf. If she was, as former records indicated, then why had she turned toward the door of my office in anticipation of it being opened moments before it actually opened! My mind raced as I concluded that I must have inadvertently glanced toward the door when I heard someone approaching. Sure, that was it . . . she must have followed my gaze. Thusly, as we continued our conversation, I was very careful about not giving any visual clues. Nonetheless, moments after I heard someone open the main door to the agency (which is about eight feet from my office door) she again turned in anticipation of someone entering. No one did, and we got back to work with nary a word exchanged about the matter. Eventually, after we had established a comfortable and enjoyable trust-level, I asked her how she knew that someone had entered the building. She wrote, "Didn't you feel the air?" "What air?" I asked. "The air from under the door," she answered. Given the fact that my office is carpeted and there is little space between door and carpet, I found myself thinking, "Wow, this is one sharp sixteen year old!"

After finishing the evaluation, I told this deaf girl that I felt it was imperative I teach her how to speak. With the wisdom of Confucius twinkling in her eyes, she said, "I've had enough of speech therapists, but you can do your thing with me if you let me teach you how to sign." In a way, I so much as said "What's that?" She showed me the manual alphabet. (See page 161.)

Being a lover of languages and intrigue, I eagerly agreed. From that point on, I played therapist for one-half hour and she functioned as teacher for the remaining half-hour of our weekly sessions. Soon I was capable of "g-o-o-d", and on my way to "g-o-o-d m-o-r-n-i-n-g".

Besides languages and intrigue, I love a challenge. Thusly, I had decided I would attempt to teach her how to voice /k/. It happened quickly enough and I was so elated tears nearly came to my eyes. If I could get her to produce /k/, a back-throat voiceless sound, then surely I could teach her anything! Most assuredly, teaching her the voiced /b/, the visible /p/, the vibrating /m/ would be a breeze!

Did I ever have something to learn!

Granted, I came to realize that I could teach her /p/, /b/ and /m/ with not too much effort. The letter/sound /s/ was a little more of a problem. If I taught it to her as /s/ in "sun" then what kind of a clue could I give her regarding the /s/ in "sugar" which is pronounced as /sh/, not /s/?

The letter/sound for "c" presented yet another true challenge. In fact, that little letter seems to have no sound of its own! My brain whirled with the realization that I would have to walk her through the entire unabridged "Webster's" in order to have her memorize that "c" in "cake" makes a /k/ sound, that "c" in "cease" makes a /s/ sound, that "c" in "control" makes a /k/ sound, that "c" in "civil" makes a /s/ sound etcetera. And then, if we ever finished that task, we could tackle the "c's" in words like "circumnavigate". She would have to learn that sometimes the "c" is pronounced differently even if in the same word! Besides that, she would have to remember, without ever hearing the word, if it was the first or second "c" that made the /s/ or /k/ sound and vice versa.

Our "therapy sessions" became an exciting adventure. She agreed to move her lips (mouth the words) so I could speechread her comments. In addition she read my lips and facial muscles. We supplemented speech-reading with some fingerspelling and note-writing when necessary. Eagerly we probed each other's brains in thirst for knowledge about the "Deaf

Manual Alphabet — Printed with permission

As it looks to the person *reading* it.   **As it looks to the person *spelling* it.**

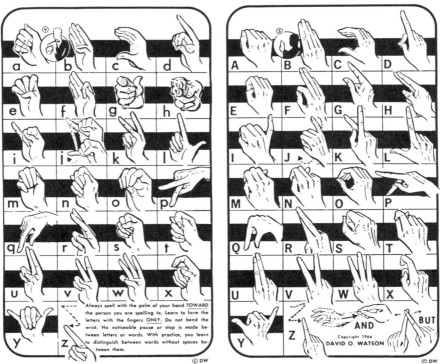

161

World" and about "Hearing Society". I had to think twice one day when she asked me to explain how a firefly sounds when it lights up.

Our conversations were exciting. However, I often felt frustrated because I would miss or misunderstand crucial things. Speechreading was too unreliable. (Some professionals say that speechreading is about 30 percent reliable in most situations. Perhaps so. However, if the subject is identified and if it is a topic that both parties are very familiar with . . . and if both parties have extensive vocabularies . . . and if both parties keep their chin up a bit more than usual . . . and if neither have beards or mustaches, and if both have nice straight clearly visible teeth . . . and if neither have thin tight lips . . . and if the lighting and background is just right . . . if, if, if, then and only then can comprehension increase significantly.)

There was another problem. Fingerspelling was cumbersome for me. My hands shook as if they were stuttering and my wrists ached. There was so much to ask, so much to tell . . . and so much time was being wasted in attempting to say it! One day, in absolute exasperation, I blurbed out, "I can't believe you haven't figured out a way to talk faster!" Again, calmly (and with that Confucius-look in her eyes) she said, "Oh, we can sign. That's faster." To that I said, "I thought that is what you taught me. Isn't that what I am doing now?!" "No, you are fingerspelling."

Within seconds, a whole new world opened up for me! Without much effort, I found myself fluently signing, "How are you?" instead of tediously spelling, "H-o-w a-r-e y-o-u?" Ahhh, three movements instead of nine! Things were getting better, indeed.

From that point on we met as often as possible so she might teach me an ever-increasing signed vocabulary. Nonetheless, our thirst for knowledge about each other's world superseded everything else. As a result, we used fingerspelling when we had the chance to talk outside of the therapy environment, but we reverted to writing (due to my signing limitations) when we really wanted to share details. At the beginning of each session, we each wrote a question on a piece of typing paper. Then we would exchange the papers and proceed to answer the other's question. In other words, we constantly had two separate conversations going at the same time. We went through an entire ream of paper in three weeks.

What happened to the speech therapy /k/, "c" and /s/ drills? They were abandoned. Because we wanted to take the "easy way out"? No, emphatically no. Rather it was because we wanted to *communicate*, to learn from each other. Articulation therapy was dropped because communicating and learning was so much more productive and enjoyable than memorizing the sounds of words (especially without time to talk about the meaning and usage of those words). Something interesting happened when we stopped focusing on the articulation drills and began focusing on communication. It was the fact that I stopped thinking of her as "the deaf girl" and started thinking of her as "Elissa". In other words, she suddenly became a personality, a person. The deafness became secondary.

162

I should add, however, that if Elissa had had true functional residual hearing and had had reasonable speech-discrimination capabilities, I would have felt a responsibility to continue focusing on the development of her speech-discrimination abilities.

But she didn't.

The results of her hearing test showed what is commonly referred to as a "left corner audiogram." This meant that she could not "hear" any frequencies at all but that she responded to very loud low frequencies because she felt the vibrations they produced. Put your hand on a drum that someone is playing. You will "hear" the vibrations, too.

If deaf or hard of hearing children or adults are asked, "Did you hear that?" they will often answer "Yes". Don't for one minute, however, think they heard that particular sound, word or sentence with the same clarity you probably do. There is a tremendous difference between *hearing* and *understanding*! If you really want your question answered accurately, then ask the deaf child in different ways, ask what the question was, ask what the child understood you to say. Remember, a hearing aid only hears (amplifies) sound. The aid cannot interpret sound into a meaningful message. It is the brain that enables the person to understand what has been heard.

I remember the first time I worked with an elderly gentleman who had gradually lost his hearing. He was so thrilled the day his hearing aid finally arrived. I reminded him that he might have to learn to re-identify the meanings of sounds. I don't think he knew what I meant at first, so I told him to go home, put his hand on the side or top of the refrigerator, and then wait until he felt the vibration of the motor starting. This would enable him to distinguish the sound of the refrigerator from other sounds in the house. Then I told him to do the same thing with the furnace, the car engine, etcetera.

Intuition I guess, caused me to feel it necessary to walk out of the agency with him as he left my office that day. He took about three steps and "stopped dead in his tracks". He glanced around with a perplexed look on his face and then proceeded a few more steps. Again he stopped. This time he looked around in a more frantic way. Then he searched my face for a reaction. He obviously was frightened. I said, "What's the matter?" He said, "What's that loud sound?" I scanned our surroundings. Nothing unusual. I said, "Do you hear it now?" He said, "No". I said, "Ok, let's take a few more steps." We did. He blurted out, "THERE IT IS AGAIN!" I said, "You are hearing your footsteps."

A very similar experience occurred one day with Elissa. We were walking out of my office when she stopped abruptly and looked around. There was a perplexing look on her face. She looked again and then asked me, "What is that sound? Where is it coming from?" I had to think a moment, had to listen . . . "Oh, there are tracks behind those trees, a train is approaching." She had felt the rumble but couldn't identify the vibration, couldn't attach meaning to it until it was defined for her.

Some months later, we spent a few days at Holiday House North in Door County (a vacation spot for people with disabilities which is operated by Holiday House of Manitowoc County, Incorporated). In part, our day together was brought about by a shared decision to clean cottages. There were several buildings to attend to. I chose to work in the "big cottage". Elissa volunteered to clean up the "yellow cottage". After working a while, she came looking for me and spotted me washing the inside of the kitchen window. From outside she asked, "Where can I find some more Spic and Span?"

I saw her lips move. I could easily read the fact that she wanted something, but I wasn't sure exactly what it was. As if by instinct, I raised the window and said, "What do you need?" (I asked the question because all I could read from her lips was, "Where an I fine uhmore bik ae ba".) My action (opening the window) startled her into silence. A question mark appeared on her face . . . a look of bewilderment . . . or was it shock? She said, in amazement, "Can't you hear through the window!?!" Uhh . . . I was as startled as she was and shook my head "No." It then dawned on me that she could.

After we had finished cleaning cottages that day in the Spring of 1970, we decided to reward ourselves with a leisurely walk in the fresh pine-scented air along the road that lead from the cottages to a special junction. We started off late in the afternoon. The sun was bright. (I gave no thought to the fact that it would start to set within the hour.) Wild flowers perked their enticing scented blooms along the roadside. We shared the scent of unfamiliar blooms. We lost sight of the fact that we were Deaf, that we were Hearing. We were simply two people enjoying the delights of nature. We paid no attention to time.

After we had walked about a mile, I said, "Why don't we go back along the beach?!" Enthusiastically, she agreed. Upon my suggestion, we slipped our shoes off. (Although I was new to "deafness", I had quickly surmised that tactile and kinesthetic experience might be particularly pleasing to people who couldn't *hear* the splashing waves of cold bay water swirling between their toes. I must have been right.) She laughed as the cool rushing waves splashed against her feet . . . so did I as the water tickled my toes. (Deaf and hearing people share more similarities than differences!)

At one point, we stopped to lift intriguing stones out of the water and studied the tiny fossils imprinted on shells. At times we ran ahead of each other in search of flat stones that would be the most likely to skip a great distance over bay waters. We laughed outloud. With exhilaration, we both laughed outloud. I suddenly realized that I was hearing Elissa's vocal voice for the first time. It was great! Except for that instance, however, I neglected to think about the fact that we were from two entirely different sensory worlds. That is, I forgot about that fact until . . .

The sun went down.

Suddenly, without warning, the sun was gone.

Rising moonlight turned her presence into a silhouette as it skipped, ran and weaved its way ahead of me through bushes and reeds along the shoreline. Abruptly, like the light of day, my vision diminished . . . disappeared. *My ability to hear her was gone. Her ability to hear me was gone.* (Just as you should not be afraid to use the word "see" with a blind person, you should not refrain from using the word "hear" with a deaf person. Deaf individuals feel comfortable in making comments like "Did you *hear* what happened to Benita last week at LIU?") But, back to our experience along the beach at Sand Bay, Wisconsin.

Clouds covered the moon. A wind began to whistle. Darkness deepened. I could barely differentiate between her silhouette and that of swaying trees. The distinctiveness of her body, facial features, hands and fingers (needed for communication) drastically and suddenly faded and fused into a mere unidentifiable darkness.

Being very familiar with the shoreline, I was vividly aware of the fact that we were approaching an area wherein a wide and deep creek veined its way between the tree-lined roadside and the ebb tide of bay waters. She had never treaded these paths before. She was not aware of the creek, much less its dangers.

I yelled at her in warning. (By instinct and habit, I should add, certainly not by any great insight on my part!) Of course, she did not respond. I screamed at her! Naturally, no response. Only then did it again occur to me that she was deaf. Ok, so she couldn't hear through her ears, but she sure could hear through her eyes. I waved my arms. Frantically I waved my arms. No response. How could I have expected and hoped that she would respond?!? The darkness had become formidable! I felt an awful chill (and it had nothing to do with the rapidly cooling temperature of the evening.) Winds were roaring in my ears . . . winds that were capable of drowning out any kinesthetic contact I might make with her. Once again I began to comprehend the fact that we came from different sensory worlds and although she sometimes acted as though she had eyes in the back of her head, it was too dark to make a difference. Ensuing years and experiences would cause me to realize that . . .

The ramifications of deafness can be profound. As additional years passed, however, I realized that this frightening experience would have hardly been any different if the individual with me had had normal hearing. (May I repeat, there are more similarities among deaf and hearing individuals than there are differences.)

When the world rumbles in storm, when roaring thunder and slashing wind makes it impossible *for anyone* to hear, and when utter darkness separates people even by a mere foot, the possibility of tactile or kinesthetic communication is drowned out by reverberations that mask any attempt at contact.

Thank heavens for lightening!

We survived that harrowing experience because the impending night, quickened by storm, splattered the darkness with brilliant flashes of light. That lightening produced opportunity for communication, for warning of the stealthy creek that lay ahead. That lightening very possibly saved a life that night.

What does this anecdotal experience have to do with education of Deaf infants, adolescents and adults? Everything! It relates to the sum and substance of everything crucial to communication and comprehension. It is the core-door through which we, as Hearing people, might begin to understand the sensory, cultural and linguistic world with which deaf individuals reside . . . and flourish.

Oh my, we had so much to learn about each other and the world's in which we lived! And it was such an exciting adventure! Let it be known from onset, that Elissa taught me far more than I was ever able to teach her in spite of the fact that I was a degreed and well-seasoned speech pathologist and she was a "mere" recent high school graduate of the Wisconsin School for the Deaf.

Are you aware that 85 percent of what you know today did not come from school experience? It came from what is called "incidental learning" . . . from over-hearing what your parents and grandparents talked about. That is how you became familiar with your heritage. Furthermore, you learned the rights and wrongs of certain behavior by over-hearing siblings, aunts and uncles, cousins and family friends. That is how you became familiar with the rules of society . . . how to express anger, how to resolve issues in an appropriate manner. And don't let anyone convince you that your primary basic belief, or disbelief, in some kind of Supreme Being came from the pulpit of some church, temple or synagogue. Not so. It came from across the breakfast table as your family members discussed what the priest, minister, rabbi or agnostic/atheist acquaintance said last week, last year. Don't deny your deaf child of that incredibly important information. Encourage your child to be a part of those conversations. Try with all your might to avoid saying "Never mind" or "It's not important" when your child says "What did that man or woman say?" Give your child time to participate, to share an opinion of his or her own.

Natural access to viable communication and language is, in my estimation, the most incredibly important key which will enable deaf children to realize their maximum potential. It is far more important than tongue-lip-teeth articulated speech. It is the thing that enables parents to joyfully relate to their children . . . it is the thing that enables the child to access *incidental learning* and, therein, become a knowledgeable person, a true family member, and a contributing member of society.

On a previous page, I mentioned that Elissa had figured out that she could be aware of people entering a building without being able to hear or see the door opening if she paid attention to the change in air pressure. Another somewhat comparable survival technique occurred after she moved in with us.

The Halvorsen family, by the way, was composed of my husband Bj and me, as well as Ingrid, Gretchen, Halvor, Bridget and Elissa. These siblings ranged in age from five to sixteen years of age. The household was not a dull place. Try peeling potatoes for a crew of seven while reminding kids to finish their work, to feed the family dog, to stop teasing each other, while simultaneously answering a doorbell that *none* of the seven seemed able to hear! It made for interesting living! We all learned a whole lot about deafness and hearingness in quick fashion. To add to the excitement, I had a grand repertoire of about 200 signs back in those days. That certainly has changed through the years but, nonetheless, I'm still not real adept at signing while doing dishes . . . soap bubbles keep running down my sleeves. But back to my example of how astute Elissa was.

I normally got up before anyone else, turned on the radio and made a pot of coffee. When Elissa got up, I'd practice my signing skills by attempting to reiterate the highlights of the morning news. One morning, as I groggily made my way to the coffee pot, she bounced into the kitchen with a different kind of smile on her face. I was still half asleep but something caused me to feel she had something up her sleeve. We started talking. Soon I realized that she was giving me the morning news. *She* was giving *me* the morning news! She was deaf! Deaf people aren't supposed to be able to hear news broadcast on a radio. How in the world . . . ?!?!? "Maybe deaf people can hear in a different way than hearing people do," I pondered to myself.

It was not until bacon, eggs, oatmeal, coffee and orange juice had wound its way from my stomach to my brain that I was able to figure it all out. Like a typical teenager, she prided herself in being able to do things on her own . . . including getting the morning news. How did she do it? By waking early and getting her hands on a morning newspaper. She beat me to the punch! Being the age I am, I grew up in the "deaf and dumb" era. Needless to say, Elissa eradicated that nonsense in quick fashion! She was no "deaf mute" either. She had plenty to say!

Recognizing the tremendous value of natural access to viable and visible communication for deaf people came easy for me. However, it took some doing before I began to realize how much language, language differences and language preferences can influence and impact life and living . . .

Elissa moved from Wisconsin to enroll in Gallaudet College (now University) about eight months after our initial meeting. Several weeks later, I flew out to see her. I was delighted to find that I had not lost my signing skills in the two months since I had seen her.

Our visit went without flaw . . . until a friend of hers stopped over. I wasn't able to understand a word the friend said. Worse yet, I couldn't understand a word Elissa was saying when *she* responded to that friend! What was going on, I wondered. The girls finished their conversation and the friend left. Elissa and I started talking again . . . with full comprehension on both sides.

A few hours later, another friend of hers stopped by. She said, "Nice-to-meet-you." I had no problems understanding that comment and felt pretty good about how carefully I had fingerspelled "H-i" to her. She asked, "When did you arrive?" I happily signed "Yesterday." Obviously, she had no trouble understanding me. (Wow, what an accomplished signer I was!) But then the scene changed . . . drastically. Elissa and friend number two began to discuss something. Again, I couldn't understand a thing . . . much to my chagrin.

Later, when Elissa and I were alone, I said "Talk to me like you talk to your friends." She said, "I am." I said, "No, you are not." We discussed the fact that my receptive signing skills were even more limited than my expressive skills and she mentioned that her friends "talked fast". I said, "I know that, but something else is going on. You talk differently to your friends than you talk to me."

Something even more thought provoking occurred the next day.

I was alone in the Gallaudet College Rathskeller when one of these same friends walked in. She came over and asked me to tell her the words to the song that was being played on the jukebox. It was not until after I interpreted (signed with rhythm) the words in that song to her that something significant dawned on me. I had not been able to understand this Gallaudet student when she and Elissa were chatting away in the dorm, but I was able to understand her in the Rathskeller!

I *had to* find out why. It became an obsession with me.

Eventually, I located a small article written by a man named Stokoe. In this article were the words "American Sign Language" and "signed English". "SO THAT'S IT!" I mused in shock. "THEY ARE SWITCHING LANGUAGES ON ME!" Elissa and her friends were using American Sign Language with one another and they were using manually-coded English when talking with me. They were bilingual. I wasn't . . . as I'm sure you have deduced by now.

Later, when I got back to Wisconsin, I asked local deaf people if they preferred American Sign or signed English. All appeared to think the question was at least peculiar if not downright weird . . . and none could give me an answer. Obviously, they were not aware of the difference between the two. How they communicated with Deaf people was how they communicated with Deaf people; and how they communicated with Hearing people was how they communicated with Hearing people. It was simple as that. Little did they realize that they were automatically switching to manually-coded English when a Hearing person walked in the room. Neither did professionals recognize that. The year, recall, was 1970.

Many people with normal hearing tend to think that sign language is universal. It is not. Many people also tend to think that it ought to be. I used to be one of those people, but the more I studied cultures and languages (both aural/oral and visuo/kinetic), the more I realized why languages are not universal and really can't be. Various attempts have been made to create an international language, however.

In 1887, Dr. L. L. Zamenof, a Polish eye doctor, invented Esperanto, an oral language for international use. In the 1940s C. K. Bliss developed a graphic communication system he hoped would promote world understanding. It is called Blissymbolics. I've used it from time to time with non-verbal hearing people. The World Federation of the Deaf compiled Gestuno, an international sign system used primarily at world conferences. I knew a bit of it at one time and that came in handy (pun intended!) during 1977 at the first National Symposium on Sign Language Research and Teaching when I was having dinner with a number of Deaf and Hearing professionals from around the world. Like Esperanto, Gestuno is an artificial communication system rather than a natural language. It is signed, whereas Esperanto is voiced.

While all of the above named communication systems are functional in certain settings, none can be considered true languages and none are commonly used in any part of the world by general society.

Sign languages differ as much as voiced languages do and native Sign Languages, created by Deaf people, definitely are not derived from voiced (aural/oral) languages. Even if they were, it would be very very difficult to create an international language stemming from one or the other. Would we pick oral Russian, French, German, Bohemian, Japanese, Chinese, Hebrew, Norwegian, Spanish or Italian etcetera? Imagine how hot the debate would become at the United Nations if such a task were demanded of the organization! The same debate would likely occur with members of the World Federation of the Deaf's Unification of Signs Commission if that organization were given the chore of selecting one Sign Language for the entire world!

Deaf citizens from around the world might be able to agree on a specific *sign* for a particular noun or verb just as Hearing citizens might agree on a specific *word*. What can't be agreed upon is the manner in which a sentence should be constructed. Should an adjective come before a noun or should it follow it? Should a sentence be constructed as, "I saw three young children yesterday" or should it be constructed as "Yesterday, I saw children three, young"? Should speakers identify what they are talking about immediately or should they leave people wondering until the end of the sentence or phrase? Example. Should we say "apple, big round and red" or should we say "big, round, red apple/ball/pillow"? Frankly, this author often wishes people would identify their subject immediately (and so do most hard of hearing people because speechreading is much easier once the topic is identified). But, unfortunately, English puts adjectives before nouns.

The difference between oral and manual languages is fascinating. English, as well as most languages hearing people are familiar with are aural/oral languages. These languages are generally received through the ear and spoken via the tongue, lips and teeth. We know that these languages are composed of *words*. In reference to the composite of words we use in these languages, we speak of *vocabulary*. We can even say that "vocabulary" exists in signed versions of those languages, but vocabulary certainly does *not* exist in any native language of Deaf people from any country. In other words . . .

THERE ARE NO WORDS, PER SE, IN AMERICAN SIGN LANGUAGE.

If American Sign Language doesn't have words . . . doesn't have vocabulary . . . what is it that we are seeing when we observe two native ASL speakers engaged in conversation? It is *viscabulary*.

REMEMBER: VISCABULARY IS NOT THE SAME AS SIGNED VOCABULARY!

There are a number of manually coded systems available for conversing in signed English (or any other oral language we might want to encode manually). The words and vocabularies of oral languages, whether transmitted in a vocal or signed manner, are static entities of those languages. The basis of American Sign Language, i.e., viscabulary, is anything but static! Viscabulary is viable meaningful motion. And how can we put meaningful motion on paper? Much like minuscule segments of a movie film, component bits of viscabulary (cheremes, as opposed to phonemes) can be frozen in space so as to capture the sketches or pictures one finds in most sign language books.

American Sign Language (ASL or Ameslan, as it is sometimes called) can be defined as a language that utilizes visuo-kinetic, and sometimes tactile, symbolization units that move in a conceptually accurate way to convey precise and very definitive thoughts or messages to the eye of the receiver.

Although a number of people, especially W. C. Stokoe and Ursula Bellugi, had conducted insightful sign language research prior to the time when American Sign Language was recognized as a legitimate language, little was known about the language until after the first National Symposium on Sign Language Research and Teaching (NSSLRT) was held in Chicago, Illinois May 30-June 3, 1977. Prior to that time, few people were cognizant of the unique differences between ASL and manually coded English. Even fewer were willing to admit that "signing" (of *any* language) would benefit deaf children. In fact, most people held the viewpoint that manual communication would be detrimental. It seemed as though they were not only putting the cart before the horse, i.e., were expecting the child to develop speech before language, but were also denying the child the right to even have a horse! In other words, they denied deaf children the right to have access to general information. Without access to information, children are seriously handicapped.

How often haven't we heard people say, "Your deaf child lives in a Hearing World. S/he must learn to speak!" To that I say, communicate with your children in a manner that enables them to comprehend; give them information in a manner that enables them to absorb it, process it, and utilize it. Only then will they acquire *something to talk about*!

Recognize the value of trying to see the world through the eyes of your child. If your child is profoundly deaf . . . if your child tests out as having nonexistent or poor speech discrimination capabilities, then don't waste endless time attempting to turn that child into a successful hearing adult. Your child can stand on its head until the cows come home . . . and it can pray fervently to all the gods of earth and all the Gods of Heaven (in order to try to please parents and professionals) but still that child will not be able to become hearing . . . no matter how strong anyone's desire is.

IT IS OKAY TO BE DEAF! ALLOW YOUR CHILD THE PRIVILEGE AND JOY OF SENSING THAT YOU TRULY AND SINCERELY BELIEVE THAT.

It truly is okay to be deaf. Deaf children can become *very successful deaf adults* if only they are allowed to become so. They cannot, however, become successful hearing adults.

Love your children as they are, and be willing to "speak their language". Hug them. Do fun things with them. Create situations wherein you can laugh together. Play baseball with them. Take them to the circus. *Let them teach you a few things instead of always feeling that you are responsible for teaching them one new sound, one more word every day of their lives . . . for the rest of your lives.* Be parents, not therapists. Communicate with your deaf children just as joyfully as you do with your other children who have normal hearing. Until you are able to sign with your deaf children, speak to them with voice at all times. They will certainly be able to comprehend the expression on your face, i.e., will be able to get the basic message you are imparting. In other words, they will be quick to discern if you are pleased or angry with something they have just done. Trust me . . . they want nothing more than to please you, to be accepted by you, *as they are.* Why? Because they cannot possibly become the hearing child most of you had expected upon their birth . . . *and they sense that!* Be very mindful of the fact that it is okay to be deaf, just as it is okay to be hearing.

Children will be children. It matters little if they are deaf or hearing, children have need to communicate and they will do so . . . by hook or crook, they will communicate. They need to be heard . . . need to be "listened to". If, however, the only way they can get their point across is by kicking you, they will do so. Therefore, don't ever attempt to talk to very young deaf children about anything out of sight. They won't have the foggiest notion what you are referring to. In other words, don't say things like "You made your Grandparents very happy (or sad) when we were at their house yesterday" or "You did a great job yesterday." These young children cannot hear well, i.e., cannot understand speech fully. They may simply be able to read your facial expression . . . will probably *not* be able to comprehend your words. In other words, they will not be able to comprehend what you are uttering . . . only what you are *showing by your actions* . . . and, therefore, they will think you are referring to something that occurred a split second ago.

Any disciplining or praise regarding the incident at the Grandparent's house, on the playground, or in school *must occur immediately at that house, the playground or school.* Never, never say something like, "Just wait until your father comes home!" (The actions of the father, when he finally gets home, will probably be understood by the deaf child as meaning "I, your father, hate you for no reason at all.") In other words, it is incredibly important that the only person who should discipline a deaf child is the very person who participated in and/or witnessed a particular misbehavior and they discipline/praise *must* be stated at the moment the behavior occurs.

Deaf individuals sometimes have a tendency to let the water run or drip from a faucet. Why? Because they cannot hear water slowly d-r-i-p-p-i-n-g (or rushing like a falls at Niagara for that matter!). There have been a number of times that I, as a professional interpreter, have been called for services by real estate owners who are irate with deaf tenants for "flooding the place!" Instead of getting upset about something like this, take time to *show* your deaf child how to use a faucet and, be sure to teach them what happens if the faucet is left running.

At onset simply turn the faucet on full blast and allow the child to see *and feel* the gushing force . . . and frown just slightly *when the child looks at you.* Turn the faucet off halfway (show how to get a proper balance between hot and cold) and allow the child to see *and feel* the difference . . . and smile *when the child looks at you.* Then have the child draw a similar flow and temperature of water on his/her own. Reward the child with a big smile and affirmative nod. Then demonstrate turning the water off only partially so that you produce a slow drip, drip, drip. *As the child looks at you,* produce a quizzical facial expression demonstrating you recognize something is wrong. Take time to point out the slow drip, then shake your head "no, no, no" *as you look at the faucet,* NOT at the child. The child needs to know you are unhappy with the faucet . . . that you are not unhappy with the child!

How often are you going to have to go through this demonstration with your deaf child? About the same number of times you have to tell hearing kids in the family to *"CLOSE THE DOOR!"* on a day when hungry flies are zooming in to taste the warm cake you have just baked and frosted.

EXPECT NO MORE *AND NO LESS* FROM YOUR DEAF CHILD THAN YOU DO FROM YOUR CHILD WITH TYPICAL HEARING. You'll succeed with this attitude and realistic expectation, I can assure you. With certainty, having Elissa become an integral part of the Halvorsen family has been one of the most exciting and rewarding experiences of life. She has gifted us all with an expanded three-dimensional and non-prejudiced view of the world. She has added an element to life that would have never been experienced without her. She has taught us to think beyond our own noses.

It usually takes most people about nine months to become parents of an infant. If my recollection is accurate, it took my husband, Bj, and me seven months to become parents of a deaf teenager! Such a privileged phenomenon is rare, indeed.

"Nine-month parents" are generally thrilled with the birth of their child and they feel very positive and excited. Quickly, however (as they spend numerous hours pacing the night's floor with a colicky baby) they begin to wonder if they are up to being good parents. Bj and I were equally excited about the arrival of Elissa. However we, too, "paced the floor". It wasn't because of colic, however.

Certainly you are aware that we are all now, in 1994, living in the "Information Era". Such was not the case in the early part of 1970. Imagine trying to provide viable support to a deaf teenager . . . and "keep track of" that teenager without access to a functional telephone! The lack of appropriate technology was a very special concern when we finally noticed that Elissa had "become of age" and should be "on her own". She did, indeed, move into an apartment of her own. But how to "keep in touch"? It was a challenge.

A telephone was installed in her apartment, but, as I said, those were the days before modern TTYs/TTs (tele*ty*pewriters/*t*ext *t*elephones) were available. I decided that there must be ways to circumvent these "technical difficulties" . . . that there must be ways to "beat the system". Thusly Elissa and I worked out a scheme.

Because I realized that Elissa was very much "in-tune" with vibration, I suggested that she put her hand on the phone in her apartment each night at 6:00. We worked out many code clues but the first involved the fact that she would not actually pick up the phone receiver. Instead, she would simply put her hand on the receiver of the phone and pay attention to whether it rang one time, two times or three times. One ring meant that I was, indeed, going to be able to stop over for a visit later. Two rings meant that I would not be able to come that evening.Three rings meant that there was a lot going on and I would stop if I possibly had the time, and if I didn't, then I would call her the following evening.

Fortunately, life is much easier for families composed of deaf and hearing members at this present point in time. Even if some family members don't have a text telephone, contact can easily be made via the state or national voice/text phone telecommunication relay service. The number of the Wisconsin Telecommunicators Relay Service is generally listed on page one of the standard phone book. As of this 1994 writing, the Wisconsin Relay Service number is 1-800-947-3529. For additional information, call toll-free (voice) 1-800-395-9877 or (TDD) 1-800-283-9877.

Elissa's education, employment history and leisure time activities have taken her from one end of the country to the other. She attended college . . . and now teaches in one. Originally she studied medical technology. Later, she became fascinated with computer technology and pursued that vocation. She married. A daughter, Benita, who is presently a college student at Long Island University in New York, routinely converses with her Mom via a personal text phone in her dorm room. Ingrid, Gretchen, Halvor and Bridget all have text telephones too. I mention this because I want to assure you that a family composed primarily of people with typical hearing and one deaf person can, indeed, live in joy-filled harmony and close contact.

Elissa owns a car and a half (her daughter's) and a three-bedroom house in a fine suburban neighborhood in Rochester, New York. She started her employment experience many years ago by working as a payroll clerk in a rehabilitation center. Later, after graduating from college, she got a job as a junior computer programmer for a large firm on the West Coast. Later she decided that she wanted to see another part of the country and, therefore, moved to the east coast after accepting a job offer from a major U.S. corporation there. This firm promoted her to the position of "Lead Systems Engineer" after a few years of employment. At present Elissa is on a "company-reluctant" leave of absence from this firm and is teaching college tech students at a well-known post-secondary institution. Her outstanding success as a professional and parent lies in the fact that she is bilingual and bicultural. I am not suggesting, however, that this means she has chosen (or is in any way *capable* of choosing) to articulate English in a voiced manner. Except for laughter or in very rare moments of extreme anger, she never emits a sound. She is, however, extremely proficient at reading and writing English. In fact, she devotes part of *every single day*, no matter how tired she is, to reading for pleasure as well as for professional and work reasons. She is, therefore, *very familiar* with the English language in written form. As a consequence, she is *extremely adept* at reading lips, i.e., speechreading. Needless to say, she is also very fluent in American Sign Language and manually-coded English.

Why do I mention the above? Because I want parents to know how much deaf children will enjoy (and thrive on) being read "bedtime stories". At onset (until you are capable of communicating with your deaf children in American Sign Language), read bedtime stories to them by simply pointing to the pictures in the book. Wait for the child to *look at you in response* and then smile or frown, show fear or anger or excitement according to the illustrations you are pointing to. By pointing out these illustrations and simultaneously demonstrating the appropriate accompanying emotion, you will be teaching your child very valuable concepts of life. You will be initiating their comprehension of "right and wrong". After you have learned a number of signs or signing techniques, go through these same story pictures and start identifying objects, i.e., point to something very specific and show its signed name. In other words, if there is a tree on the page, point to it and when *the child looks at you*, sign "tree". As your signing skills increase, go through the same book again and add adjectives and other information such as "tree-leaves-green-trunk-brown." This process is called "labeling". Labeling is not as fulfilling as true communicating but it certainly can be an exciting avenue that leads to true dialogue and comprehension.

Remember the story about Helen Keller and that particular moment when her teacher Annie Sullivan was holding Helen's hand under the water pump so that Helen might feel the gushing water? Ms. Sullivan signed "water" . . . and eventually Helen grasped the concept of names-for-things . . . and Helen grasped the concept of water itself . . . and eventually Helen grasped the full concept of true communication and therein, got beyond the limitations of "labeling." There are other deaf people who have done as well, such as Elissa and . . .

I am reminded of the story about the Hearing professional who married a Deaf colleague. At one point in this couple's life, they had the obligation of

174

going to a party composed entirely of Hearing people (except, of course, for the Deaf wife). After a while, the hearing husband started to "tip a few too many". His deaf wife decided simply to stand back and observe the whole scene. Later, on their way home, the Deaf wife said to her Hearing husband, "Jane (wife of John) and Robert (husband of Susan) are having an affair." Her husband replied, "Oh, that can't be! What makes you think that! Where'd you ever hear that!" His wife replied, "Oh gosh, sometimes I think you are blind!"

Deaf individuals may deal with the world in slightly different ways than people with typical hearing do, but their uniqueness should never be equated with inferior. In fact, astute and well-educated deaf/Deaf people can sometimes be far more perceptive about the dynamics of life than Hearing people are. Deafness is neither sin nor crime. It certainly is nothing to feel guilty about. And no parent should feel responsible for it! No single individual has the power, in and of herself/himself, to create hearingness or deafness. What each person have, however, is the power and capacity to love . . . to enjoy . . . to nurture . . . and to learn from others. In truth, we can learn from our children (deaf or hearing) if only we take time to listen carefully to their actions as well as to their words.

Focus on the child, not on the deafness. Be forever mindful that deaf children are much more similar to their hearing siblings than they are different. Deaf children can, indeed, do it all . . . albeit, in a sight-ly different way.

As you know, people with typical hearing are born, and they go to school. Some like to sing and dance while others prefer to hunt or fish. Some are happiest at being innovative leaders while other prefer to follow the guidelines of very stringent and definitive job descriptions. These hearing individuals may or may not hold a driver's license . . . may, or may not own a "rattle-trap" or a Mercedes Benz. They may or may not be graduated from grade school, high school or college. They may or may not choose to stay single, marry, or divorce. They may or may not select to have biological or adopted children. These hearing individuals will have specific personalities, interests, and hobbies. At times these people will be healthy and strong . . . at other times they will be sick and frail. They may have a lot of money . . . or be pauper poor. They will be young for a while and then they will become older. They will be "on top of the world" at times and "down in the dumps" at other times. They certainly will feel joy at some points in their life and pain at other times. They will have dreams and they will have disappointments. Fortunately, they will learn to love and unfortunately, they will learn to hate. They will succeed in their work at times and they will fail on other occasions. In the final analysis, they will laugh and they will cry . . . they will live and they will die.

IT IS NO DIFFERENT FOR CHILDREN AND ADULTS WHO ARE DEAF OR HARD OF HEARING. Expect no more and no less of deaf infants and adults as they travel through the various dynamic paths of life's passages.

Encourage children to use interpreters as soon as you and they feel comfortable about the matter. By so doing, you will be encouraging independence. At about the same age that you might drop your hearing child off at the dentist's office for an exam or cleaning, do likewise for your deaf child. Do not think that the use of an interpreter fosters dependency. Just the opposite is true! *Deaf children will quickly learn to THINK FOR THEM-SELVES when they are held responsible for answering questions without Mom or Dad in the room.*

Elissa has chosen the "sense-able" route in life. It was a wise choice that led (and continues to lead) to a very productive, successful and contributing life for herself and her entire familial and acquired family members. As parents of a deaf child, follow Elissa's philosophical footsteps and be guided by the words of John Wooden who once said, "DO NOT LET WHAT YOU CANNOT DO, INTERFERE WITH WHAT YOU CAN DO."

• • • • •

Educational Interpreters

Since Section 504 of the Rehabilitation Act of 1973 and Public Law 94-142 (the Education of All Handicapped Children of 1975), as many as 50 percent of the hearing impaired children have been mainstreamed in public schools with interpreters. These interpreters are expected to use a manual code for English.

Success of this support program depends upon the training of the interpreters and how the school district perceives their role. Often the interpreter is the only person with whom the student can communicate. Interpreters are asked to teach and evaluate the student. This is the role of the teacher, not the interpreter.

All this raised the need to stipulate the specific activities and role of the interpreter. So in 1988 a National Task Force studied the training and employment, and developed guidelines for educational interpreters. This study questioned 45 training centers and learned that few programs offered sufficient course work for interpreters working in the educational setting. The requirements developed were to cover all school levels including postsecondary programs. The training should include educational vocabulary and sign invention, mainstreaming issues, and an understanding of deaf education and culture. Interpreters must understand normal language development.

As of 1992 Wisconsin requires Educational Interpreters to have an 884-License. This license stipulates the job requirements. There is still work to be done on the level of skill. Now every five years the interpreters must earn six additional credits to maintain and up grade their skill. Today Wisconsin has approximately 140 educational interpreters.

Registry of Interpreters for the Deaf:
Manual and Oral Interpreters

For years the Manual Interpreters for the Deaf built the organization, the Registry of Interpreters for the Deaf, Inc. (RID) to guide the members and establish a code of ethics. In 1976 it became apparent that there was a growing need to help the oral and hard of hearing population. Alexander Graham Bell Association for the Deaf took the lead in developing Oral Interpreting.

Joining this study was the National Technical Institute for the Deaf. Together they developed guidelines and training for Oral Interpreters.

Today Oral Interpreters are members of the RID with the same standards of confidentiality and accommodation, and required level of skills.

A Manual Interpreter can stand in front of an audience and be "read" by all present. However, the Oral Interpreter must be near the client. While hand movements can be enlarged, this is not so for the lip and facial movements of the Oral Interpreter. Any exaggeration or mouthing of the speech distorts it.

An added requirement for the Oral Interpreter is that she/he has an understanding of phonetics—how words look. The interpreter needs to know what sounds and words look alike, must be able to select the more visible word or rephrase as necessary. The oral interpreters must wear a plain shirt or blouse or smock and not move her hands. It goes without saying that the Oral Interpreter must have mobile lips, good dentitiion and expressive face and eyes.

All interpreters must convey the intent of the speaker. They may not interject personal feelings, nor give advice.

· · · · · ·

What is Sign Language?

Throughout many of these stories and articles sign languages are mentioned. The differences among the various sign languages are stressed. The Deaf, representing the Deaf Culture, claim American Sign Language-ASL-is their natural language. Time and time again writers say that it does not follow English, but it has a grammar of its own. How did it evolve? It has to be visually explicit. It must convey, in many cases, a picture of the thought. Every country has a natural form, all different as the signs grew out of the basic needs of the deaf population within a culture.

Other forms used in the United States copy the basic motions of American Sign Language, but put these "glosses" in English word order.

Basically the "motions" of simple everyday actions are very suggestive of that activity. Here are a few concepts:

cry	draw the index fingers down the cheeks to represent tears
hit	motion of hitting with the fists
walk	move the hands, palm down, to represent walking forward
catch	motion of catching an object
smile	draw a smile on the lips
sleep	draw the fingers down over the face to show shutting the eyes
eat	fingers pressed against the mouth as though putting something in your mouth
home	two movements that suggest where one sleeps and eats. The sign for bed is the palm against the cheek and then the sign for eat
put	motion moving the hands, curved, forward as though placing something forward
push	pushing forward with both open hands
work	make fists and pound the right one on the back of the left fist
banana	appear to peal the fruit, index finger representing the banana
more	put finger tips of both hands together several times
milk	both hands mimicking milking a cow

As you can see by these simple examples that many of the action words mimic the activity. Toddlers readily understand and mimic these simple actions.

Of course abstract words require a movement that is not readily recognized. However, even these ideas retain some iconic characteristic or likeness to the root meaning. For instance, signs concerning the mind: know, think, wisdom, forget, understand, and imagine are made about the forehead. Words to express feelings are formed touching the chest.

To learn sign language one has to work witha person who can show you how to produce the signs. There are thousands of signs so they must become very stylized and exacting. Now as to the order of the signs—ASL has its own grammar. You have to learn ASL from a knowledgeable signer. And then it takes practice and more practice. As with learning any foreign language, one has to use it, depend upon it. To become fluent, you must use it in everyday conversation with deaf people. It isn't yours until you can think in signs. The Deaf include facial expressions and body language to convey the full meaning.

One can learn to sign, but it is more difficult to read what is signed to you. And especially demanding is the work of an interpreter who must follow closely what others are saying either in sign or speech. That is, the interpreter may need to sign what a speaker is saying and then in turn speak what the deaf person has signed.

Parents and care givers will need to enroll in classes to learn to produce the proper placement of the signs. You need to work with an instructor. After you have a start it will help to have a text book and videos that explain how to form the concepts of both ASL and Signed English. These pictures of how to form the signs do not tell you the grammar of any method. That you must learn from a knowledgeable person.

Children learn faster than adults—the younger, the better.

(The following numbers and basic signs appear in a pamphlet published by Wisconsin Department of Health and Social Services, Division of Vocational Rehabilitation, Bureau for Sensory Disabilities. 5/91)

Numbers

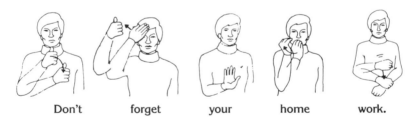

You will be looking at the back of your hand.

A teacher reminds her students: *Don't forget your homework.*

Don't   forget   your   home   work.

Following are other basic signs. There are books and videos to help parents and students. However, one must study with a knowledgeable instructor. These are only the "glosses". One must have instruction for the language of ASL.

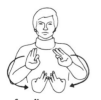

family
2 'f shapes
circle away from body

father
5 handshape
on forehead

mother
5 shape
touches the chin

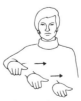

child, children
Use palm to pat the heads
of imaginary children

yes
Nod 's' or 'y'

no
Close 2 fingers
and thumb

please
Circle palm on chest

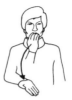

thankyou
Open right 'B' handshape
moves from
mouth outward

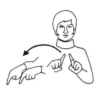

go
Index fingers rotate
around each other and
go out from body

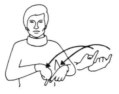

come
Index fingers rotate
around each other
and move towards body

good
Touch lips with fingers
and move hand down
and away from mouth
with palm up

bad
Touch lips with open palm
then turn palm down and
away from mouth

medicine
Right middle finger
makes circular motion
while touching open
palm of left hand

more
Fingers of both hands
move in and touch

time
Index finger to
opposite wrist

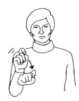

need
Nod 'x' shape twice

bathroom, toilet
Shake right 't'
handshape

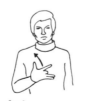

feel
Open hand, middle
finger extended brushes
up over heart area

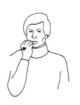

food
Closed 'o' shape
gestures like eating

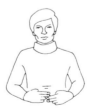

name
Tap the sides of two
'h' shapes

180

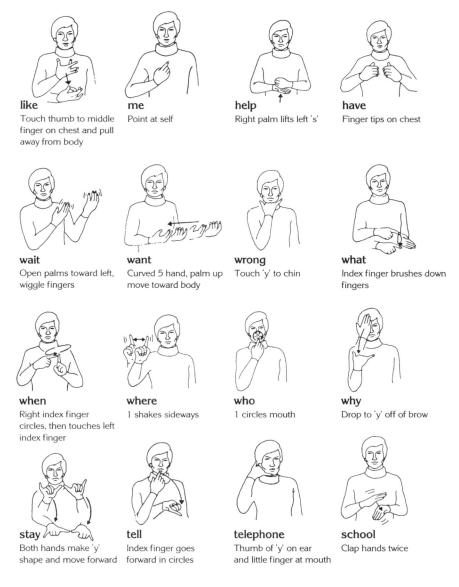

like — Touch thumb to middle finger on chest and pull away from body

me — Point at self

help — Right palm lifts left 's'

have — Finger tips on chest

wait — Open palms toward left, wiggle fingers

want — Curved 5 hand, palm up move toward body

wrong — Touch 'y' to chin

what — Index finger brushes down fingers

when — Right index finger circles, then touches left index finger

where — 1 shakes sideways

who — 1 circles mouth

why — Drop to 'y' off of brow

stay — Both hands make 'y' shape and move forward

tell — Index finger goes forward in circles

telephone — Thumb of 'y' on ear and little finger at mouth

school — Clap hands twice

Deaf students, even Gallaudet University students, are not kind to "oral" deaf even when they sign.

American Sign Language is the only language children learn from children when they go to a residential school that accepts sign language. Only about ten percent have deaf parents as models. Deaf parents often have hearing children who also learn signing naturally.

Children learning to sign from one another cannot be expected to use "correct ASL". Therefore it is recommended that it be taught in school in proper form. This is the heart of the Bi-lingual/Bi-cultural movement that several large residential schools are developing. The contention is that children can become proficient in ASL and with that language background can more easily learn English as a second language—even if only to read and write English.

Schools using Total Communication, using signs in English word order, still have a language problem. You cannot sign every which way. English grammar is very demanding.

What is the literacy rating of our deaf students? Recent research paints a picture that challenges teachers to improve teaching methods.

Is the Bi-lingual/Bi-cultural approach the answer or is it merely returning to an old method? The schools initiating this approach are keeping records to form a body of research. However, it will take years of follow-up studies to ascertain if their premise is valid.

• • • • •

Total Communication

1960's

Wisconsin day classes for deaf and hard of hearing children were oral from their introduction in 1888. Students were taught to lipread and speak. The class work was individualized as various aged children were in a class. Milwaukee had a sufficient number of students to group them in grades, but most programs had only one to three classes. There were 28 such day classes in the 40s and the teachers had to adapt the regular texts.

Individual hearing aids were heavy and children were not fitted with them. However, the classrooms did have auditory trainers. The one used in my class was donated by a service club in 1934. Heavy head sets were wired to the desks or a rack. Some classes had an audio loop (induction loop) with a mike suspended from the ceiling. A boom allowed it to move over the desks. Day classes were self contained classes usually held in elementary buildings.

The children who could integrate returned to their neighborhood schools usually a year below their age level. It was felt the students needed that extra year to adjust. And except for help from Speech Correctionists (the terms Speech Pathologist or Speech Therapist were not in use), the student was seated in the front row and expected to "make the grade". Few made it through high school and college.

Children of deaf parents entered The Wisconsin School for the Deaf— perhaps it was the "ol' school spirit". These children learned sign language in the home. Often the day school children who were 12 or so begged to go to Delavan as they knew there were after school activities, a social life they did not find in their home settings.

It was in the late 60s that the day classes gradually began to accept sign language in the schools. A task force developed a book of signs called *Wisconsin Instructional Signs* hoping to develop a standard throughout the state. This Signed English used ASL glosses (signs) but in English word order. See Leslie Halvorsen's article about Sign Languages. There are several manually coded English methods.

One difficulty was that there were no oral teachers who were fluent signers. Consequently teachers and students had to learn together. Today the young teachers graduating in the program are fluent in both Signed English and American Sign Language.

However, many young teachers today are not given sufficient background in speech development. They depend upon the speech therapists to teach and maintain speech. There is not time enough in the college curriculum to make them specialists in all areas. In fact their education is generic—with certification for all grades. Unlike the regular teachers who must have an academic major—they do not necessarily do so. It would be unrealistic to think they could have even minors in math, science and social sciences. Therefore the junior and high school regular teachers are better prepared in the academic fields. So the day classes mainstream their students in the academics and the teachers of the hearing impaired act as resource teachers. FM systems and interpreters accompany the students into regular classes. Hopefully all the staff working with the hearing impaired collaborate and work from the same curriculum. The IEP should require this cooperation.

This use of speech and lipreading, signs and fingerspelling is known as Total Communication (TC). The goal is to use a combination of methods to reach the child. Fit the system to the child, not the child to the system.

The program for Lindsey Becker, a junior high student in the Appleton Public Schools, illustrates the supportive staff necessary to make it possible for a profoundly deaf student to not only keep up to grade, but be on the honor roll.

Which ever method parents decide to select, they must follow through. Speech requires constant encouragement, help with lipreading, and gentle reminders how to pronounce and use new words. Parents must see that the child is included in all family conversations. *Remember that the child can watch only one person at a time. This is true for both lipreading and watching signs.*

If signing is used at school, parents must not only take basic signing classes, but continue to learn through the years. Children learn quickly and if the parents do not keep up, they are signing like a second grader and the students need conversation at ever advancing levels.

Most communities have sign language classes, however, for those families not living near such centers, there are excellent video libraries teaching sign language. The Oshkosh Department for the Hearing Impaired received a DPI grant allowing them to have fall and spring classes for parents and the purchase of a vast video library for the parents to borrow and continue to learn sign language on various topics.

Practice is the name of the game. Constant conversations with your child will build your skill. Sad to relate, it is reported that over 50 percent of hearing parents do not sign.

March 1990 Senate Bill 336 in the Wisconsin legislature became law that permits high schools to offer American Sign Language to regular students for foreign language credit. American Sign Language (ASL) does not follow English grammer. It is a recognized language and does have a grammar that makes it easy on vision. Presently the Department of Public Instruction is trying to work out a college curriculum that will qualify high school teachers to be instructors in ASL. This is the method that most adult deaf prefer, but is not the issue in the educational setting where the goal is to develop English—the language of the working and every day world.

Day classes and educational interpreters for mainstreamed students use a form of manually signed English. The philosophy of signed English is that it leads into reading the English language.

1990—Total Communication Today

Today Total Communication incorporates modern technology. Hearing impaired students wear hearing aids in conjunction with FM systems in special classes as well as in mainstreamed settings.

The teacher wears a lavaliere mike-transmitter, or one clipped to one's blouse or tie. The student's hearing aid picks up the voice. The FM system is set at a certain frequency and has a range of 300 feet. If another student is in a near-by class, his FM system is set at another frequency. And it is possible for as many as three student groups to function in the same room as each group FM set is on a different frequency.

Today not only the hearing impaired students, but all students, are computer literate. And with the use of modems, the classes can communicate with students in other locations. The student can work at his/her own pace on programs set to improve learning, challenge creative thinking and give the necessary drill.

The educational movies are captioned. Like old time silent movies, the dialogue is on the screen. And today's technology is becoming very creative with the print—in color, on different parts of the screen. (Forty percent of separate decoders purchased to date are by people learning English as a second language.) As of July 1, 1993 all televisions 13 inch or larger sold in the United States must have built in decoder circuity as stipulated by the 1990 Television Decoder Circuity Act. Closed Captioning appears on the T.V. screen, but many situations require captioning to be added to existing videos. For instance, hospitals show videos before one has surgery. These existing videos can be captioned by *QuickCaption*, (copyrighted) process which shows the captions on a regular T.V. without the decoder. There are a myriad uses in schools, libraries, and training programs in business.

The use of the telephone has been impossible for deaf people, and very difficult for hard of hearing persons. However, volume controls have helped the hard of hearing.

A recent development of Telecommunication Devices for the Deaf (TDD), which couples a typewriter and phone, allows two deaf parties to communicate. These machines are now known as Telecommunication Texts (TT) as people with speech problems can use them—not only the deaf. But each has to have a TT. This still does not give the deaf person access to phoning and many were forced to ask family and friends or even strangers to make calls for them.

Gradually relay services were established which had operators who could take TT messages and transfer them to a hearing party. Or take messages from a hearing person who wished to contact a deaf friend. But this system was available in only a few localities and delays were long. And the service was only week days from 7:00 a.m. to 7:00 p.m. at best.

With the passage of the Americans With Disabilities Act of 1990 all states must set up a central Telecommunications Relay System (TRS). Wisconsin now has this TRS in Madison with 80 or more operators and the system is 24 hours a day, every day. The TRS has an 800 number and all calls move swiftly. Operators are versed in ASL so that the incoming call or the out-going call is easily understood. Added to this service for the hearing impaired who speak fluently, there is what is called Voice Carry Over (VCO) which means that the message appears on his TT, but the hearing impaired caller may speak.

The nature of the call can be the same that anyone makes—friendly, ordering a pizza, calling a doctor's office with no limitations on time. Local calls are charged as local calls even though they move through the TRS. And the TT user gets a reduced rate as such calls are longer.

Now hotels and airports have them and of course police and fire departments. Public phones must be hearing aid compatible. And at least one phone in a bank of phones must have volume control. And airports now have at least one in a bank that is equipped with TTs. If a caller dials a TT phone, the TT comes out in a drawer. Desk sized TTs are used in homes and offices, and smaller ones are portable.

A new use for an existing technology is computer notetaking. This requires a computer with a special program showing larger letters than is usual. The typing moves through a projection panel placed on an overhead that projects the printing on a screen visible to a room full of people. This requires a skilled typist as it is used at meetings where the typist keeps up with the speaker. Real-time captioning requires a stenographer and a computer that transcribes the printing immediately.

And deaf people rely on interpreters. Registered Interpreters for the Deaf

(RID) are in great demand and are just now developing skill requirements and pay scales. There are more educational interpreters than teachers for the hearing impaired as they move into many classes. The DPI is working on tests for skill levels. The school board sets the wages.

There are many organizations to help hearing impaired children, parents, and adults. The Division for Vocational Rehabilitation takes hearing impaired students under its wing at age 14 (as of 1994). A listing of some organizations follows this article. Do locate parent organizations, both local and state.

Total Communication today really means "Total Communication". It strives to open the world to our hearing impaired children and adults. Today, as never before, our work places and social milieu are more understanding and open to our hearing impaired adults. They have many talents to share. And the Americans with Disabilities Act (ADA) of 1990 is opening doors.

However, for a handicapped person to be accepted in the work place, he has to be "qualified" for the job. The school has the responsibility to educate our deaf and hard of hearing youths so they can enjoy a bright future.

Organizations

Alexander Graham Bell Association for the Deaf, Inc., 3417 Volta Place NW, Washington, DC 20007

National Information Center on Deafness. Gallaudet University, 800 Florida Avenue NE, Washington, DC 20002-3695

Self Help for Hard of Hearing People. Inc., 7910 Woodmont Avenue, Ste. 1200, Bethesda, MD 20814

. . . . .

Cued Speech

In 1967 R.O. Cornett developed a system of hand cues to be placed near the mouth to aid in lipreading for the consonants that look-alike such as /b/p/m/, and vowels that can be confused. However, if the child has residual hearing, then hearing aids are more reliable. Nor does cueing show phrasing and stress as the child would hear with an aid.

There are only 12 hand positions that are easy to learn, four positions indicate vowels and eight positions for the look alike consonants. For instance, /p/b/m/ appear the same on the lips. The cue merely indicates whether a consonant is voiced, non-voiced, or nasal. The system has to be learned and used by both the person speaking and the hearing impaired child. The individuals cueing must be fluent so that normal rate of speech can be maintained. And special attention must be given to each sound in the words. It adds an additional visual load for the child lipreading.

Perhaps Cornett observed that many teachers of deaf children (not speech therapists who came up through different experiences) used a number of hand signals to cue for voiced, non-voiced and nasal sounds by merely pointing to the area of the face or chest. These were not formalized movements, but they did alert the child as to what was required. These mannerisms were for aiding speech, not lipreading as Cued Speech is expected to do.

* * * * *

XIII
YOUNG ADULTS

Young Adults

Many young adults from other backgrounds and educational experiences were invited to write their stories. Each exemplifies his or her ability to cope in the Deaf Culture and the Hearing World. While many hold positions in the services for the Deaf, it is their personal stories that are so important in understanding "growing up Deaf". Remember too that these adults are in their thirties and forties and educational and employment options have changed for the better.

Today, where would Mary Morois, a child who lost her hearing at age 11, be best served?

What was the secret that gave Vincent Holmes and his wife Pam the ability to succeed in regular grades with no support systems?

Jeanie Coltart was the child today's literature calls the "forgotten child", the hard of hearing child whose family and regular school had no understanding of her needs. She found such joy in the residential school. A word to understand why she found the language classes such a bore—she did not need language development as she had acquired it in a normal fashion.

Then there is Heidi Mischo who managed the oral program in a day class and stands firm for the need for speech. Today with two deaf toddlers, she understnds what is necessary to function in the hearing world. She speaks of her professional challenges.

And Sara Rhoades has a reliable job in a bank. One sees that success is there for those with ability who pursue further education and technical training.

See how the age of on-set of a hearing loss is all important. Only Heidi Mischo and Sara Rhoades were born with severe to profound losses. And Jeanie Coltart was only "hard of hearing" as a child, but her loss progressed in adulthood as did Vincent Holmes' loss.

Parents may see that many roads lead to a fulfilling life, successful careers, marriage and families.

Their stories are as written so that parents may see why "acquiring English language" is such a challenge for our hearing impaired children.

· · · · ·

Seven Times Seven
Personal Reflections Growing Up Deaf

By Mary J. Morois

Sit back for a moment and picture a familiar scene, one which you played a role every year, kindergarten through twelfth grade. It is the first day of school. Students, both apprehensive and excited, are milling around the school grounds, greeting friends, renewing acquaintances severed at the end of the last school year, and excitedly telling and re-telling tales of the best summer vacation they ever had. Then the peal of the school bell efficiently signals the moment of definition: the exact moment that clamor slips into organization. And the students head toward the school doors with barely audible sighs of resignation: the new school year has officially begun.

Now move to the classroom, recall the sound of the teacher calling out names in alphabetical order and assigning seats. Chances are in all of your classes students acknowledged their names and took the assigned seats in an uneventful manner. But in some schools and, particularly for some students, the first day of school is not so smooth. As the teacher proceeds through the role call she calls out this name: Morois, Mary Jo, who earlier had surreptitiously surveyed her classmates, calling to mind names and arranging them in alphabetical order so as to guess when her name will be called, recognizes it with a hand raised in acknowledgement and moves to take the assigned seat. Even as she does, her mind is awhirl: "I was off by only one name." Almost simultaneously the teacher realizes alphabetical order for Mary Jo is at the end of the row, too far removed. She rushes to get Mary Jo's attention gesturing to the seat in the front of the next row. And Mary Jo seeing a movement of lips but still unwaware of the reason for the commotion, heads for the new seat. Then with a sudden twinge of chagrin sits down to the realization that she is the reason for the commotion: alphabetical order has been disrupted because of her deafness. The need to lipread requires that she sit in front of the room as close to the teacher as possible.

This is an easy class for Mary Jo. The teacher has assumed some reponsibility for the extra-ordinary communication need and made appropriate changes. But this is not the end. The thirteen-year-old is still considerably agitated, almost impatiently waiting for the end of the class. For it is only then that she will have the opportunity to approach the teacher with the important request: "Please don't write on the blackboard and talk at the same time. I can't lipread when your back is to me. And walking back and forth across the room doesn't help either." Unfamiliar with this type of request and certainly unused to methodology criticism, Mary Jo's teacher is taken aback. But she promises to oblige, wondering at the alacrity, the surprising amount of self-possession evident in this student. The bell rings and students head toward their next class. Mary Jo prepares to face another teacher, this time one who has not been told he will have a deaf student in his class. Again Mary Jo is at the end of a row (there's something about last names beginning with "M") but she waits until the end of the class to approach this teacher. "I just wanted to tell you that I'm deaf and need to sit in the front row so I can lipread you. Didn't anyone tell you I'm deaf?" Seven times in one day, seven different teachers, seven different reactions.

Today I am 27 years old and "Mary Jo" has long been shortened to Mary. In the 14 years since then, I have graduated from Gallaudett College and have been employed by the State of Wisconsin, Office for Hearing Impaired for the past three years as one of six coordinators of Hearing Impaired Services. Looking back, I am amazed I had the presence of mind to advocate for myself at such an early age. I had no training whatsoever: my only memory is of being told I had to sit in front in order to lipread. But advocate I did, class after class, year after year. Today I am paid to be an advocate with hearing impaired people in a variety of settings but it is no longer as easy as it was when I was thirteen years old. At that age your experience with people in different settings isn't very broad. And most thirteen-year-olds haven't faced enough adverse reactions to become conditioned to the knowledge that extra-ordinary requests of people can result in a lot of rejection. They don't know that most people will not understand and will probably not honor your request. But it doesn't take long for that reality to sink in. It doesn't take long to be conditioned to fear making a scene. And yet, to live an ordinary life with as few physical and communiction barriers as possible, disabled people must not let conditioned fear prevent them from making their needs known. Neither should their family and friends.

I became deaf at age eleven from what doctors termed a viral infection "of some kind". It wasn't the sudden overnight loss "Yesterday I could hear, today I can't." Instead it was a progressive loss over a period of time, one which had no clear beginning, but a most definite end: I could no longer hear. At the time I was enrolled in Catholic parochial school: Wisconsin School for the Deaf officials told my parents it would be better to leave me in my current class than to uproot me to WSD, taking me away from home in the process. After all I didn't know sign language, English is my first language and I was at or above the appropriate level for my age group. *For educational purposes I am sure that was the best decision. My social and emotional needs were an entirely different matter. I think they are just as important as educational needs. Hindsight tells me they were not met in even the smallest way.* Someone should have recognized it and taken action. Someone should have made and accepted suggestions about meeting other deaf adolescents, if only a weekend at WSD: or we could have been told where to go to meet deaf adults. The rule of life has us learning appropriate behavior and mannerisms from adult role models; tell me then, *how can a deaf child become a deaf adult without role models?* That, it seems was my destiny.

Instead of having a rounded educational, social and emotional atmosphere in school and out, I had an excellent education minus communication and what appeared to be a well rounded social and emotional atmosphere. On the outside there were a few neighborhood friends, yes, but when I went to school I went for school and I came home immediately afterwards.

In a nutshell, sixth through twelfth grade was a most isolating and lonely period. Sure, there were people around me and before I became deaf I had friends at school. After I became deaf a wall was slowly but surely constructed between us: my friends did not know how to handle the fact

191

that ordinary methods of communication were no longer adequate. And I did not know how to explain much less handle the fact that I could no longer hear and therefore could not understand anyone. But everyone else could understand me just fine, the first of many paradoxes. You can imagine how quickly attempts at conversation, whether on my part or theirs, failed. Why keep trying when it doesn't work and this thing called lipreading certainly is not quickly becoming an adequate substitute for auditory stimuli—hearing. It would be three years before I could lipread enough to understand my family—people I knew better than anyone else. Finally one day the last brick was in place; the wall was complete. The friends at school had backed away and I let them go.

In addition to being isolating and lonely, the six years were an extended identity crisis. Who am I? Where do I belong? Why am I so different from everyone else? Isn't anyone else like me? Doesn't anyone else have experiences like mine? Why is communication so difficult? Imagine having to depend on others, mainly your parents, to make telephone calls to friends or having to ask friends to call your parents to pick you up and this at an age when the natural sequence of events leads to independence. I don't know what was worse, depending upon people to make phone calls, or watching them make the call the way they thought it should be made, rather than representing the way I wanted the information conveyed. Sometimes I think those experiences had a lot to do with the subsequent over-dependence and then a strong tendency to avoid depending on people. Either other people did things better than I did or they couldn't be depended on to take my best interests in mind. There was never a happy medium because I didn't know how to fashion one. Finally I decided people weren't worth depending on: the best thing was to be as independent as possible. I especially learned not to depend on people for emotional needs, and that was a mistake I'll live with all my life. It seems like a no fault situation: neither the people nor the opportunity to develop intimate relationships were present. So I lived in an emotional vacuum which no one could crack.

It seems that after about my sophomore year things were "Okay". By that time there was a group of people whom I called friends and they pretty much returned the favor, but I never felt like I really belonged, partly because communication was so difficult. I could never reassure myself going into any situation by saying, "Oh, I know this will be easy". It never was. Either it was too dark to lipread, or so noisy I couldn't raise my voice above the din. Or there were too many people talking and I'd get lost early on, never really catching on after that. But the other reason I felt like I didn't belong was because I didn't. No matter how many times I told myself it wasn't true, the truth is, I was different. No one else faced the communication problems I faced every day and as a result I began to hate it. *It wasn't pleasant being different in our society ten years ago, and it's still not always pleasant now (1988). But when I was in high school I didn't know any other deaf person. Perhaps that was why I had so much trouble accepting my difference, why I resented it so.*

When I look back on the next turn of events, I feel very fortunate. In my junior year at least three people brought to my attention that there is a college especially for deaf people, then called Gallaudet College, in Washington, D.C. I was intrigued. In the span of a year I sent off for catalogs three different times, hungry for more information about this place where students and teachers alike use sign language and a barrier-free, total communication education is provided. I started to learn some signs with the goal of attending. The more I thought about it, the more sure I became. I did not want to attend the colleges my friends were going to attend. I was determined to attend Gallaudet, meet other deaf people and get as much out of the post-secondary education as I could. I also think I was naive! Most high school seniors might have quaked in their boots at the thought of taking an uncharted journey into unfamiliar, totally unfamiliar, territory. We had no relatives out East. I didn't know anyone from Wisconsin planning to attend Gallaudet. And Washington, D.C. is definitely not Marinette, Wisconsin, population 11,965. Guess who balked? Guess who quaked in their boots?

My parents faced all the fears with the experience of parents who have watched three other children grow up and leave home. Obviously, their 17-year-old's experience could not compare with theirs. Understandably, then, they said, "No". To which I replied, "Yes". My parents argued, "The school here at the UW-Extension Center is just as good. Why can't you stay home with us for at least two years and then decide? It will be much cheaper." I think I countered with, "It'll be a lot lonelier and harder too" or some such rebuttal. I don't remember how long the battle lasted but one day it was okay. I never dug down to find the real reason for their change of heart. I don't think the reason is important. The permission to leave is itself the focal point because it allowed me to move on. It said non-verbally, "We understand even as we don't understand. This is what you have to do. We will support it." Who I am today is largely a result of my parents' generosity and pain in watching the last child leave the nest.

One paragraph, no not even one chapter could begin to explain the Gallaudet experience. Because that is what it is—an experience. You have to go there, stay for awhile, live it. Feel it and think about how it feels. Meet the people, sink into the experience and simply start to swim. A friend of mine went there some time ago as part of his training in Deaf Ministry, when he wrote to me about it, his first sentence said "Hello from your world." He could not have put it more aptly for I knew and still know that Gallaudet is the place where I and most hearing impaired students can be most at home. Even more homey than Marinette. There are few if any communication barriers at Gallaudet. There we can and do go about our business communicating as freely as anyone else. "Hello from your world" told me as a barometer tells the weather, how authentic my friend's experience of Gallaudet had become. He could see my experience in the hearing world in light of his own experience in the deaf world and knew that for me the latter is infinitely better. Not all the time, but a lot of the time.

For that is what it was, infinitely better than my experience the previous six years. Sadly so on the one hand but excitedly so on the other. The impressions that stand out most are, "Boy, have I got a lot to learn", when my first encounter with American Sign Language turned out to be as frustrating as the experience of trying to lipread. And then, "Gee, they're all deaf like me but we still can't talk, can't carry on a conversation!" but there was hope. Those of us with what is considered a basically oral education and upbringing, depending only on residual hearing, speech and lipreading to communicate, were enrolled in sign language classes. There were quite a few of us in the class of 1982. Mainly due to my minimal sign skills, proficient signers and I kept a careful distance when we met. But those of us with the same background fulfilled the old adage, "Birds of a feather flock together." While we did branch out after our sign skills improved, nontheless, one of my closest friends today is the first deaf person I met when I entered Gallaudet—herself also a non-signer.

Despite the initial frustration of not being able to sign enough to communicate, deep down inside I must have known that Gallaudet was it, the end of the line. To be sure, I needed a lot more sign skill and exposure to deafness and deaf culture but I knew I couldn't back out. Besides, I was having too much fun with experiences like making my first telephone call via TDD without help from my parents! I knew I would either have to rise to the challenge and improve or end up back in Marinette. Quitting because of lack of sign and social skills wasn't an option. Moreover, half the students in that semester's English 205 (an honors course reserved for those with better English backgrounds) had the same problem! Mrs. Stevens, deaf herself, deserves a medal for the delicate but sure way she handled our diversity. It was in that class that I met my closest friend, someone with whom I've kept in touch ever since. Our distinct memory of '205' is understanding questions and being able to recall answers, but not being able to say it in sign! Subsequently, we kept our mouths shut a lot and saved Mrs. Stevens the problem of talkative students.

Some Advice For Parents of Hearing Impaired Children

From the hindsight that only comes from experience, the first thing I would suggest to parents of hearing impaired children is to allow, even insist that your child have exposure to other hearing impaired people, both children and adults. There is no better peer than someone with the same disability, someone who's been there and back. But at the same time don't limit your child to only hearing impaired peers. Make an effort to find activities he or she enjoys that the general population participates in. Some people will be very uncomfortable upon meeting your child and it may make your child equally uncomfortable to feel singled out. But with time both hearing impaired and hearing people can get over the hump. If they don't, look for something else. One day the situation will be right. The result will be that other people may be less uncomfortable the next time they meet a hearing impaired person and your child may have found friends for life.

I'm single. It's easy for me to tell you to make the time to give your child exposure to deaf adults and peers but I realize too that the demands of reality, for example, other family members, a two occupation household, etc, don't always allow for it. I don't have a pat answer but I do have a suggestion: look for single hearing impaired adults willing to share a day, an afternoon or an evening with your child. Or ask a deaf adult to babysit for you. Someone who can be an example of a successful hearing impaired adult (aren't we all?) yet someone who can share reality, the down times and the up times. Your child needs to see physical evidence that hearing impaired people can and do cope, even though we have bad days when the future seems dark. And at the same time it is still okay. Sometimes we have to ride out the waves, the crests as well as the troughs. There are deaf adults out there, single and married, whose lives would be brightened by the innocence and fresh outlook of a child. Said, that is, from the point of view of one who doesn't have a child all day every day! It is easy for me, for example, to get all caught up with life and forget how uncomplicated it can be. But after spending some time with a child my outlook often becomes more relaxed, more playful.

Accelerate on acceptance: don't be afraid to have a heavy foot. I can't emphasis acceptance enough. Your child is growing up in a society that has come a long way, but not far enough. We are a society that views difference not as something new and exciting, but as a threat, as wrong. And not only that, but there are plenty of people out there who cannot deal with a disabled person comfortably, who do not know how to treat a disabled person as their peer. On the surface, yes, but deep down inside? Manifesting itself in different ways, sometimes it seems as if we Americans have been inbred with a gene that directs us to treat anyone different as just that, different and unequal. It may sound cynical put this way, but for the most part it is true. More often than not I face people who panic when they find out I'm deaf. That has been termed "shock-withdrawal syndrome" with good reason. Your child will face this reaction too. If continued exposure to circumstances like that aren't a sure way to influence self-esteem, the way panic selling influences the stock market, I don't know what is.

Your child needs to be prepared to face a society that is not always accepting, needs to have enough self-esteem, confidence and acceptance of him/herself to get through it and still come out intact. This may be hard if you yourself have not yet accepted your child's deafness to the point where you can see your child as child first, disabled second. It may be that you need to work on your acceptance first before you find ways to instill in your child a self-esteem that can go hand in hand with hearing impairment.

It is okay to be deaf. You're still a good person. There are perhaps many things you may not be able to do as well as others, but there are some things you can do better. Your child can show the world that it is okay to be different. You and your child can show people what it's like to be accepting, of yourself and of others. Granted, these don't have to be and won't always be specific goals, but people will see it even if the only sign is self-confidence. Teach your child to be his or her own source of acceptance, even when everyone else is uncomfortable. Let your child know he or she doesn't have to and, in fact, shouldn't let others' acceptance or rejection be an indication of self-worth. For some children this may come easy: for others it might be a struggle. In fact, I'm one of those who up until recently used other peoples' reactions as a barometer for my self-worth. I thought I had accepted all the implications of my adventitious hearing loss. But I still had to let go of one more thing: my own subtle acceptance and belief in society's stereotype that to be different is to be less of a person.

Also, do not be afraid to stand up for what you believe in. Do not be afraid to fight, even to be nasty sometimes, for accessibility for your children. There are people out there who will tell you you're wrong or offer a less acceptable but easier and quicker solution. Don't listen to them unless deep down inside you realize you're being unrealistic. Chances are you won't be but people will try to make you feel as though you are. Treat them as a detour to go around rather than a permanent barrier. Sometimes results are gotten by being nice: other times you have to be nasty, make a scene and find that people don't like you. Well, we can't be liked by everyone and it's the goal that's important. Some of the people out to prove you wrong won't hesitate to be nasty to get their point across. You'll have to do the same. Teach your children these same things. As they mature bring them with you when you advocate for better services. Then on graduation day they will have had preparation for life on their own at college or on the job. They will not have to rely on mom and dad to fight them any longer.

Finally, it might be painful to cut the strings and let your child spread his or her wings, but it is also very important. Yes, you do cut strings by teaching your child independent living skills. But at the same time, no less than any hearing person, your child needs to be given free reign to develop him or herself.

Each child, hearing or hearing impaired, has the right to become an authentic and mature member of society.

* * * * *

At the time Miss Morois wrote this article she was the Coordinator for Hearing Impaired Services at one of the six regional Offices for the Hearing Impaired (OHI). The Green Bay office serves the many counties in north eastern Wisconsin.

The mission statement for the OHI: To ensure that the needs of the hearing impaired are identified; to ensure that all programs, services and privileges accorded to hearing people are also available to hearing impaired individuals in a manner that is adequate and fully accessible; and, to advocate on behalf of Wisconsin's hearing impaired individuals.

As coordinator Miss Morois organized a committee that assisted her office in presenting numerous workshops for parents, hard of hearing adults, as well as deaf organizations. A newsletter kept all groups in touch. She was open to problems of schools and agencies that served the hearing impaired.

Several Years Later

Miss Morois left that position in 1988 to attend Smith College for her Masters Degree in Human Services.

She writes:

Today I'm a social worker at an outpatient, not-for-profit, mental health clinic in Salam, Massachusetts. I work a case load of about 30 Deaf, Hard of Hearing, and Late-Deafened or Asphasic children, adults, and families. Some are multi-handicapped with the additional diagnosis of Mental Retardation. As part of my job providing therapy I have to travel to nine satellite offices/schools each week, about 440 miles a month, because ours is a low incidence, scattered population.

· · · · ·

The Beginning

By Vincent Holmes
District Director
Wisconsin Division of Vocational Rehabilitation

It is hard to pinpoint the exact time when I began having trouble hearing things that "hearing" people take for granted. I remember having German measles when I was five, also, the worried expressions exhibited on the faces of my relatives. Following this illness everything appeared and sounded normal. I could still hear my little 45 rpm phonograph and distinguish the words sung in such popular songs of 1957 like "Hound Dog" and "Great Balls of Fire". Since we lived in Tampa, Florida, a city with a large Cuban community, the song, "La Bamba" was played so many times I could recite the Spanish lyrics.

Florida has a great and beautiful variety of birds, each with its own distinctive song. If my 1957 primitive record player reminds me that I once heard speech from an electronic medium, the call of Florida's birds cued me to an exquisite natural environment which I still remember. There were mourning doves that sounded as if they had lost their religion, mockingbirds that tried to imitate them and blue jays that sounded so awful that we tried to shoot each one with BB guns.

When I was six, my elementary school, Ballast Point, gave hearing evaluations to all first graders. Here it was discovered that I had a mild hearing impairment. I could still hear the school public address system. One statement I remember hearing and has been fixated on my mind since, was: "Miss Burns, would you please send Vincent Holmes to the principal's office!"

My hearing impairment was insignificant until I was 8 years old, the same year I received my first hearing aid. After the initial curiosity about the object in my ear, other children did not treat me differently than before. As long as nothing interfered with our pursuit of playing little league baseball and football games, and giving each other bruises, everything would be fine. As I grew older, my hearing loss became progressively worse. It was somewhere during the sixth grade when my functional hearing was gone and I began sitting nearer to the teacher. Fortunately, I enjoyed reading and found quite early that most teachers were not creative enough to deviate from a textbook. As long as I read, I would manage. Even if it was just half of what was required.

I enjoyed Ballast Point Elementary School. Of the six teachers I had there, all except one made an effort to insure that I understood my assignments and appropriately, as they would for anyone else, made my life hell when I did not complete them. But life really begins in the seventh grade or junior high school. Chronologically and biologically, the South Tampa gang and I had been elevated to the exalted status of a teenager.

Rude and Pleasant Awakenings

In Tampa, Florida, junior high starts when you reach the seventh grade. I believe that the Hillsborough County Public School System deliberately planned for seventh graders to be initiated into the junior high mainstream in a similar fashion Marine recruits are at Parris Island, South Carolina. Whether you are hearing or deaf, your first day in the seventh grade is also the first step to adulthood.

Instead of one teacher for six courses, you have six teachers for six courses. You have to bring your gym shorts for mandatory physical education class; then expose your privates in the locker room when you change into them.

Riding a bike to school was an uncool thing to do. We had to dress right, get the right haircut, come up with some savvy lines and savvier tales. Along with the snowballing flow of problems that accumulated such as becoming Clearsil addicted zit factories, the seventh grade boys had to learn how to deal with "gurls". I was wearing a very uncool box for a hearing aid because my functional hearing was gone when I arrived at Monroe Junior High, but, I had less zits than most people.

Most of my Ballast Point friends, many of whom I had known since first grade, were in the Monroe Junior High district. The others, who lived north of Gandy Boulevard went to Madison Junior High, would be reunited later at Robinson High School. Other students needed me as much as I needed them. One of the first lessons a deaf, or hearing person needs to learn is that life will be much easier if you give as much as you take. My survival depended on my classmates keeping me informed of what was happening on the streets and letting me borrow notes but there were a few people who depended on me to edit, or even write, their project papers. Math was my bad subject. I found that I could not lipread the back of teacher's heads when they demonstrated solutions to mathematical problems on the blackboard. My mother decided early to hire a tutor for me. The guy could explain algebraic equations and geometric postulates better than most teachers, therefore, I would relay his process for solving difficult mathematical problems to some of my classmates.

Much to the chagrin of my competent tutor, I never made an 'A' in any math course. The people I helped did. Most of them were unaware that I had a tutor through the 12th grade and attributed these fantastic problem solving feats to my own intellectual abilities.

I survived on borrowed class notes and most of the students were very good about keeping me informed of what was happening in school, and in the neighborhood. Sitting near the teacher helped but I still could not understand everything that was being said. I had to ask teachers again to confirm my understanding of the details involved in certain assignments.

Some teachers could care less about the little communication problems I was having in their classes. Every profession has its bad apples. Such bad apples had little time for the hearing students and much less for the one who is deaf. The majority, however, did very well and were helpful when needed.

I entered the eighth grade and I was into my second year of running track, dealing with bad teachers, one rotten coach from Mississippi, and being sent to the principal's office for swearing and various other sins I swear I never committed. I aced a few courses, but during one report period, when I was not concentrating on my work, received a 'D' in math. I guess the amazing discovery that year was that "gurls" became "girls."

My last year at Monroe Junior High was uneventful in the classroom. My grades were still good enough not to arouse the concern of special education officials. There was still some concern about whether I was receiving maximum educational benefits by remaining in a regular school setting. However, after exploring the available options, it was felt that I would remain at Monroe with the few hundred people I felt comfortable with.

Another important reason for this decision was track. Social acceptance in South Tampa was heavily reliant on spectacular athletic achievements. I participated in little league baseball for nine years, made an idiot of myself dribbling on the basketball team and dabbled some on the football field, but I found that track was the one true sport that tested my physical and mental preparation.

Before track, I thought football was hard. After experiencing my first track drills, football became as physically and psychologically stressful as a game of chess. We had a good track coach who focused on building a base of stamina, oxygen depth and developing innate natural running speed into an explosive competitive force. To obtain the best results on the track, I had to participate in, and religiously comply with, a strict training program.

Of several track coaches, I especially remember Coach Valdez. The man knew every malingering trick our adolescent minds conceived. Nothing short of an obituary would get you excused from track practice. He was also one of the few people who, when they spoke directly to me, I could lip read every word.

There were periods when I completely forgot about my deafness. Sports, especially track, gave me a sense of equality with my hearing peers and even adults. I did, however, encounter situations where I had to learn new coping maneuvers as I began to be relied on by the team to place in my track events. It felt great to have this responsibility and devastating when my deafness caused me to miss the starting official's gun during an important track meet. The coach, and other members of the team, were never concerned about my hearing impairment. When a 14 year old runs 100 yards under 10.3 seconds and broad jumps 20 feet, nothing can go wrong. At least until those anxious moments when the starter's pistol has a weak blank.

In the correct starting pose I had my head down, fingers on the white line and my mind on using what little residual hearing I had to catch the shock of the starter's pistol. I know I was in a fanatic trance and hell bent, along with the rest of my teammates, on pulverizing the rejects from Madison Junior High. After an unusually long period of waiting for the pistol to fire, I noticed the other runners where ten feet out of their blocks.

I felt like an F-4 fighter pilot being shot down over DaNang: somewhat embarrassed, but not completely demoralized or without lifesaving options. I admit though that the ejection seat is a more attractive option than the schemes I would have to devise to avoid a repetition of such incidents.

Monroe was part of South Tampa, and the mecca of great Tampa street fighters and schemers. We called ourselves the "Junior Mafia" and settled our differences in "Bad Ass Alley." We were just a bunch of Italian, Greek, Cuban, Jewish, African-Americans trying to survive puberty in a sea of redneck sharks. I still get newspaper clippings about them. Good and bad news.

Robinson High School:
"You Weren't The Only One Who Had A Rough Time"

In October 1989 I flew to Tampa to attend a work related meeting in Clearwater. Upon arriving I rented a car and drove to meet an old friend for lunch. We were both excited about our Robinson High School 20 year class reunion. Steve and I went to this Italian restaurant. Thank God for Tampa restaurants. Whatever the place, the food is usually good.

After Steve gave me updates on the old gang, I mentioned how I could appreciate them better after seeing how isolated some deaf people felt while they attended public schools. Steve's reply was an enlightenment that directed me to a totally new perspective:

"Most people who grew up in South Tampa went through some rough times."

"How rough," I wondered. The only thing I needed to do to answer that question was to review the Robinson High School Annuals. There were teenagers that had to work to supplement their family income. Many had a bad home environment. The deafness related problems during my sophomore, junior or senior years seem minuscule when I recall some of the advantages and opportunities I had that were beyond the reach of most of my hearing peers.

While attending high school I thought studying was synonymous with having a root canal procedure without using an anesthetic. Only when I needed to keep my head above water, I would sacrifice a few hours with a text book. Otherwise I read my Frank Yearby and Leon Uris novels. This attitude resulted in a few bad report cards and raises questions about the prudence of my college admissions officer.

Before the days of closed captioned decoders my favorite entertainment was paperback books. I must have read two or three books each week. I would read stories like "Exodus" on the bus while traveling to a track meet while my teammates wondered how in the hell a 600 page book could hold anyone's interest. Miraculously, I developed an interest in using the dictionary as well. This is the only reason I have never been intimidated by any type of written material.

Considering my ability to absorb written information and my understanding of how most teachers seldom taught anything unavailable in written form, any poor grades I received were my fault.

At Robinson, people continued to give me what assistance I needed. Most of the teachers were understanding. Again, there were a few bozos I wanted to get even with. One disgrace to the teaching profession, who I still think is the "missing link" between apes and humans, would give the class calling quizzes. This is when the teacher verbally cites the questions while the class listens, then writes answers.

This guy had teeth that could not be reconstructed with all of the steel holding up the Triborough, Brooklyn, Golden Gate and Sunshine Skyway bridges combined. Further, he was in serious need of an introduction to a large can of Right Guard which was probably invented for his exclusive use. The distraction of the smell and the waywardness of the teeth forbade me from lip reading Bozo. When I could not lip read him, he refused to repeat the question.

Other students must have had problems with Bozo too. One day, as he drove his car to work, the carburetor, which someone filled with BB's, completely devastated three pistons and the head gasket. We know who did it, we still ain't telling and the statute of limitations has expired.

There were other hobbies besides revenge. If you could not absorb or counteract a bombardment of teasing, practical jokes and being thrown in the shower, or swimming pools, fully clothed (sometimes in a tuxedo) you might as well be a pariah. When I recall the grief rendered from my actions or imagination, the inevitable awkward moments I endured were well deserved. I thought I had a good sense of humor, at least until T.C. arrived.

Theo had just moved into town and was hammering more nails into his coffin each day. Besides calling Speedy a spic, he flipped my behind-the-ear hearing aid off of my ear where it dangled by the tube holding it to the earmold. The next day Theo decided to imitate the way I mispronounce some words that I have difficulty lip reading because of their hidden phonetics.

Everyone has a saturation point. Mine was reached one afternoon on the basketball court. The beating rendered upon Theo almost made him a candidate for plastic surgery. Theo was tall, lanky and uncoordinated. I really felt guilty afterwards but the butthead had flipped my hearing aid again. This was the absolute one and only physical altercation involving my deafness.

Theo's troubles were just beginning. A few months later, Speedy provided further facial, and attitude adjustment. After the punches were thrown and our adolescent energy expended, we all became good friends.

Track: Winning Is Everything

High school track was not as strenuous as it seemed in junior high. The drills were more intense and sophisticated, but after three years of experience I was used to them. Although I did the broad jump and was primarily a sprinter, I still had to maintain a decent base of stamina. You never knew when the coach might decide to make you run in the 440 yard dash or one mile events.

Competition was fierce and Robinson High, like Monroe Junior High, was a track powerhouse. We did everything we could to win. This attitude, and my fear of missing the starter's pistol, lead to an explosive incident.

It was one of those times the coach was feeling like the sprinters were not getting enough work during a track meet, therefore assigned each of us to run in a middle distance event such as the 440, or 880 yard dash. I got the 440.

There was a man on each lane of the track. To make up for the distance variations, one started a certain distance ahead of the other, i.e. the runners in the lane nearer to the rail started somewhat behind the others. I was in the lane nearest to the rail.

The starting official had already given me permission to watch as he fired the gun. He was going to be positioned at least 10 yards ahead of the runner farthest from the rail and almost 25 yards ahead of me.

We all got into our starting blocks, put our hands on the white line and braced for the gun.

Since the starter was so far ahead, and the other runners were required to listen for the sound with their heads down, I saw the sparks emitted from the gun, was out of the block and at least ten yards into the race before the reverberation traveled to the ears of the other runners.

I did not see the official fire a second shot to indicate that I jumped the gun so I continued into the race. With such a great start, naturally, I won the race, but lost the war.

The other schools filed a protest. We were allowed to keep the points earned from my first place finish but it was the last time I would be able to watch the starting official fire his pistol.

If I could not watch the official fire his pistol, I could always resort to predicting when he was about to pull the trigger. This is a dangerous feat and not recommended in races that mean the difference between winning and losing a track meet.

During a regional track meet where so many schools participated that every point counted, two of my teammates and I were too anxious to get out of the starting block. We were doing the 100 yard dash and each of us was good for at least three points. All three of us were disqualified for false starts, or "jumping the gun."

Instead of having someone stand behind me, or asking the starter to come closer so I would not miss the gun, I decided to try to predict the exact millisecond he squeezed the trigger.

I miscalculated two times, i.e., I jumped the gun twice and was disqualified. Our team lost the regional meet by two points, and lost another badge for our letter jackets.

Some compensation is necessary for a person to cope with deafness; however, you do not have to go to extremes.

Vocabulary Tests

High school teachers were as creative as elementary school teachers. They rarely taught anything other than what was in their text books. Since studying was among my short list of assets during that period, I seldom aced a course. However, I did determine how to study in a way that I had a perfect system for making an 'A' on English vocabulary tests—without hearing or lipreading any of the words.

We had to learn a total of 20 new vocabulary words each week. When the teacher recited these words during the test, there were times when I knew the word but not how it sounded or how it should be lip read. There is a limit to how many times you can ask the teacher to repeat a word without driving her and the rest of the class insane. Heretofore, the V.A. Holmes Vocabulary Study System for the Hearing Impaired was created. I think this system aggravated the teacher more than having to repeat words like "symposium" and "crypt" seven times.

First, take the 20 words. Memorize each one of them, their definition and correct spelling. Be sure you remember each word by heart so you can write them without having to review the list. I always thought someone with the memory of a low grade chimpanzee could remember 20 words. It beats having to memorize the 5000 lines in Hamlet any day.

The first time I strutted into class, sat down at my front row seat, all ready for such a test there was the usual teacher paranoia about such things:

"What in the hell are you doing?" Mrs. Lavoris stated as I started writing each word, with its appropriate definition.

"The vocabulary test," I innocently replied.

"But, we have not finished number two yet and you are—what?—on number 12. Vincent, you cannot do that!"

I can too buttbreath. This was one of the more pleasant thoughts I was having at the moment.

Mrs. Lavoris continued to give the class the rest of the test while I finished mine somewhere between the time she was waiting for them to complete number seven. I am still confused about why she was so disappointed when she found I had made 100 percent with this fail safe system.

The Dating Game

All true American boys and girls are faced with that time when they have to go out with members of the opposite sex. Deaf kids in hearing schools are equal in this respect.

I grew up participating in every available organized sport in the neighborhood. The opportunities to meet people were numerous on the baseball diamond, football field, basketball court and track. But this is 1967 and girls did not do these things yet. Along with others, I had to meet them in the classroom or on "Teen Night" at the Interbay Community Center.

One technique suitable for deaf people trying to get a date in a hearing world was discovered as a result of a minor disaster. I will call this one "The Leo Matassini Guide to Getting the Right Date." Leo is still in Tampa and one of the few people with a losing record against me (in every sport).

One day Leo's phone broke down. You might equate this to pulling the heart-lung pump out on a transplant patient. In a mad desperate scramble to secure a date for the Junior-Senior Prom, Leo rode a bicycle to the girl's house, whereby, he popped the question.

Getting dates was a real pain. The girls (they were girls then) at Robinson High were "nice girls". They usually went out when I asked. I did, however, envy guys like Leo who pulled out a little red book with a list of telephone numbers, then commenced calling each girl until he got a date.

Normally I would ask them in class or in the halls since the telephone was an impossible instrument. I distinctly remember resorting to the Leo

Matassini technique which meant an unexpected visit to a girl's house; but I did not use a bicycle to deliver the question.

We all needed a date for the "Night of Knights" dance. I was sitting at home the weekend prior to the dance without a date and aggravated because I could not call a list of girls in a little red book like Leo, especially this particular girl in my government class who I swore was Miss February.

I am at home. I am bored. I am deaf. I am mad. I had to be crazy for not asking her at school. All the girl can do is say no and then there are at least 500 more left to ask. However, it is much easier handling rejection over a telephone. In a typical reaction to such serious problems, I put on my running shoes and went for a run. Straight to her house.

She answered the door. I was wondering why they always had to be home at such times.

"Uh, I need some water," I asked grasping for oxygen while contemplating the return trip which was five miles.

"Vincent, you're crazy," she said walking to the kitchen to pour me a glass of iced water. Since I removed my hearing aid prior to embarking on this aerobic sojourn, I was completely deaf and having to channel 100 percent of my communicative capabilities to lipreading. What's wrong with the hearing aid industry? Producing a sweat proof hearing aid for deaf runners is still an impossibility!

I needed to ask right away, otherwise I would seem like a complete idiot trying to lip read her slow southern drawl.

"Um, Are you going to the dance next week?" I asked, also fighting the need to go to the bathroom.

"No," she says. "Are you?"

"Well, suppose I pick you up at six-thirty Saturday?" I asked, hoping my anatomical dam holds.

"Sure!"

With this important mission accomplished, I was rewarded with permission to use the bathroom. Miss February offered me a ride home. If we were friends before, we were good friends afterwards.

There were other occasions when my shyness and fear of rejection forced me to build a brick wall and safe distance from certain girls I wanted to date. I worried about being able to communicate with them, whether they would be tolerate of my hearing impairment. While there was anxiety about whether an individual would understand the little nuisances associated with being deaf, it was still up to me to venture a friendly gesture or inform hearing students, and everyone else, that I accepted them as well. Such an enlightened perception came during my first 10 year Robinson High Reunion.

As I was busy eating the rubber chicken, the girl who I (and everyone else) had thought was the 1970 Miss Playmate-of-the-Year ambled over to my table. After we exchanged the usual information about what we were doing and how many kids we had, she introduced me to her uncomfortable ex-marine husband, then exclaimed for all to hear:

"Vincent, I really wanted to go to our graduation dance with you. I was going to ask you but you were such a stuck up S.O.B."

People who hold their noses too high in the air are liable to get in it.

Seeing Them Again: 1990 Robinson Class of 1970 Reunion

Our 20 year reunion had an interesting effect on me. I flew down to Tampa from Madison, Wisconsin in what I thought was the longest plane ride ever. I couldn't sit still. The pilot must have been flying that thing at stalling speed. I refused the lunch offered on the plane. In accordance with our prearranged plan, my buddy Dennis Baptiste was going to meet me at the Tampa International Airport with a foot long Cuban Sandwich to be washed down with Cuban coffee strong enough to be sliced with a hacksaw.

Everyone I wanted to see was there. We were all a little older, but I was happy no one had changed too much. On the plane I wasted plenty of time worrying about whether I would still be able to understand everyone. This was a venture, re-entering a world where I never used sign language or had an interpreter. Naturally I was somewhat tense about this. What made me more tense was the fact I was in a room with 300 other people and knew most of them by name.

Some people did well in their lives, and some didn't. Some were lawyers, one a doctor, quite a few recovering alcoholics could be found and the list would not be complete without a jailbird report. Whatever they are, I love every one of them. They're home.

I continue to keep in touch with people in Tampa, and I admit, I still have not been completely comfortable with anyone like I am with my Tampa friends. They were, and still are, the absolute best. If anyone wishes to dispute this most accurate assessment, they should arrange to meet me in Bad Ass Alley. Just state a day and time.

· · · · ·

TT (Phone) Conversation With Vincent Holmes

Ferris: Glad you are in this morning. I can type your story so I can put it on a disk.

Holmes: I was trying to find time to do another portion of the story for after the reunion. I am busy with this new position (District Director of the Wisconsin Division of Vocational Rehabilitation) with 16 people to supervise. I think I am the first deaf person in such a position. And spending time taking my two boys everywhere.

Ferris: I have some more questions. Did you meet your wife Pam at Gallaudet?

Holmes: Yes. Our first conversation concerned my having to wash clothes and how I put everything in together.

Ferris: Love it! What is Pam's job?

Holmes: She is Director of Consumer and Regulatory Relations for ULTRATEC, Inc.

Ferris: Do you and Pam wear hearing aids?

Holmes: Yes we both wear hearing aids. We both have profound hearing impairments. The hearing aids help us both tremendously in our lipreading. Not so much for large groups, but mostly for one-on-one situations.

Ferris: I gather Pam came from an oral program.

Holmes: No, we both went to regular run of the mill neighborhood schools.

Ferris: Do both of your boys have normal hearing?

Holmes: Yes.

Ferris: I was impressed how well they answered the TDD. Do you sign at home?

Holmes: Not really. But both boys want to take sign language in high school because it will be easier for them. One son, Jason who is ten, signs, because he wants to learn. But it is not absolutely necessary. He just likes to use his new skill. Brian and Jason both play with the computer so they have some typing skills.

Ferris: Now the big question—What about ASL as a starting language for deaf toddlers?

Holmes: I don't know. All of these outfits say their method is the best. The Cued Speech gang say theirs is best for toddlers. Then there's the Coded English group that thinks they created the earth, then there's the ASL people who say they are the Messiah, then there's the Oral group who speak for everybody. At this point, having not been indocrinated by anyone, I remain noncommited.

Ferris: Your wonderful gift at writing shows in this message. May I quote you?

Holmes: Yes.

Ferris: What did you and Pam do at Gallaudet? Did you sign? You must have had to learn to sign some method.

Holmes: Oh, my hearing aids broke and I was too lazy to send them to be fixed, and just started picking up sign language during the first three or four months there. It wasn't that difficult when you are around deaf people. There were plenty of people that came from the same background as we did so we were not alone. During the first few days at Gallaudet my main mission in life was to learn all of the more colorful signs. Exactly how to tell people what they were, where they could go, what I thought about them and what they could do. Those signs came in very handy.

Ferris: I know how you felt. I was sitting at the speakers table at a convention. At the table right below our table were the Deaf and the interpreters who were carrying on a lively conversation in sign. I wanted to use my "school teacher" favorite signs. "Be quiet. Pay attention."

Holmes: I got along fine with the ASL users. But I had a quick temper with some of the faculty. I thought they were a little too patronizing and paternalistic at times. I wrote a few articles in the *Buff and Blue* newspaper that lit their fuses.

Ferris: Wonderful. And that is exactly why the deaf want to run their own show. And more power to them. One former Gallaudet student said that the only thing we can't do is hear. However, at a college you do not have mentally retarded or hyperactive students. You have the cream of the crop.

Holmes: Yes. People tend to forget that at Gallaudet the student body represents less than one percent of the people who applied for acceptance. Gallaudet was a good experience. I was arrogant and mean when I arrived and left a little more arrogant but somewhat nicer.

Ferris: As at all colleges only half who enter graduate.

Holmes: Yes. That is right. It is the same for Gallaudet.

Ferris: Did you get your Masters Degree there?

Holmes: No. I did my southern duty and paid homage to my home state by attending that divine institution called the University of Georgia where others destined for heaven attend.

Ferris: Did Pam go on?

Holmes: She got her MA at this college called the University of Tennessee.

Ferris: You are the only one who uses humor and it is delightful.

Holmes: That goes with growing up down south. We all had such a Godawful hard time keeping our heads above water that we had to learn to make fun of everything. That was especially true in Florida where I grew up. In south Tampa we didn't have a cent, but we sure did have fun. I hope those cops have retired.

Ferris: Let's hope so. Maybe I will make up a different name for you.

Holmes: No. The statute of limitations has run out. Tampa was unique. You really had to grow up there to understand what was going on. All the nonverbal stuff. I had a good time at the reunion, better than I thought I would. But then those guys know how to throw a party. They also are still a bunch of con artists. I got suckered in to buying the drinks.

Ferris: I won't try to re-write this. I could never catch your humor. Must say good bye. Best to you and Pam.

Holmes: You are welcome. Thanks for calling. Good-bye. sk

* * * * *

Education For The Hearing Environment

Heidi Immell Mischo
DVR Counselor

I grew up with two other members who also are profoundly deaf: my Dad and brother, Bob. All of us were brought up in the hearing world that we were required to learn how to speak and get along with hearing environment daily.

I am very grateful for what my parents did for me, even though, being an oralist for a profoundly deaf was a struggle. However, going through my struggling to cope with hearing world is greatly rewarding.

I will mention why I said "a greatly rewarding" in the next paragraph.

While I was growing up, I was sent to a private school for six years. I received speech and speech reading training daily to learn to speak and lipread. At times with this intensive training, I got fed up with this training (getting so tired of same routine therapy). It was included in the public schools where I went. My parents requested them to provide me speech therapy one hour three times a week during my period. I had to give up my social time with friends. Later, I didn't mind a new therapist who replaced one that I did not like. She allowed me to suggest any therapy method therefore, I could enjoy myself. It had worked out so well.

I learned how to sign after I graduated from high school. After one year of learning how to sign, I thought I had a good knowledge in my signing skill until I went to Gallaudet University. I was in a deaf culture shock for sometimes, because I was brought up in the hearing world. I had to continue to learn more signing and their deaf culture. I did not accept deaf culture because someways they were brought up in State Schools for the Deaf very differently. I have learned to get along with them.

I again, really appreciated what I went through in public schools in spite of my frustrations. I can see this benefit for myself in the hearing world. I enjoy myself by getting along with them on daily living besides in the deaf community and I can communicate with anyone with very little difficulties. The only difficulties I have with hearing persons is a lot of noisy backgrounds. I do not speak loud enough according to the level of noises they hear. (Probably Heidi refers to talking in factories or offices where she is communicating with the employer where her VR client is going to work.)

Senate Bill 336, high school credit for a course in American Sign Language (ASL) as a foreign language. High school kids can take it to learn how to communicate with hearing impaired. In my feelings, I prefer to see this bill pass only if it is a Sign English class. (The bill did pass, but the problem is finding certified high school teachers who are also certified in teaching ASL.)

Sign English language will help in developing the deaf's skills in language. Therefore, it would be a lot better for accessibility to the hearing world for the hearing and deafened to understand what they are talking about. I will be leading this discussion with parents vs their hearing impaired child to—talk as much as possible, and have a speech therapist to work with him as long as they can. If a child cannot learn how to speak fluently, I would suggest Total Communication with signing English.

Education related, I would suggest at the same time to have a speech therapist, the hearing impaired child should go to public school or to mainstream with hearing impaired program.

From my point of view in State School for the Deaf, the hearing impaired children tend to learn to stick together as a group. It means that they feel that they have nothing to do with the hearing environment at all. How could they learn to cope with this situation well after they leave school. I am not saying that all of them are that way. I have seen a few exceptions that don't mind to be blended with hearing environment.

Signing since I was 20 years old, I have noticed that I have trouble with both hands for the last seven years. Two years ago my hands were diagnosed as having Carpel Tunnel Syndrome. This is common among mechanics, dentists, interpreters and signers. I had surgery that time, however, it wasn't successful. At times I could not sign due to pain in both wrists. Recently I was told by my doctor that surgery will not help and I may have a form of arthritis. I was referred to an orthopedic specialist to have biopsy to find out what is going on with both my wrists. *I am so glad that I have learned how to speak.* If it is arthritis, I may not be able to use sign language in the future when it gets worse. If I have to communicate with the hearing impaired on my job as a vocational rehabilitation counselor, I may as well have an interpreter to sign for me. I will wait and see what happens.

Author's Comment
Keith Mischo—Age 4, 1965
In going over my records of the summer I made home visits (1965), I find

I visited the Mischo family who then lived in Sheboygan. My record reads, "The Mischo family must decide to move either to Green Bay or Oshkosh area rather than put the child in a boarding home. Keith is very co-operative and thoroughly enjoyed our working together." The family did move to Green Bay. It was an oral program too.

· · · · ·

Heidi and Keith Mischo

Keith Mischo is a draftsman. Presently he is a "house husband" caring for their two toddlers.

Both Heidi and Keith are deaf and their two children are deaf. Misti is now almost three years old.

Mrs. Mischo writes: Misti, her last hearing test in September had changed since she's older and more responsive to the sounds. She has 75dB loss in her left ear and 120dB in her right ear. This exam is already exactly when she had her ABR. Since she has a unilateral loss, she wears only one hearing aid.

Heidi Continues

Blake is only three months old. The test result is unknown as the ABR malfunctioned. At the hospital he failed the test as he didn't respond to 40 dB, and did respond at 90 dBs. Therefore his loss may range from moderate to severe. My observation on Blake at 15 weeks, he more likely has a severe loss around 70-80 dB. He has another test next week.

Both Judy Gaines, a speech pathologist and Donna Glasheen, a teacher of the hearing impaired are taking turns every week to work with Misti.

We believe our kids are to be raised in Total Communication as well as our mandating them to continue speech therapy on a daily basis till they finish high school.

The purpose for them to learn to sign is to build up the vocabulary they need to know. From our personal experiences in our lives we learned increasing knowledge of vocabulary through signing!!

Also since I've been a VR Counselor, I have found a lot of deaf oralists (they have nothing to do with the Deaf community) have limited knowledge of vocabularies. That was the biggest surprising fact for me. But I know there are some exceptional deaf oralists do have success in their lives. I believe they have special gifts or have the talents to learn early.

Here are some of the services I provide for Hard of Hearing and Deaf population . . .

Number one—To educate the supervisor about the best and worst needs for deaf and hard of hearing employees.

Worst: Phone
         Noisy background
         Group discussions

Best: Focus on job duties due to limited communication.

However, low functioning people are the most difficult to work with because they don't either understand or care for work policies.

We educate on the needs of the individual since each individual is different. I know what to look for each individual.

Right now my case loads are most hard of hearing clients. I don't have that many deaf on my case loads. Don't ask me why, but the only thing I see different between deaf and hard of hearing . . . *deaf can live on social security while hard of hearing people are not eligible for social security. Therefore, hard of hearing people must find a job to work in order to support themselves!*

I also provide hearing aids, TDDs, and various devices, except Closed Captioning. I only will be willing to purchase a closed captioned device for only for a person who is deaf and multiple disabled as a home maker. I only did one in 5½ years. This person could not work again after a serious health problem occurred.

Oh, Grrr! Misti just pulled both shoe strings out! I better get going since she is pestering for her own mommy's attention.

So long,

. . . . .

The Making of An Activist

By Jeanie Sullivan Coltart
Pres., Wisconsin Deaf, Deaf-Blind,
 and Hard-of-Hearing Alliance, Inc.
Member-at-Large, Wisconsin Association of the Deaf
Member, Self Help for Hard-of-Hearing People (SHHH)
Political Science Student, University of Wisconsin

In writing my story I hope to help create a positive awareness of the physical limitations of the group of people commonly referred to as "handicapped", and Deaf and Hard/Hearing people in particular. In the wake

212

of passage of the Americans With Disabilities Act (ADA), great changes and new ways of thinking are taking place as never before. Never again will "handicapped" people be satisfied with things "the way they are". Never again will "handicapped" people be satisfied with second-class citizenship. We will continue to go only forward. My story here is a reflection of the old style of thinking toward "handicapped" people which inadvertently made them even more handicapped than they were already. Hopefully from here on out, since passage of the ADA, more parents will view raising their "handicapped" children as a POSTIVE CHALLENGE, rather than a NEGATIVE BURDEN. Yes, let us all quickly put the dark ages behind us!

Before going on with my story, I would also like to point out that many people with physical limitations do not like the term "handicapped" applied to them. It has a very negative connotation. A better term is "differently-abled". Also, the term "hearing impairment" has come to be seen in a negative light by a large number of Deaf and Hard/Hearing people. The group of people with less than normal hearing is a very large and diverse one; a huge gray area made up of people with varying degrees of hearing ability who share the common bond of less than normal hearing, yet have many different needs in different situations. Deaf people have different needs than Hard/Hearing people. In addition, two deaf people may seem to a hearing person to have the same need, yet they may have different needs (one person may use American Sign Language, the other may not know sign language). By the same token, to assume two hard/hearing people would have the same need is also erroneous (one person may benefit greatly through use of assistive listening devices, the other might benefit more from sign language). The term "hearing loss" is also not always correct. If a person was once hearing, but through disease or accident developed less hearing, then that is "hearing loss". But if a person was born deaf or hard/hearing, "hearing limited" would be a more correct term since a person cannot lose something they never had in the first place. In any case, I myself prefer to use the terms "differently-abled", "hearing limited, limitation", "deaf", and "hard/hearing". They are more positive and accurate than "handicapped" and "hearing impaired". And in most cases we can do everything, except hear or hear well.

My hearing limitation is one of which there is no known explanation. My mother was not stricken with rubella when pregnant with me, nor is there any record of deafness in my family. I have no idea if there is a hereditary factor involved. In any case, I have no hearing in my right ear and have only about 35-40 percent hearing in my left ear. My hearing level was higher at one time but dropped after age 16. With a hearing aid I am hard/hearing, but without it I am functionally deaf. I have trouble with sound discrimination, difficulty understanding people's words even though they might be speaking loudly enough. It depends on the person I am listening to. Without a hearing aid I have difficulty hearing people's voices at all and understanding their words, and cannot hear things like the telephone, doorbell, or television. Depending on how one looks at it, I suppose in some ways I could be considered lucky, being able to "turn my hearing on and off" at will, like electric lights in a house! If I have a house full of kids, for instance, I simply don't wear my hearing aid, for reasons most parents would know (and which most hearing parents would envy)!

My aunts, uncles, and grandparents first noticed something was different when I start talking. I did not always respond when called, did not pronounce the "s" or "z" sounds, and had some comprehension difficulties in what was said to me. Even today I do not pronounce the letter "z". As time went on my speech difference became more noticeable. My parents suspected something different too, but I'm told they felt guilty, as though it was all their fault. Not knowing what caused my hearing to be less than normal contributed to their guilt feelings, so my parents pretended nothing was wrong. The "ignore the problem and it will go away" syndrome. Also, there was the stigma factor . . . this was back in 1948 when it was "not quite the thing" to have any physical difference, and there was a social stigma attached to being deaf or hard/hearing. Support groups for parents of deaf and hard/hearing children were scarce, and schools for the deaf were still regarded more as "institutions" rather than bona fide schools, as far as a major segment of the hearing population was concerned. My grandfather's elder sister, who was my godmother and doted on me, would not admit to any problem either. I'm told she was a rather forceful and overbearing individual. She and my parents would not accept the fact that I might have a hearing limitation, and passed off my hearing comprehension difficulties and my speech as "not paying attention" and "babytalk". Time was to prove them wrong. My parents are no longer living, so I am going on my own memories, and what my aunts and uncles told me later on. My parents never, ever discussed my hearing limitation with me, nor my grandparents. It was like a "conspiracy of silence".

I attended a regular nursery school. The teachers there noticed something was different with my hearing and tried to discuss this with my parents. Eventually my mother and father brought me to see a doctor. I vaguely remember the visit and playing with the doctor's stethoscope, but not what was said of course, since I was only three or four years old. He must have been testing my hearing, because the following year instead of going into regular kindergarten, I had a private teacher all to myself. My teacher, Judy, was a student at the local teacher's college. She worked with me on my pronunciation and we played word games and went on field trips. One day Judy took me over to her dormitory building to introduce me to her friends. When we got there the girls were working on a huge jigsaw puzzle on the floor. They talked with me, and then Judy took me around to some classrooms. Judy was a lot of fun and I really enjoyed being with her, but I had no interaction with other children my age, much less other hearing-limited children.

Then came first grade. I don't know whether my parents prepared me for entering first grade or not, but they must have said something. At any rate, my mother brought me over to school the first day, said she would see me later, and then left. I promptly panicked and started to howl at the sight of her leaving me, but the teacher talked to me and quieted me down. She introduced me to some other girls in my class, and then school began.

I can remember having trouble understanding all that my teacher said, and as a result fell behind and had to have help to catch up. I remember conversations going on all around me and not understanding any of what was said unless people talking were sitting next to me. I never understood my classmates' replies to our teacher's questions. Sometimes I would be asked a question, misunderstand the words, and as a result, give an inappropriate answer. Of course snickering from my classmates would follow. This made me afraid to answer at all. Eventually my teacher never called on me unless I raised my hand for fear I might not understand what she was saying. My teachers were not intentionally mean to me or anything, but they themselves were not trained to deal with children with hearing limitations, plus in my case they had to deal with my parents, who themselves were not broad-minded about my hearing. None of my teachers in public school were trained to deal with this. For some reason my math was particularly bad. My reading and reading comprehension were very good however, in fact, way above my grade level, at a fourth grade level at beginning of first grade. But math was "the pits". My father, who had graduated from college with an engineering degree, couldn't believe I could have that much trouble with my math. I guess he figured if he was good at it I should be too! I remember my father trying to help me with my math homework. He was not at all patient and would shout at me if I couldn't seem to grasp something; then I would become frustrated and start crying. I wonder if the fact that I couldn't hear everything my teacher said ever entered his head, that it might have something to do with the difficulties I had in school. The end result of this was that I hate math to this day. It continues to be a difficult and unpleasant subject for me. As I got older I did pretty well in all subjects in school, with the help of my teacher and classmates, except for math. Math was always something I needed help with. But sometimes I would fall behind in something to the point that I had to sit in another class with younger children to catch up. This was very embarrassing for me, and I felt stupid as a result. A special class or a special tutor would have saved my self-esteem, but this was not standard procedure in the public school system I was in, I guess.

I read a lot, loved going to the library which my mother and I visited often. My mother read to me a great deal, and I grew up surrounded by books. I was in a Brownie troop, of which my mother was one of the leaders, had friends in the neighborhood, went to birthday parties, and had parties myself. But I also enjoyed spending time alone, reading, playing with my dolls, and making up poems and stories. I used to like to sit and listen to my mother play the piano. She was very good with music, and apparently had written some in her younger years, but did not attempt to teach me any. I tended to feel most comfortable in the company of adults, and with just one friend my age at a time rather than a group. When I was with two or more girls my age, I tended to get "left out" since I didn't hear everything that was being said by them. So I would end up pushing my way into the conversation in order to become a more active part of the group, raising my voice to overcome theirs in my effort to be heard. This would sometimes start fights, as my friends were too young to understand why I was being so pushy. Sometimes though, if I was in a group of girls, things would go along fine. It just depended on the situation and the girls involved, I guess. Being around adults a lot gave me a certain maturity in some ways, but I was very immature in other ways. When there were arguments between me and my friends my parents always intervened for me. It wasn't until I went away to school that I learned to fight my own battles and stand on my own two feet with my friends. Also, because I was not comfortable with my hearing limitation, I did not discuss this with my friends, and instead tried to pretend I had normal hearing like them. They did not bring up the subject, and I don't know if anyone ever discussed it with them. Sometimes kids would comment "You talk funny". I think we all somehow picked up on the sense that my hearing "problem" was a shameful thing, not to be mentioned. Children are afraid of things they do not understand. I remember once when I was seven years old, playing outside at a friend's house. Suddenly my girlfriend turned to me and said, "Your mother is calling you." I went home and asked my mother why my friends could hear her calling me but I could not. Instead of seizing the perfect opportunity to explain my hearing limitation to me she said, "You'll understand when you get older." Had I been raised to feel more comfortable and matter-of-fact about my hearing limitation, and had it been brought out in the open in a casual manner with kids my age, my assimilation into group activity would have been easier and much more pleasant, and my own self-esteem would have been healthier. As it was, I was labelled "a difficult child", because I was obstinate, easily frustrated, and given to temper tantrums. Nobody ever bothered to find out why, or if some people did know, there was not much they could do about it because of my parents, I guess.

When I was nine years old my mother was striken with cancer and I went to live with an aunt and uncle for a while, my mother's older brother and his wife. My Aunt Dot worked with me a lot on my speech using flash cards. She was, and still is, wonderful with children, and had no children of her own at the time. She was careful to make sure I understood her when she spoke. I went to school and made friends with the children in the neighborhood. My Uncle Jack and I had a ritual of walking his dog every evening after dinner. We would clean my uncle's huge tropical fish aquarium together, with me getting in the way more often than actually being helpful, but Uncle Jack had a lot of patience. My aunt's elderly mother, Aunt Polly, lived with them. When my aunt and uncle went off to work Aunt Polly looked after me. I would pound away on their piano, an ancient upright affair, with happy abandon. The noise never bothered Aunt Polly since she was very hard of hearing herself. Aunt Polly was the only other person I ever knew of who had limited hearing. My aunt and uncle let me play the piano when they were around too, but not for as long a period of time as Aunt Polly did. They were very tactful people, even with children. They would listen to my piano playing in suffering silence for a certain length of time, then suggest that I "might like to give it a rest for a while." Had something to do with the piano keys being "old and brittle!"

I also spent a lot of time with my maternal grandparents who lived in New York. They took me with them in the summers to a farm resort in the Catskills. The same people would go year after year, so some of the children got to know each other fairly well. We would take hikes, play games, go horseback riding, and walk through cornfields carrying huge inner tubes to get to an old-fashioned "swimming hole." The water was rather shallow for any real swimming, but perfect for sliding down slippery rocks and riding huge inner tubes. We would find fossil rocks. In the evenings just before dinner we would watch the farmer and his helpers get the cows in from the fields and milk them. People played badminton and croquet, cards, and chess and checkers together. During the school year at two-week breaks for holidays, I also went to stay with my grandparents. They would take me all over New York City, to see various museums, the Barnum & Bailey Circus, movies, Radio City Music Hall, and other points of interest within the city, the World's Fair, and once we went on a boat ride around Manhattan Island. We visited other relatives in New York, cousins in New Jersey, etc.

I also spent some time living with my maternal grandfather's cousin and his wife, Uncle John and Aunt Margaret, who lived not far from us in Connecticut. Uncle John and Aunt Margaret were rather well-off people who owned and lived on several choice acres of Connecticut property. They had a "winter house" and a "summer house" on the property, a large garage, and a storage shed. The property was high up on a hill, overlooking the valley below, and the view was spectacular. Aunt Margaret's hobby was gardening . . . she had beautiful flower beds and rose bushes, and she also enjoyed growing vegetables. Across the road from them was a farm, where there were several horses. My favorite horse there was named "Lucky." Aunt Margaret used to give me sugar cubes to feed Lucky, and sometimes the farmer and his wife would allow me to ride Lucky. Well anyway, from nine years old on, it seems I spent more time in other relatives' homes in addition to going to boarding school at age thirteen, than I spent in my own home anymore. However, I felt comfortable with all the relatives I stayed with, and they did not act at all as though they minded taking care of me. I very much enjoyed being around them. My hearing was, however, never discussed.

When I was ten years old my parents finally decided to have me take speech therapy lessons. That was all well and good, but there was no follow-up on the lessons at home, and still no hearing aid, or any discussion with me about my hearing limitation. I hated the speech therapy, and felt frustrated at my attempts to pronounce "s", "z", etc. My mother was not in good health, which didn't make things any easier. Then when I was eleven years old, still without any discussion of my hearing, my parents told me I would be getting a hearing aid. I reacted to the news adversely since I was at a self-conscious age. I did not want to wear a "box with wires", was quite frankly very shy about my hearing limitation, and still did not know any other children with hearing like mine. As much as I loved her, I did not enjoy being "lumped together" with Aunt Polly, who was by then old and feeble, and wore a hearing aid . . . a "box with wires". My parents failed to get me to wear a hearing aid, and they couldn't understand why I didn't want to wear it! What my parents should have done was come to terms with their own difficulty in dealing with my hearing limitation. Along with that they should have helped me accept my hearing and worked on helping me develop better self-esteem, before trying so hard to get me to use a hearing aid. They were trying to "put the cart before the horse" in this situation. Probably at this point my parents and I would have benefited greatly through family therapy. Too bad that never happened!

Then when I was twelve years old my mother died of cancer. I knew she had been sick a long time, but was not prepared for her death, and my father would not tell me what she died of. Other people did. My father just would not level with me. My mother's wake was a nightmare for me, and I became hysterical at the wake and had to be taken out of the room by my grandfather. My family decided it might be best if I did not attend the funeral, so I stayed with close friends of my aunt's and uncle's on the day of the funeral. I continued to attend public school for a year after my mother died, but I was falling behind. My father was an alcoholic, and he would be out all hours of the night, coming home sometimes as late as 2 a.m. I would sometimes not see him, really, for one or two days at a time since he was out all night after work drinking. His drinking problem apparently started before I was even born, so did not stem from my mother's death. I was alone in a big house many nights, so frightened that I would sit on the floor in the kitchen by the telephone until my father finally came stumbling in. Only then would I feel safe enough to go to bed. I was pretty much "on my own". We had several housekeepers who came and went, but they had no control over me. A number of weeks after my mother's death I met the woman who was to become my stepmother, who I liked very much. I didn't like any of my father's other girlfriends, who tended to come and go frequently. My father was put under pressure by my family, my future stepmother, the neighbors, and the local school authorities to send me away to school because he left me home alone too much for my age. He looked at a number of private schools for girls. At one school the woman interviewing me "tested" my hearing by putting her hand up to her mouth while she spoke to me, to gauge how well I could hear her! My father told me I would have to go to "the school for the deaf". He made it sound more like a threat than a positive prospect! My future stepmother, on the other hand, talked to me about the school in a more positive light. So the following fall I went off to the American School for the Deaf in West Hartford, Connecticut (ASD).

My school in West Hartford is a beautiful school . . . the oldest school for the deaf in the United States, founded in 1817 by Thomas Hopkins Gallaudet, Laurent Clerc, and Mason Cogswell. At that time, tall old elm trees lined the two very long driveways from the road to the main building. They have since fallen victim to Dutch Elm disease, have been removed and replaced by another variety, maples I think. The American School is oriented toward sign language, along with teaching lip reading and speech. At the time I entered the school I had never seen nor heard of sign language before, and had no idea what anyone was talking about, but it was not long before I began to become conversant in it. It was the first time in my life that I had contact with other hearing limited children, and the first time that I felt I fit in with my classmates. My school grades improved dramatically and I was at the head of my class the whole four years I went there. The American School for the Deaf was just like other Connecticut boarding schools, and it is privately endowed. Some of the kids went home every weekend, some less often, and others were day students since they lived close enough by. Most of the students were from Connecticut, but some of them came from Vermont, New Hampshire, Massachusetts, Maine, and Rhode Island. Governor Baxter School for the Deaf in Maine did not have a high school department at that time, but does now. Other schools for the deaf in New England were oriented toward the oral method and discouraged use of sign language.

Some of my teachers at ASD, deaf, hard/hearing, and normal hearing, were very influential with me and encouraged me to strive to the best of my abilities in everything. Several come to mind, but one teacher in particular who I had the most admiration and respect for was Loy E. Golladay, who taught literature and poetry. Mr. Golladay eventually went to join the faculty at National Technical Institute of the Deaf (NTID) in Rochester, New York, retiring there in 1980 as NTID's first Professor Emeritus. He became deaf himself in childhood, had graduated from Gallaudet College at age 20, taught at the West Virginia School for the Deaf and Blind in addition to ASD, and was editor of two school publications, "The West Virginia Tablet", and "The American Era".

In geography/civics class, taught by Paul Peterson, we used to discuss current events. In fact, current events was the main part of this class, really. As a result, we were very well informed about what was happening in the world around us. Of course, like teenagers everywhere, some of us were more interested than others! We discussed the Russian and American space programs, watched Alan Shepard's flight into space, and watched the tragedy and its aftermath of President Kennedy's assassination on television at school. The 1960's was a volatile era, and the time of the black civil rights demonstrations. My awareness of prejudice and hatred toward people who were "different" was sharpened then. Even though my parents themselves were prejudiced toward black people, I was not. There were a few black students in our school, and they did not seem to me to be much different than anyone else. The injustice of prejudice was strongly pointed out to me on our senior class trip, when in Virginia at the school for the deaf there, our black classmates had to stay in a segregated area, separate from the rest of us. That surprised me. So I became very interested in the civil rights movement of the black people. It impressed me that those people had to struggle for their basic civil rights . . . rights that white people took for granted, and that the black people were willing to confront authorities, at the risk of their very lives, to attain those rights. My respect for people like Martin Luther King grew more and more as time went on.

The only class I did not like was English, which was basically just English grammar. In itself the class, in a school for the deaf, can and should be a beneficial one. It is especially important today, in a fast-changing world, that deaf people acquire a good command of English skills and good reading comprehension. This is true of anyone, deaf or not. Otherwise people who do not acquire these skills will be left behind. Good English and reading skills are much more important today than they were even just thirty years ago! Well, at the time I went to ASD, the English class was repetitive and excruciatingly boring. The same stuff was taught over and over again each year. No account was taken of the different English skills level of the students in each class. My own grammar skills far exceeded the class level. Even the students who would normally stand to benefit the most from the class were bored. As a result, I had to endure sitting through three years' worth of English classes in which I learned absolutely nothing I did not already know, lost respect for my English instructor, who I had a basic personality conflict with to begin with, and slacked off. My English teacher and I were at constant loggerheads. She did not like me, I did not like her. What a waste! A complete, revolutionary overhaul of teaching methods for that particular class was desperately needed! This was back at the time I went to ASD . . . probably teaching methods for English are a lot better today.

Dr. Edmund Boatner, the headmaster of the school, was also very influential with me. He used to give me books to read out of his personal library, and I used to drop by his office once in a while. Dr. Boatner was hearing, and he had a rather peculiar way of signing. He would start off in the usual way, with hands about chest level, but when he came to a word that had to spelled manually, he would slowly continue to move his hand out away from him sideways, the last few letters of the word fading out on his fingers, like a person's voice trailing off toward the end of a sentence. However, we were used to his signing, and usually were able to fathom what he was saying! Dr. Boatner's fondness for his students was obvious and genuine, and I remember one time he attempted to teach my class in the art of playing golf in the yard of his home next to the school.

Dr. Boatner was one of the pioneers of captioned films for the deaf, and the students watched captioned movies every Sunday night at school. In the 1950's Dr. Boatner and J. Pierre Rakow, the head of the vocational department at ASD, had worked together on this. With a $5,000 grant from the Junior League of Hartford, Boatner and Rakow studied different methods of captioning films, decided the superimposed method was most satisfactory and feasible, and established Captioned Films for the Deaf. The project became very successful and snowballed to the point where it became too big on a private basis. It was decided to try for a government-sponsored program to take over the project. Dr. Boatner approached U.S. Senator William Purtell of Connecticut, who agreed to sponsor a bill in Congress for Captioned Films for the Deaf to become a government subsidized program. In

September, 1958 the bill became federal law, and Captioned Films for the Deaf fell under jurisdiction of the U.S. Department of Education.

Dr. Boatner's wife, Dr. Maxine Tull Boatner, was an author, and once she had some of my classmates and other students at our school help her with one of her books. This book was part of a project of which Maxine was project director. Dr. Maxine Boatner had received a research grant from the Vocational Rehabilitation Administration of the Department of Health, Education, and Welfare for this project. The name of the book is *A Dictionary of Idioms for the Deaf*. Maxine had us help her go through and sort out the idioms and do some of the typing. I was one of the typists for the project and am listed in the book credentials under my maiden name of Sullivan. Maxine Boatner also authored *Voice of the Deaf; a Biography of Edward Miner Gallaudet* in 1959, and she edited *As It Looks to the Angels and Other Essays*, by Henry A. Perkins, 1954.

School life at ASD in the 1960's was much like that in any other boarding school in Connecticut . . . strict rules, dress code, monitor system (older honor students became supervisors' assistants), waiting on tables, chores, using the dormitory phones to call home once in a while, Sports Day, head girls/boys at dining room tables, societies and clubs, football, basketball, soccer, and swimming at the YMCA in downtown Hartford. However, the school now has an indoor pool. There were small woods and a cottage on several acres in back of the school where some nature hikes and scouting activities were conducted. In addition to the main building at ASD there were also some primary buildings, vocational building, several gymnasiums, and beyond the football field in back of the property was a small housing complex for teachers, staff and their families. ASD also owns an island estate retreat, called Isola Bella, in Connecticut. It had been bequeathed to the school by a wealthy family, and the property includes a huge stone and wood "cottage" with some stained glass windows, beautiful panelling, numerous small bedrooms, and a "great room" with two huge fireplaces, one at each end of the room. The island provides for great swimming and fishing. My first class reunion, complete with our spouses and children, was held there over a long weekend in 1975.

We kids at school got into the usual scrapes and cutups that teenagers normally do. We also used to like to order out for pizza and grinders once in a while. The pizza parlors in Hartford loved to have us call them since there was a nice profit to be made from the sheer number of our orders! The boys and girls would make their orders the same night, so it took more than one delivery van to make the trip. There was also a strict dress code at our school during the 1960's . . . girls had to wear dresses and skirts in class and in the dining room, and boys were not allowed to wear jeans to class. Of course, the rebels among us (of which I was always one) would "push" on this rule, but our teachers and dorm supervisors were unmoving. If we showed up in class in "improper dress" we had to go back to the dormitory and change. Eventually we girls succeeded in getting the rule bent to allow culottes. The Beatles and Beach Boys craze was at its height then too . . . and the dorm supervisors fought a losing battle with the students over keeping Beatles and Beach Boys posters on the dorm walls. They felt these groups were a "bad influence", that the Beatles' hair was too long, and their pants were too tight! Eventually the supervisors gave up on this battle altogether.

One of my classmates, Jane Wilson (now Jane Golightly), and I once did some part-time volunteer work at the Mark Twain House in Hartford. We would take one of the school cars to drive over to our volunteer job. Since Jane was older and had more driving experience than I, she got to drive and I didn't. Of course, to my teenage mind I thought this wasn't fair, and said so. But our dean, Gladys MacDonald, was adamant . . . Jane would drive, period. So that was that!

Gladys MacDonald, the Dean of Girls, was very strict. We did not dare answer her back. Even though she was hardly popular with us at the time, most of the girls would agree today that she probably should have gotten a medal, just for accepting the job. It could not have been an easy one, being in charge of 80-100 teenagers! Ditto for the Dean of Boys! New supervisors were always "put to the test", and tended to come and go fairly quickly and often, with the exception of several long-time older people, like Miss Annela Kaczynski, who had been a student of ASD herself, and Miss Geraldine Coughlin. Miss MacDonald was a graduate of Gallaudet College, and was dean of girls at the school for several decades, and had very interesting stories to tell of her experiences on the job! One of Miss MacDonald's, as well as the rest of the school staff's, most tense times on the job, was during the Cuban Missile Crisis of 1962, when the United States and Russia were literally at the very brink of nuclear war. Bomber planes from a military base in Connecticut flew right over our school to their fighting destinations. We older students at school were all aware of the seriousness of the situation, and were also tense, and we were kept informed by hearing staff of updates of radio and television broadcasts (this was before they had closed captioning on television), and our teachers, and by reading the newspapers. The responsibility for the welfare of the students weighed heavily on Dr. Boatner and his staff at that time. After all, Connecticut was one of the prime targets for missiles because of the Navy yard in Groton, and other defense industries in the state. Very fortunately, Kennedy and Krushchev were finally able to come to more or less agreeable terms and diffuse the two-week stand off, so war did not develop, and everyone breathed a sigh of relief when the crisis passed!

Pets were not allowed in the dormitories. One time my roommates and I were secretly taking care of two pet hamsters for another classmate, Vincent. The cage was kept hidden on the floor under our dressing table in our room. One day the hamsters got loose. We searched all over but couldn't find them. Then one of us heard a loud scream down the hall. We ran down to see what the yelling was about. Miss MacDonald had been sitting at her desk going over some paperwork, when she opened her top drawer and found two beady eyes staring back at her. The hamsters had gotten into her desk! It was difficult for us to keep a straight face, while Miss MacDonald's eyes bored into us with a stony stare, accompanied by "pregnant silence", as she watched us retrieve the rodents from her desk drawers! At times various "secret pets" also included guinea pigs, mice, and one time one of the girls arrived back from a weekend visit home and smuggled in two huge horseshoe crabs, which the night watchman discovered and saw fit to confiscate! Miss MacDonald was not without a sense of humor . . . she may have been strict, but she was also a very perceptive and a very kind person.

In the 1960's the older students' dormitories were completely in the main building, a huge old brick structure. Girls' dormitories and boys' dormitories occupied opposite ends of the building, with classrooms, offices, dining rooms, library, infirmary, private apartments, and everything else of that ilk in between. Sometimes some of the kids would sneak up to the attic to smoke, unbeknownst to their dorm supervisors or the deans. I'm surprised the building is still standing! We did our ironing up there, and even had a tanning light, for suntans in the winter. The building is sort of a square-shaped "C", so some of the boys' and girls' dormitory room windows faced each other, and thus sign language was a big advantage in "long-distance communication"! During mid-morning class breaks we would go back to the dormitories for refreshments . . . cakes, rolls, doughnuts, juices, and milk. Most of the time the school food was good, but we had our pet peeves . . . one dish in particular which most everyone hated was chipped beef and hard boil eggs in some kind of cream sauce! Another was the tapioca pudding (called "fish eyes and glue")!

As mentioned earlier, we had many extracurricular activities, including dances, parties, and special holiday activities and customs. We would go shopping and to the movies in West Hartford. The hearing public was not as familiar with sign language as it is now, and we were stared at with curiosity, and sometimes with derision by hearing people. The movie theatre charged us only partial admission because most of us could not hear the movie dialogue.

For my 16th birthday my father and stepmother threw a party for me and my friends at school at an expensive West Hartford restaurant. Dr. Boatner and his wife Maxine were also at my party, and they gave me a beautiful gold bracelet which I still have today.

My class took a fabulous senior class trip . . . Virginia, Washington D.C., Pennsylvania, New Jersey, etc. We had raised money for this trip by fundraising activities over a period of several years. My years at ASD were happy, and I made lifelong friends there, two of whom are godparents to two of my children.

I was very, very close to my stepmother, and she was one of the most influential people in my life. My stepbrother and sister-in-law were also extremely close to me. They did a lot to help me try to accept wearing a hearing aid. It was an uphill battle. My stepfamily had a matter-of-fact attitude about my hearing, but with my biological family it continued to be a "conspiracy of silence", never discussed with me by my family. Aunt Dot

223

came closest to it by going over flash cards with me, and did try to discuss it. But I was not permanently living with her, and consequently she was not able to make any inroad with me over this. By this time I had deep-rooted feelings of shame about my hearing limitation, and this sort of situation does not get easily resolved in short-term visits. Both my aunt and uncle were much more open-minded about my hearing than the rest of the family, and had they gotten permanent custody of me after my mother died, they would have been, I feel, very good about changing my attitude about it and raising my self-esteem. I appreciate now what Aunt Dot tried to do, and thank her for it.

My father was becoming a much more distant figure. When I did go home for visits he took me to fancy restaurants for dinner, but for the most part our relationship was strained. My father gave me things, and always made sure I had plenty of spending money for school (gave me too much money actually), but he did not give me that much time. He was older when I was born, and was more of an "uncle" rather than a father. I was brought up primarily by my grandparents, aunt and uncle, stepfamily, and boarding school, and did not see much of my father after age twelve. His alcoholic problem, along with his unspoken attitude toward my hearing limitation, was the biggest contributor to our strained relationship. Other factors, which are too painful for me to discuss, contributed to this as well. I will only say I was never physically abused by my father in any way, that is all. Needless to say, as I got older our relationship deteriorated completely. When he and my stepmother separated I remained with my stepmother, and did not see my father again for almost seven years. By the time he died in December, 1977 we were essentially strangers. It is very difficult for me to talk about him today.

I passed an entrance examination for Gallaudet College at age sixteen, scoring high enough to place directly as a freshman and bypass the preparatory year most Gallaudet students start out with. However, I did not go to Gallaudet. I was young, immature, and did not know what I wanted to do with my life. My parents were caught up in their own problems, and they did not sit down with me and help me find a road to follow, or push me to go to Gallaudet anyway, just take courses there at first, and declare a major later. My stepmother encouraged me to try business school to learn about computers. After that I started working for Kimberly-Clark Corp. in New Milford, Connecticut. Two years later I met my future husband there.

My husband and I have been married 22 years and have three children, a daughter 18 and two sons 16 and 14. My husband and children all have normal hearing, and have taken basic sign language classes to make conversation easier at home. We were transferred to Wisconsin from Connecticut in 1984. A few years later I joined SHHH (Self Help for Hard of Hearing People) and WAD (Wisconsin Assoc. of the Deaf), and in 1989 was one of the founders of the Wisconsin Deaf, Deaf-Blind, and Hard/Hearing Alliance, Inc.

There are several factors which contributed to my interest and involvement with political activism. My overprotected childhood, and lack of communication by my parents with me regarding my hearing are one. My background left me with anger and frustration. My parents had gotten so wrapped up in their feelings of guilt that they could not "see the forest for the trees", and this was very detrimental to my feelings of self-esteem and confidence. They never taught me how to handle problems. I was around adults a lot and did not learn the give-and-take in peer relationships very well until I went off to school. Low self-esteem and lack of confidence gave me many problems in adulthood later on. It was not until I was in my late thirties and had become involved with SHHH, WAD, and the Alliance that I really fully accepted my hearing limitations and became aware of abilities I never realized I had. Before coming to Wisconsin I was involved in the hearing community, but never felt completely accepted and treated as an equal on par with hearing people in general, although I do have some very close hearing friends. In a crowd hearing people will tend to gravitate toward other hearing people, subconsciously pushing the hearing limited person aside.

The second factor that drives me in my advocacy pursuits is the difficulties I had in my jobs because of erroneous perception by employers and coworkers of people with hearing limitations. I was discriminated against, bypassed for cross-training, and passed over for promotion all because of my hearing. One time my work phone was tampered with, to make it look like I could not handle the job, for instance.

The third factor is the patronizing attitude of some hearing people toward deaf and hard/hearing people, and other "differently-abled" people. When the Deaf President Now movement started up at Gallaudet University in 1988, it "woke something up inside of me". Memories of the black civil rights movement of the 1960's came into focus again, and I saw that the present "handicapped rights movement" closely parallels that of the black civil rights movement. Then in early 1989 I attended a political process workshop in Madison, Wisconsin. Various deaf and hard/hearing groups, like SHHH, WAD, and others were at the meeting, along with a hard/hearing activist from Virginia, and a lobbyist for WAD, James Wahner, who is a former legislator and had served as House Majority Leader for a time. We all started talking about the importance of banding together into a coalition to gain political power instead of each group just acting on its own. I ended up being on the ad hoc committee, which drew up the bylaws for the new alliance, and which organized the groups. In October, 1989 the Alliance became official, and I am presently completing my second term as president. The Alliance is an organization made up of the various deaf and hard/hearing, related groups, and interested individuals and professionals from around Wisconsin. Its purpose is for educating and advocating for the needs and rights of deaf, deaf-blind, and hard/hearing consumers in the state. I'm also majoring in political science at the University of Wisconsin, and have an interest in eventually becoming a civil rights attorney, specializing in ADA cases. I will be continuing my education at the University of Maine, since my husband has very recently accepted a position with a company in the Augusta, Maine area, and we will be moving there in October of 1992.

Some people can move on in spite of early obstacles, others cannot. Parents of deaf and hard/hearing children, while they may have "guilt feelings" over their child's hearing limitations (or other difference), should try not to let these feelings get in the way of the well-being of the child. Also, there are many support groups available now for parents, to draw from for advice and guidance. From the 1960's up to the present, enormous social changes and awareness pertaining to differently-abled people have taken place, more than at any other time in history. My parents did not have the support groups to help them alleviate their feelings of guilt and inability to cope, to help them "open up their minds". The choices facing hearing parents of non-hearing children, when they know next to nothing about hearing limitations at all, are overwhelming. I think more parents are aware today, and seek out these groups and other people who can help them. Also, the "social stigma" is rapidly being eradicated today, which is also a help. Very unfortunately, as an older hearing limited adult, my story is all too common. The only things my parents did right by me in regard to my hearing limitation were: (1) my mother read to me a great deal and encouraged my interest in books, and (2) after my mother's death my father sent me away to the American School for the Deaf. It was the influence of my grandparents, aunt and uncle, stepfamily, and some people at school who had the greatest direct impact on me in my growing up years. Although my father's influence was more negative than positive, he ironically made the biggest overall impact on my life in the long run simply by deciding to send me to ASD!

In conclusion I have provided the following poem by Merv Garretson, from the book *Perspectives on Deafness; A Deaf American Monograph,* (1991), which I would like to think might reflect my parents' attitude today toward my hearing limitation, as opposed to that of years ago . . .

"Words From A Mother To Her Deaf Child"

The river of time has reached the sea
the sun has turned crimson in its setting
the leaves have bronzed that once were green.

As I look back into my yesterdays
when all your life was spring
and mine had summered into fall

When I return to your dormant years
to the struggling hours of your silence
within your world that was all glass

Oh, to forget those memories of rejection
of your deafness, of your difference
a need for a mirror of my hearing world

226

You who desperately yearned for my love
for me to accept and to come into your world
for my hands to talk to you, for my sign

Across the years I've learned the beauty
of your difference, the joy and wonder
of your being your own unique self

I beg of each deaf child of this world
and of all worlds translucent in their silence
Dear child I love, please forgive my guilt.

—Merv Garretson

Bibliography
The Making Of An Activist

1. Boatner, Maxine Tull, John E. Edwards, ed. *A Dictionary of Idioms for the Deaf.* Washington D.C.: National Association of the Deaf, 1969: page viii.

2. Boatner, Maxine Tull. *Voice of the Deaf; a biography of Edward Miner Gallaudet.* Public Affairs Press, 1959.

3. Gannon, Jack R. *Deaf Heritage.* Silver Spring, Maryland: National Association of the Deaf, 1981: pages 16, 41, 58, 267-268, 318.

4. Garretson, Mervin D., ed. *Perspectives on Deafness; a Deaf American Monograph.* Silver Spring, Maryland: National Association of the Deaf, 1991: Vol. 41, Nos. 1-2: page 6.

5. Perkins, Henry A., Maxine Tull Boatner, ed. *As It Looks to the Angels and Other Essays.* American School Press, 1954 (limited edition of 300 copies).

Also, many thanks to Roselle Weiner, LRC/Library Services Coordinator, American School for the Deaf, for her help in researching book titles of Dr. Maxine Tull Boatner.

* * * * *

Sara Rhoades

Miss Rhoades is 39 now. When she was a child audiometric testing was not as sophisticated as it is today, nor did hearing aids have the potential to assist the severely hearing impaired. So for years it was thought that Sara had no residual hearing, but recent tests prove that she does.

Miss Rhoades wrote her story in 1988. And her hope that hospitals would be more understanding of communication with deaf patients is now closer to reality under the Americans With Disabilities Act (ADA).

My Story by Sara Rhoades

My parent found that I was deaf when I was little girl. I played on drive way by our house. So my dad came home by way thru drive way. He honked and honked. And noticed me not to hear any honks. I was one year old. They took me to special doctor for test hearing. Doctor found that I was deaf. And told my parents that I was deaf. I have no nerves in my ears. I was two years old and went to Webster Stanley School in Oshkosh (Wisconsin).

There was very good program to me to make alot of learn-speech-read-write-listen spelling words. I am glad I can use lip read and understand from them to learn. Then I was 14 years old to transfer to Wisconsin School for the Deaf in Delavan. Because that time it (Oshkosh) doesn't have graduate for deaf people and also easy for me from class. But now it is time so much better for them, they can go to different classes with hearing and deaf students.

Anyway I was glad for me to learn alot classes from Delavan. I was enjoyed cheerleader-clubs Jr and secretary—many things to do there. Also I took all subject classes. I learned how to type and key punch. I never learned how to sign language when I was in (Oshkosh) school. So I had to learn how to sign language from students and teachers alots in few weeks. I finally got sign language to use. I was really interested and learned alots from there. I was cheerleader for three years for basketball and football games. It made me use voice for cheers. Keep me to lip read also sign language. I knew few deaf people cant use voice and lip read. I had learned to read from them cuz not use lip read and most use sign language so fast than me. Finally I learned alot but I still take patience with them.

Until I was graduated from there (Delavan) then I got a job in Wausaukee. I was worked as Kitchen Aid of Staff during the summer. I was alone with all hearing staffs. I was so lucky that few staffs and girls can use sign language and finger-spell but they thought I cant able to lip read. They were surprised that I can lip read as well. I really love to work and talk with together from staffs. Alot of fun with them.

After camp it was over and came home. I looked another job and hard to find and wrote some application forms for Bank of Neenah opened door last time ago. I went to there and looked around if I can work at bank. So I had waited for long time and decided to go to Fox Valley Technical in Oshkosh.

I learned alot of different machines for key punch and type over year. My teacher noticed I did very good to type. She said to me that I should get quick job. She knew that some company wont hire deaf person to work. Finally I got a job at bank in Neenah. I told them to try test on me during I

228

work how do fast. They found out that I do best to work job. They keep me at bank. I work for 15 years now, I am working account now. Before I was worked proof operator and bookkeeping and CRT machine. I am glad that employees are so good to me and patient with me alot. They use to talk with me for awhile and now understand. If I would say big word so I have to write down to them. Most time I dont write as much. They never complained to me. They always take patience. They use to talk as normal to me. If they use so fast to talk to me so I tell them to slow down to talk to make me understand. So I let you know Deaf person should tell whose work any company or etc that he or she try to see and test how do job if slow so can release. Dont be afraid to tell person.

My family of brothers & sisters are different because my brothers dont learn how to sign language to me and my sisters can use sign language. But most time I understand family use lip read for all life to raise. Sometime I get difficult with my mom when she gets sick or very weak to talk with me as alike tired talk. So I have to try to read mom lip read. If she feels fine so she will lip read as good to me to make me understand.

I had a tty and caption closed (T.V.) myself. I really love to use them alot. Caption Closed on tv to make me understand and laugh what they be funny or talk funny.

I use my hearing aid to listen noise and hear when someone call my name. I can hear when phone rings and door bell rings. Most time I able to hear many things. I went to hearing test at Dr. Kile. He is so good and helps me alot. I feel so much better to use a hearing aid cuz I TIRED of employees, they always use rubber band to me as alike call my name. So now they can call me and feel better "Ha" I was appreciated them to take patience with me alot. They always care and tell me.

TTY is so important to help for deaf to call for emergency. I am glad that Theda Clark Memorial Hospital and Nicolet Clinic and Library. But I need for fire station and police station.

I gave you a happened story few years ago. I knew it is so important to use sign language to help some deaf people. One time my girlfriend came to me from hospital because she couldnt understand a lady who was sick when she used sign language without lip read. Tube was in her throat. So her sisters need me so bad and I went to hospital to help her sisters understand what did sick lady said. Finally I helped with her for many hours to make sure she felt ok and comfortable with me to tell to her sisters what she said. She need alike as three ways first to me then I tell sisters then they tell me and I tell sick lady what her sisters said. I really got experience to learn and help alot. I love kind of job and wish someone call or need to help.

I still hope and pray for nurses and doctors need to learn to use sign language for safe people. It is very important to use sign language to make them understand when they get sick or tubes in throat and cant talk. HOPEFULLY it will be successful soon.

• • • • •

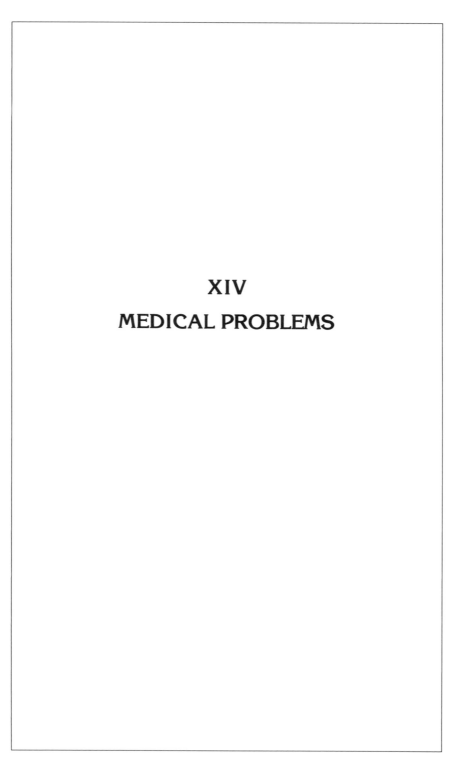

XIV

MEDICAL PROBLEMS

Forum: Questions About Hearing Loss

Responses developed by members of the audiology staff
Department of Otorhinolaryngology,
Albert Einstein College of Medicine, Bronx, New York.

Reprinted with permission from: *The Volta Review,* Volume 81, No. 3,
"Forum: Questions about Hearing Loss," pp. 169-172. Copyright 1979,
by the Alexander Graham Bell Association for the Deaf,
3417 Volta Place, Washington, DC 20007.

This permission exists for this publication only.

Question: What caused the hearing loss?

Response: Janie Chobot

Hearing losses are generally categorized as either conductive, sensori-neural, or mixed (a combination of the two) and they are caused by many factors.

A *conductive impairment* is characterized by an interference in the transmission of sound from the outer canal to the inner ear. Thus, only the outer and/or middle ear are involved. Some of the more common disorders associated with conductive hearing loss are: 1) Perforation of the eardrum (tympanic membrane); 2) Otitis media—middle ear infection, fluid; 3) Growth in the middle ear (e.g. cholesteatoma); 4) Wax (cerumen) or obstruction in the ear canal; 5) Cleft palate—deformities of lip and/or palate that may cause recurrent episodes of otitis media; 6) Malformation and/or abnormalities of outer and middle ear structures at birth; and 7) Hereditary hearing loss caused by a chromosomal defect.

A *sensorineural impairment* occurs when damage has been sustained by the cochlea or auditory nerve. Some of the more common causes for nonhereditary sensorineural hearing loss include: 1) Drug induced loss; 2) Cochlear trauma (skull fracture); 3) Congenital syphilis; 4) Rh incompatibility; 5) Acoustic nerve tumors; 6) Meniere's syndrome; and 7) Viral disease. Both prenatal and postnatal infections have been found to cause hearing loss. Prenatally, maternal rubella has played a large role in creating hearing impairment. Postnatally, viruses have caused early acquired deafness, such as infectious meningitis. Other viruses occurring later in the postnatal period, such as measles, influenza, chicken pox, and mumps, can also cause hearing problems. There are also cases of sudden sensorineural losses of unknown etiology.

A large number of hearing losses are attributed to *hereditary factors*. Chromosomal defects are known to cause a hereditary hearing loss that may manifest itself at birth, during childhood, or later in life. Congenital malformation or abnormalities (i.e., those present at birth) of the inner ear can cause a hearing problem. The loss may be genetic or due to a change produced before birth from outside causes, such as the rubella virus.

Question: Will my other children have a hearing loss? Is hearing loss hereditary?

Response: Deborah Guthermann

Hereditary material is carried as genes on chromosomes. The chromosomes occur in 23 pairs. One member of each pair is inherited from each parent. Generally speaking, 53 percent of congenital hearing loss (i.e., that present at birth) is due to hereditary (genetic) factors that are passed on through different transmission patterns.

Dominant inheritance accounts for approximately ten percent of congenital hearing losses. Only one dominant gene for a particular trait need be present in order for that trait to occur. The recipient of that trait (the hearing impaired child), in turn, has a 50 percent chance of transmitting the chromosome containing that gene to his or her offspring. Dominant inheritance can usually be anticipated as one parent of the hearing impaired child will also have the trait to some degree.

Such is not the case with *recessive inheritance*. In most cases, the parents have no family history of the trait because recessive characteristics are manifested only when the individual has *two matching* affected genes. If only one such gene is present, its "carrier" has the potential to pass that gene on to his or her offspring. When two carriers with the identical recessive gene mate, they have a 25 percent chance of producing an affected child (who inherits one such affected gene from each parent). Likewise, they have a 50 percent chance of producing a carrier offspring (who inherits only one affected gene) and a 25 percent chance of producing children who are genetically normal with regard to that particular trait.

Recessive inheritance accounts for 40 percent of all congenital hearing losses. Unfortunately, persons with the potential to transmit recessive hearing loss usually cannot be identified until they have produced hearing-impaired children since they, themselves have normal hearing. Couples with recent common ancestors have an increased chance of passing on recessive hearing losses to their children, as the existence of a common ancestor increases the probability that the two parents have inherited the identical recessive gene.

Sex-linked inheritance is the third method of genetic transmission. It is involved in approximately three percent of congenital hearing loss cases. Sex is determined by a combination of "X" and "Y" chromosomes. In cases of sex-linked inheritance the gene for a particular trait is located on the X (sex) chromosome. Only male individuals can manifest the trait, however, since they possess one X and one Y chromosome (females possess two X chromosomes). If the X chromosome is affected in males, it is genetically unopposed as no second normal X chromosome can be present to counterbalance the effect.

Factors other than heredity, such as prenatal environmental factors and events during birth, are also responsible for a significant number (47 percent) of congenital hearing losses.

If you are the parent of a hearing-impaired child who is concerned about the likelihood of having additional children with the same problem, do seek a genetic counselor. The otologist can recommend the genetic counselor services in your area.

Author's Comments
The rest of the April 1979 article tells us that only the outer and middle ear may be treated medically. This shows how far medical treatment has progressed in these few years.

* * * * *

Today's Medical Progress

Today over 2,000 children have had cochlear implants. Central Institute for the Deaf, an oral residential school in St. Louis, Missouri, has 24 students with cochlear implants.

The following summary comes from the *Okay Kids Magazine*, Fall 1993. This is also an Alexander Graham Bell Association for the Deaf publication.

Caitlin Parton, the child of "60 Minutes" was one of the first children to receive a 22 channel cochlear implant. Caitlin was 22 months old when she had meningitis. She had the implant at age four. Her parents say she is something new: "a profoundly deaf, hearing child." Her parents chose this procedure even though it was still in investigative status with the FDA.

Despite the objections by the National Association of the Deaf—NAD, choice, no matter how difficult, must exist. Mark Ross recently wrote, "By not trying oralism and broader means of language used by the majority of the country (you) take away a future choice for these children."

* * * * *

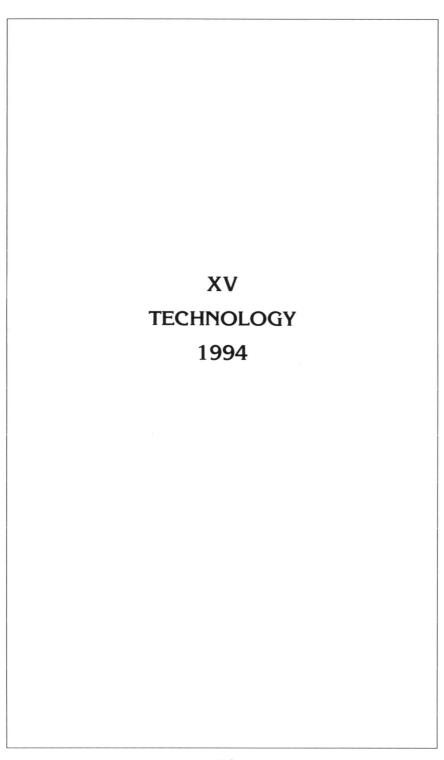

XV

TECHNOLOGY

1994

Technology

The advances in technology are opening the world for our hearing impaired children and adults. New devices are coming on line at an ever increasing pace.

Briefly listed are the many assistive devices now available.

Telephone

Telephone handset has a built-in amplifier and adjustable volume control, inductive receiver and modular plug. This handset can plug in to regular phones. All public phones must be compatable with hearing aids that have "T" switches. Americans with Disabilities Act (ADA) of 1990 required that if there is a bank of public phones, at least one must have a volume control.

Videophones are soon to be introduced. They offer full color, full motion that comes over regular phone lines. What a boon for deaf customers who can read sign language directly.

Telecommunications Text

This TT device allows a person to contact directly a person who also has a TT. The conversation is transmitted (not spoken) through one typewriter to another typewriter. Desk model is portable, but is generally connected to an electrical outlet. Now small ones are available which fit in a briefcase, purse, or child's back-pack. These run on batteries. All phone handsets are compatable. Some models have a readout tape.

These phones are limited to people and places that have TTs. The new law, ADA, now requires each state to operate a Telecommunication Relay System (TRS) so that the hearing impaired may have complete accessibility to all phones. Operators man the service 24 hours a day, every day. The operator receives the TT message and speaks to the listener, or the other way—transcribes the voiced message to the TT user.

Television Listening Devices

Infra-red System: This is a wireless amplifying device consisting of a transmitter and receiver. The transmitter is placed on top of the television. User wearing a small portable receiver can sit anywhere in the room. Receiver picks up the infra-red signal and transfers it into a clear, amplified audio signal. Receiver has a separate volume adjustment control. Does not affect the sound for regular listeners.

Caption Decoding: As of July 1993, all new televisions 13 inches and larger must have a decoder built in the set. A switch allows the print to appear on the screen. Many innovative ways are being developed—some print in color and not necessarily at the bottom of the screen. Music literally dances. In the past, 40 percent of separate decoders were purchased by people learning English as a second language. And for all children to improve reading skills.

Personal FM Systems

These systems are on frequencies set aside for such transmissions. They will not have interference from radio stations. They have a radius of 300 feet. If more than one program is being presented in a building—different classes—each frequency has a separate crystal which sets its frequency. As many as three classes can function in one room with different crystals.

The speaker or teacher wears the microphone (transmitter). The child or other hearing impaired person wears an earset or telecoil loop and "T" switch on the hearing aid. The FM systems use regular 9 volt batteries. Classroom systems use re-chargeable batteries. No connecting wires. Reduces background noise that is so troublesome in a classroom. School systems are more sophisticated than those used in a church or theater, travel tour or family automobile.

If installed in churches and meeting places, the transmitter is connected directly to the PA system and is a permanent component of that system.

Pocketalkers

These devices are merely amplifiers. The microphone is part of the small box about the size of a small radio. The wire goes to an ear piece. It is only a few feet long. This device is excellent for one-on-one conversation for a doctor and patient, a social worker and client, and also for a TV amplification. The person wearing the ear piece must sit close to the television—as far as the wire allows. That person can adjust the volume without bothering the control for normal listeners.

Infra-red System

This system is preferable in theaters especially where there is a row of small theaters. This system requires direct visual contact between the transmitter and the receiver worn by the individual. The advantage is that the amplified message does not leak out of the room. The ADA requires theaters to be accessible.

Portable Induction Loop Amplification System

A coil of electrical wire around a room creates a magnetic field that can transmit sound. A wire is attached to the amplifier. Speaker must use a microphone. Use with a "T" switch on the hearing aid, or if no hearing aid, there is a hand held device. This system eliminates background noise. These loops may be installed in classrooms, churches and meeting rooms.

Alerting Devices

A variety of visual and tactile alerting devices and systems are available to warn hearing impaired people of a baby's cry, a telephone or doorbell, a door knock, or smoke alarm signal: there are also many vibrating or light-connected alarm clocks on the market. These devices allow the hearing impaired person to function independently and feel a sense of security.

Computers

We are now in the Information Age and no office or school, factory or store is without computers. All sorts of educational programs are in use. Math, language, and reading and all school subjects can be on disks at grade levels.

Video Libraries

The Oshkosh Department for Hearing Impaired Children received a grant from the Department of Public Education (DPI) to give parents classes in fall and spring in manual coded English, and a library of videos on many topics for parents to borrow. Residential schools, Gallaudet University have free lending libraries.

Computer Notetaking

Computer notetaking is helpful for hearing impaired adults who do not sign. Also useful in educational programs at the junior and senior high school level as well as technical schools and colleges. A typist follows the speaker. The typing flows from the computer through a projection panel that sets on an overhead projector. The printing is projected upon a screen in large letters that can be read in the classroom or meeting room. An inexpensive program is entered into the computer to enlarge the print. There is a Self Help for Hard of Hearing People, Inc. program, and also WordPerfect has a method.

New Technology

Innovations have rapidly come on the market that make the computer a versatile tool. A modem allows messages to move to other locations through telephone lines. Computers correct spelling and language. Printouts make messages ready for mailing or publishing. Children are taught keyboarding by third grade. They are growing up in a work world that demands the knowledge of new devices.

Basic to the use of technology is a good command of English. The schools have a challenge to educate our hearing impaired children to live and work in today's world.

· · · · ·

Places to Purchase Listening Devices

Any store selling televisions

AT&T Special Needs Center

Radio Shack

Most large retail stores

Audiologists and Hearing Aid Dealers. They should have catalogues listing at least 40 dealers and outlets.

Sound Systems & Equipment

Check libraries for other companies

For listings and prices for Educational Materials:
— Alexander Graham Bell Association for the Deaf, Inc.
— Self Help for Hard of Hearing People, Inc.
— Gallaudet University, Press

Parents may ask for help in purchasing hearing aids for their children through the Department of Health and Social Services (DHSS) if they qualify at the 150 percent poverty level.[1]

1. Schools are responsible for FM systems, interpreters, notetakers, captioned instructional videos and films.

. . . . .

XVI
A SHORT HISTORY OF DEAF EDUCATION

Bright Silence

Year of Our Lord 1550

In the year 1550 spring came late to the hills along the Ebro River near Oña in northern Spain. Wildflowers spotted the green hills, and the sun shown warmly, yet the breeze bore a chill as it came over the distant mountain range. Brother Pedro Ponce de Leon, dressed in coarse woolen trousers and a heavy sweater with rough brogans, walked over the rocky hills. After the students at the Monastery San Salvador left for Holy Week, he sought solace in the archives of the monastery. Still he experienced a restlessness that even prayer did not dispel. Today, finally, he found renewal from the countryside—shepherds taking their flocks of sheep to high pastures, the farmers working their terraced fields, the farm wives in their black aprons, and the children playing in the sunshine.

Brother Ponce de Leon breathed deeply and quickened his pace back to the monastery. He rapidly climbed the many steps to the church, but turned to the right and entered the building that housed the monks' cells. He would change into his black monk's garb and again become an exemplary member of the Order of Benedictine Brothers.

Brother Jose, the Abbot's secretary, met him in the hall. "Brother Pedro, Father Abbot requests to see you immediately. He said it is most urgent."

It was not often that Abbot Philip Lopez made such a request, for he was a methodical man who made appointments well in advance. So Brother Pedro went directly to the Abbot's study. His rap was immediately answered.

"Come in, Brother Pedro. I see you have been out walking. The hills are beautiful this time of year," the Abbot conceded. "I must content myself with my cloistered garden."

Brother Pedro stood silently waiting.

Father Abbot had been a robust man in his youth, but now his habit hung loosely from his shoulders. His lined face looked as though he did not need one more concern. The winds of reform threatened the equanimity of his Benedictine Order. Brother Pedro's roaming the countryside dressed like a sheepherder was one of his irritations, but today he had need to make a special request of Pedro Ponce de Leon.

Finally he spoke. "Tell me, Brother Pedro, did you instruct a deaf-mute lad, one Gaspard Burges, to both read and write?"

"Yes, Father Abbot, several years ago. The lad was about six years old when an illness left him deaf. He had normal speech and language, but at that age no instruction in reading or writing."

"He must be the lad that the Marques de Velasco and his wife, Dona Marie, spoke of when they came to see me this morning. They have not one, but two young sons who are deaf-mutes. They fear, and rightly so, that their sons'

240

futures will be blighted by their inability to hear and speak. The sons will not be recognized under the law which means they will not be able to inherit property."

"Unfortunately that is so, Father Abbot, nor can they learn the doctrines of Christianity."

"The de Velasco family made an earnest plea for education for their sons." The Abbot paused, then added, "You are aware that the de Velasco family has given generously for the re-construction of the chancel. We must try to help their sons."

Brother Pedro considered the implication of Father Abbot's remarks. "How old are the de Velasco sons?"

The Abbot looked at his notation. "Pedro is five and Francisco is seven."

"It is time to begin their education," Brother Pedro nodded.

"I knew you would agree that steps must be taken immediately. Marques de Velasco will send his carriage for you this afternoon. Appraise the situation and report your evaluation to me within a week." The Abbot sounded hopeful, but he had misgivings.

Brother Pedro had taught one deaf-mute to read and write—a lad who had acquired speech and language in a normal fashion. The de Velasco children were born deaf.

As Brother Pedro turned to go, the Abbot said, "God be with you, Brother Pedro."

The de Velasco carriage drew up into the courtyard of the great house, the wheels clicking on the cobblestones. A lackey opened the carriage door and Brother Ponce de Leon stepped down. He wore a cloak over his black habit and a wide brimmed hat. However, he did not follow the young man, but stood in the courtyard watching several boys playing a lively game with sticks and a stone. Lines were scratched on the courtyard, and each tried to drive the stone across the others' line. As Brother Pedro watched, he became aware of a younger lad who threw stones at the players. They paid no heed until he ran up and grabbed one of the sticks. With that a larger lad gave him a shove. At that instant a woman in peasant's dress shouted, "Leon, no!"

The lad withdrew sulking. With the interruption of the game, the lad dressed in lace cuffs and collar sent the stone over the line. He laughed at the other players. They threw down their sticks and ran off.

Ah, thought the monk, I do indeed have my work cut out. He then mounted the steps while a servant held open the carved doors and said, "Dona de Velasco will see you in the great room."

A fragile woman rose to greet him. The only adornment on her plain dark dress was a delicate lace collar held by a large gold brooch. Her hair was pulled back severely under a lace cap. She had a timid, fearful expression.

However, she spoke with sincerity. "We are most grateful that you have come to recommend education for our sons, Pedro and Francisco. They are spirited, and I fear, completely unmanageable. Forgive us, but what can we do? There is no way to explain things to them. Their nurse, dear woman, has her hands full."

At that moment, children's screams, followed by raised voices, could be heard from back in the house.

"That's the cook. No doubt the boys snatched food from her tables," and Dona de Velasco sighed.

Still screaming, the two boys ran through the hall, each carrying a large sweet.

The Brother knew that discipline would have to come first. He spoke to Dona de Velasco, hoping his voice and face showed no reaction to the boys' behavior. "I will see your sons in their rooms tomorrow morning at nine."

"Nurse will try. Nurse will try," lamented Dona de Velasco.

"At nine," the Brother repeated.

The dinner hour was quiet as the boys were fed in their rooms much earlier. The Marques de Velasco was a jovial man, perhaps in his early forties, his hair very gray. A deep scar showed beneath his full beard, and he had a slight limp. He had served his king in his youth.

He was saying, "Dona Marie has faith, faith for both of us, that Francisco and Pedro can learn. She says that they have to be smart to get into so much mischief, don't you, my dear?"

He addressed Brother Pedro. "I am sure the good Lord understands their problem, but not so the courts. My estate is vast, and now I have interest in a shipping company going to the New World. All my property will go to my cousins, scoundrels, every last one of them."

"I understand your concern, Marques, and within the week I should be able to judge if your sons are capable of being educated."

The suckling lamb was good and the port wine, rich in color and taste, was from the de Velasco vineyards. Brother de Leon retired immediately after the meal.

He lit a candle and knelt at the altar in his room. He rose feeling regenerated and prepared to work with the lads.

Pedro Ponce de Leon entered the boys' rooms at nine the next morning. Young Pedro did not wish to put on the suit the nurse set out for him. He ran screaming from the room, nearly shoving the monk against the door. His wail echoed throughout the great house. Francisco allowed himself to be dressed. Bits and pieces of their morning meal were strewn about the floor.

Brother Pedro paid no attention to this disorder. He found a wooden

242

bench and several stools which he set in a clear area of the room. In a corner he found some small, exquisitely carved horses. Several had legs broken off, tails missing, or were headless, but he did manage to find four in fairly good condition. At least they could stand alone. He set them on the bench in a straight line.

Francisco watched him with cold, but curious eyes. At that moment Pedro ran back into the room, and gave the horses a furious swat which sent them flying across the room. Then he hid behind nurse's skirt.

The monk continued to sit on one of the stools and waited. Slowly Francisco gathered up the horses and set them in a row just as Brother Pedro had done. Then he too moved away.

Brother Pedro counted the horses, speaking directly to the boys, and using his fingers to count: uno, dos, tres, cuatro. Then he took up the horses and replaced them one by one, again counting each as he had before. He removed them again, spoke, and used his finger to indicate one. He paused and looked directly at Francisco. Slowly Francisco came forward, picked up a horse, stood it on the bench, and indicated two fingers. Brother Pedro flashed him a smile and a nod of approval.

All this Pedro watched. Suddenly he came forward, snatched a horse, placed it in the row, and showed three fingers.

The monk barely nodded. He was not about to approve of young Pedro's general behavior.

He then turned to the nurse. "Do the boys have slates?"

"Yes." Eventually she found one.

Brother Pedro drew four stick horses. He placed a carved horse over the first drawing and wrote the number one under it. Then he motioned for Francisco to place another one. Without hesitation Francisco did, but Pedro threw his against the wall.

Without a flicker of expression, Brother Pedro wrote on top of the slate "los caballos", indicating all the horses. He again counted them. Then he rubbed out the numbers, and repeated the exercise. This time he wrote the numbers under all but the first one, then handed the marker to Francisco. And Francisco put a "1" under the first horse.

Brother Pedro nodded approval, got up and left the room.

He returned to his quarters and made a detailed report of the time with the de Velasco boys, also a description of the room, and what the nurse did. Then he went to see Dona de Velasco.

"I will see Pedro and Francisco again tomorrow morning at the same time."

"Thank you, Brother Pedro. I am most grateful."

"This afternoon perhaps you would enjoy a ride over the countryside. We have some excellent riding horses."

"That sounds most pleasant. I would enjoy a spirited mount. Could a groom accompany me to show me the extent of your estate?"

And so it was arranged that Brother Pedro rode each afternoon.

By the end of the week, Brother Pedro found the boys dressed and they themselves brought the stools and bench. The boys did not tire of counting. They counted toy soldiers, caps, sweets, stones, and whatever articles they could find. Brother Pedro convinced the nurse to put out simple clothing that the boys could put on themselves. He had to smile when some articles were on backwards or wrong side out. Obviously the boys had never dressed themselves.

Brother Pedro wore his simple black habit. He did retain his gold Cross on a chain from his belt. His goal, in addition to that of the Marques, was to bring Pedro and Francisco to Christianity.

Together they acted out commands. March. Gallop. Sit down. Stand up. Come. Walk. Pray. Each he wrote on the slate with stick figures showing the action. In the courtyard where the boys had a cart with wooden wheels they learned: Push. Pull. Ride. Stop. Take turns. He got the other lads to join the games.

Dona de Velasco stood on the balcony overlooking the courtyard. She smiled as she watched her children comply and enjoy the exercises.

When the week was over, Brother Pedro gave his report to Father Abbot. When Abbot Lopez read it, he looked intently at Brother Pedro. He spoke slowly. "You believe you can teach these two unruly, spoiled de Velasco boys?"

"Father Abbot, I see two intelligent lads encased in silence. They are physically sound and eager to learn. Even in the few days I spent with them, they became more compliant."

"That may be, but what about speech?"

"Fortunately Castilian is a very phonetic language. Surely I will find a way to teach speech."

"You expect a miracle," the Abbot sighed.

"No, Father Abbot, only endurance."

"Then go. And God be with you."

The monk gathered his few possessions, his missal, his goose quill pens, and ink. He would miss the archives where he spent much of his time, but he knew he was to do God's work.

Francisco and Pedro were playing with the servants' children in the courtyard when his carriage arrived. The lackey, Manuel, opened the carriage door and greeted Brother Pedro.

"We are pleased to see you again. Look, here come the lads."

All the boys stood in a line and watched the monk. He approached the lads, nodded and spoke to each in turn: "Buenos dias, Leon. Buenos dias, Francisco. Buenos dias, Ricardo. Buenos dias, Pedro." With that the boys ran off.

After settling in his quarters, he went in search of Don Rolando, the Marques' secretary. He found him in the study doing accounts. Don Rolando looked annoyed at being interrupted.

"I am in need of a sheaf of heavy paper," Brother Pedro said, ignoring the displeasure on the secretary's face.

"Monk, are you not aware that paper, all paper, is very dear? I have none to spare."

"I am here at the request of the Marques de Velasco. I am to educate his sons. The Marques assured me that materials would be made available."

"You are not a man of the world, Monk, or you would know that deaf-mutes are not worthy of your efforts. They cannot learn."

Brother Pedro's thin features were set as he stared back at the secretary, and he bit off his words, "I will expect the paper to be sent to my quarters."

"As you say, Monk. However, it may take sometime to obtain the paper you request."

Brother Pedro Ponce de Leon regretted being so sharp, and tried to make amends. "Thank you, Don Rolando. I will see that the sons of de Velasco use the paper sparingly. I have my own quills and ink."

He then found a servant to ask if he might speak with Dona de Velasco. Soon he was summoned to her sitting room.

"Brother Pedro, we are most grateful that you returned. I know the boys missed you. After your few days with them, we all could see they became more attentive."

"Your sons need a very regular routine. Education cannot be fun all the time. They will need much drill and repetition. I will meet with them each morning during the heat of the summer, and report their progress to you each week. I am most confident your sons can learn, but you must be patient. Progress will be slow."

Gradually Francisco and Pedro recognized the written words of objects without the illustrations. Brother Pedro began to draw attention to initial sounds. A puff of air breathed on the lads' hands helped them recognize /p/ and /f/. Francisco quickly related the /f/ to his name under the stick drawing of a boy with long, straight hair. Pedro looked at Francisco's happy face and suddenly he pointed to the drawing of the boy with curly hair, then to himself and to the /p/ under his picture.

Drills on consonants and vowels soon enabled the boys to say whole words and a few simple phrases. Brother Pedro was pleased with their progress. But he knew that the Marques and Dona de Velasco expected their sons to "talk like the other children."

When the boys became more tractable and willing to follow directions, the Marques selected ponies for them. The groom showed them how to hold the reins, and then he guided the ponies about the field. Soon the boys could do it themselves. Brother Pedro often joined them.

When fall brought cooler weather, Brother Pedro took the boys for rides over the hills. They watched a vulture devour a stray lamb, they watched the trout in the streams, they found berries to eat, and learned to sit still to watch the rabbits.

It was along the river one afternoon that the monk's horse missed its step and threw him to the ground where he lay stunned. Pedro and Francisco dismounted and ran to him, and entreated him to get up. The lads communicated with each other with gestures and spoken words. "Fell. Fra hurt. Sleep. Home. Help." But they did not know which way to go.

Francisco felt the monk again. He seemed cold, so the boys took off their small capes to cover him. They sat nearby on a large rock for some time. The horse and the ponies grazed near by. As the shadows lengthened, Francisco said, "Man." He pointed back over the hills. He remembered passing a man with sheep. Both boys ran back over the hills to a hut.

The old shepherd wore a leather cape against the weather. The boys gestured, but the shepherd did not understand.

"Speak up, lads." He was puzzled that two young children were alone on the hills, and without garments in the evening chill. "What do you want?"

"Come," said Francisco in his best speech.

The shepherd understood, but where?

Francisco said, "Fra fell. Hurt. Come."

The shepherd thought, their voices sound strange, but they talk. Could these be the deaf and dumb sons of the Marques de Velasco?

He followed the boys back over the hills to where the monk was now sitting, rubbing his head. Brother Pedro was alarmed that the boys had disappeared.

The old shepherd fetched some water which the monk gratefully accepted. Brother Pedro then asked, "How did you understand the boys?"

"They spoke," said the shepherd. "They said 'Fra hurt. Come. Help.' And they pulled me along. But I understood them. They spoke."

Brother Pedro's headache vanished with that good news. "I think I can ride now. Help me up on the saddle, and the boys, too."

"Thank you. What is your name, good shepherd?"

"Alfredo, Brother," the simple shepherd answered.

"The Marques de Velasco will reward you, Alfredo."

As the monk and the boys rode slowly toward the great house, they met the groom and several servants galloping toward them carrying torches.

"The Marques and Dona de Velasco are worried. They sent us to find you," said the groom.

"All is fine now. I was thrown from my horse and hit my head. Francisco and Pedro went for help. Alfredo, the shepherd came to our rescue."

The Marques and Dona de Velasco stood in the courtyard as they rode up. The children slid off their ponies and ran to their mother.

"Fell," Francisco said and pointed to Brother Pedro.

"Help," he added. "Man come. Help."

"Man help Fra," Pedro chimed in, wanting to also tell the story.

Dona de Velasco put her arms around her children and looked up at Brother Pedro. Tears of gratitude glistened in her eyes.

That evening at prayer, Brother Pedro Ponce de Leon praised the Lord. Francisco and Pedro knew the value of speech. Silent their world would always be, but they need not be alone. Their future was bright.

Author's Note

Intermarriage among the nobility and upper class resulted in an increase of deaf offspring. Pedro Ponce de Leon wrote in a legal document in the year 1578: "In this house in Oña, I have had for my pupils, who were deaf and dumb from birth, sons of great lords and notable people, whom I have taught to speak, read, write, and reckon: to pray, to assist at Mass, and to know the doctrines of Christianity."[1]

It is clearly established that Pedro Ponce de Leon, a Benedictine monk, was the first oral teacher of the deaf.

· · · · ·

1. *Turning Points in the Education of Deaf People* by Edward L. Scouten of the National Institute of Technology, Rochester, N.Y. 1984. Pages 14-15.

Short History of Deaf Education

The President of the International Congress of 1880 reported that 263 out of the 338 institutions for the deaf in Europe employ the Pure Oral System. This was in a flyer from the Private School Number 7, S Merrick Street, Philadelphia, Pennsylvania.

Early in 1812 John Braidwood arrived in America for the purpose of founding a school. In 1815 Rev. Thomas Hopkins Gallaudet embarked for England with the expressed purpose of learning the Oral Method of Deaf Instruction. Unable to spend the three months in London to learn the Oral Method, Gallaudet went to Paris, where he had been invited by Abbe Sicard, who had developed the de l' Epee sign language. After several months Gallaudet returned to America, bringing with him Laurent Cleric, "a walking dictionary of signs", the most distinguished pupil of Sicard. They opened a school in 1817.

In 1864 the Deaf-Mute College (later named Gallaudet, now Gallaudet University) was established by Congress. The charter was signed by President Lincoln.

The Wisconsin School For The Deaf

In 1850, Miss Wealthy Hawes, a graduate of the New York Institution for the Deaf and Dumb, came to the farm home of Ebenezer Cheseboro, two and a half miles west of Delavan on the Janesville road, to teach the deaf daughter, Ariadna, who had been a pupil of the New York Institution before the Cheseboro family immigrated to Delavan. The following year there were eight students. Lack of funds caused the circulation of a petition to take enough money from the state school funds to enable each deaf child in the state to be taught free of charge. On April 15, 1852 a bill was signed by Governor Leonard J. Farewell becoming Chapter 481 of the Laws of 1852.

The first classes were taught by the sign method, however, speech was introduced in 1857. Both methods were used, and for many years the oral department was the larger.

The legislature of 1858 set the age of enrollment "not under ten and not over twenty-five". Soon we read: "It is seldom that such pupils can make any material progress in mastering the difficulties of written language. The mental facilities, after so long neglect, have lost to a very great extent, the keeness and susceptibility of earlier years." By 1919 there was a statutory provision for admission of deaf pupils between the ages of eight and twenty-five.

The need for industrial training at this institution was recognized almost immediately. A course in cabinet making was begun in 1858. Other trades followed such as type-setting, and a new building for manual training. Cooking and sewing were opened for the girls. Also rug weaving, chair caning, and brush making were offered. Cobblers, carpenters and painters received training at the school.

Extra-curricular activities began to play a large part in developing self respect. In 1933 the basketball team was the champion deaf team in the United States. Boy Scouts and Girl Scouts were thriving organizations.

Day Classes in Wisconsin

In 1878 a class of four students in Milwaukee started. Instruction was in the German language and the oral method was used.

It was in 1885 that Alexander Graham Bell spent two weeks in Madison in the state legislature to encourage the establishment of day classes. It was thus that "Wisconsin startled the world" with a public day school for the deaf. In 1936 there were twenty-three day classes with 542 pupils.

After World War II when transportation again became feasible the trend was to establish centers where children could be grouped as to ages and grades.

Today, in the 1990's with mainstreaming and integration taking place throughout the state, there are now 42 school districts that have either day classes or have hearing impaired students mainstreamed and offer support staff and/or interpreters.

The 1988-89 summary sheet shows 795 students in public schools and 175 at the Wisconsin School for the Deaf at Delavan. The 12 CESA districts service or keep track of a total 254 students. CESA stands for Cooperative Educational Services Agency, a separate system, not under the jurisdiction of any school district, but under the Department of Public Instruction (DPI).

National Enrollment

The following data is reported by the Center for Assessment and Demographic Studies, Gallaudet University, from the annual survey of hearing impaired children and youth. The year 1975 showed 47,000 students in 2500 programs. The year 1985 showed an increase of students being served to 51,000 and the programs grew dramatically to approximately 8600.

The year 1984-85 shows that hearing impaired students with one or more additional handicapping condition in 60 residential schools totaled 30.6 percent.

Sign language used in schools of adolescents ages 12 through 20: Special schools =95 percent; Mainstream settings =76 percent. Families using sign language: Special schools = 36 percent; Mainstream settings = 35 percent.

The Rubella epidemic in 1964-65 caused a dramatic increase in the number of hearing impaired students. This group has now passed through the school systems. Some may still attend technical schools and colleges to up-grade their skills. Now in addition to Gallaudet University 150 colleges and technical schools offer services for hearing impaired students.

State Charter
For Oshkosh School For Deaf-Mutes
September 15, 1888

Office of State Superintendent,
Madison, Wisconsin.

To the Mayor and Common Council
of the City of Oshkosh, Wisconsin.

Upon application, hereto
attached; from the Mayor and Common
Council of the City of Oshkosh, in
accordance with the provisions of Chapter
315, Laws of 1885, permission, by and
with the consent of the State Board of
Supervisors, is hereby granted to the City
of Oshkosh, to establish and maintain
within its corporate limits, one or more
schools for the instruction of deaf mutes,
residents of Wisconsin.

Given under my hand and
seal of office this fifteenth
day of September, A.D. 1888.

J. B. Thayer,
State Supt.

One Hundred Years Ago
In *The Neenah Daily Times*
Page 4, Twin City News Record, September 21, 1988

Glancing Backward to the Date: September 21, 1888

Harry Reed, of this city, will teach the new deaf and dumb school in Oshkosh. Reed's wife is also a mute, and is a daughter of Mr. Andrews of Shawano, a prominent citizen of that place. Mr. and Mrs. Reed have a daughter that talks. It is expected that about a dozen living in Oshkosh and vicinity will avail themselves of the privilege of the deaf/mute school, and as Mr. Reed will receive $100 from the state for each pupil instructed for the period of nine months in a year he will have a fair competency out of the enterprise.

Note: My starting salary my first year teaching in 1942 in Appleton, Wisconsin, (25 miles from Oshkosh) was $1200 for nine months. An additional $85 for cost of living.

* * * * *

XVII

RESEARCH TODAY
16-18 YEAR OLD DEAF STUDENTS

Factors Predictive
of The Development of Literacy
In Profoundly Hearing-Impaired Adolescents

Ann Geers and Jean Moog's Volta Review *article*
Reprinted with permission from: *The Volta Review,* Volume 91, No. 2
"Factors Predictive of the Development of Literacy
  in Profoundly Hearing-Impaired Adolescents," pp. 69-86.
Copyright 1989, by the Alexander Graham Bell Association for the Deaf
3417 Volta Place, NW, Washington, DC 20007

Review of article

In 1984 the National Institute of Health (NIH) awarded contracts to investigate factors that predict the development of reading and writing skills in congenitally (from birth or early childhood before acquiring speech) and profoundly hearing impaired 16- and 17-year olds. Three separate groups were studied:

Children who had been educated orally,

Children of normal hearing parents who had been educated in total communication programs,

Children of hearing impaired parents.

Central Institute for the Deaf (CID) (an oral residential school) in St. Louis tested 100 adolescents from oral programs.

Gallaudet University in Washington, D.C. tested both other groups.

CID and Gallaudet designed the battery of tests.

The 100 oral students came from 26 states and 3 provinces of Canada.

Previous research to date shows "a plateau in performance on about the 3rd grade level at 15 years of age and continues through age 18."

The more academically successful profoundly hearing impaired students are mainstreamed at younger ages and are therefore not represented in the above demographic studies.

It should be noted that the low scores for older hearing impaired students may result in additional and more severely handicapping characteristics.

Generally the population reflects a delay of 2-5 years.

This study's purposes:

Obtain literacy levels of orally trained students.

What factors in the environment, background, and abilities are predictive of reading and writing competence.

Students who were selected for the study:

Better ear—85-128 dB loss,

253

Given WAIS (Wechsler Adult Intelligence Scale) both verbal and
performance,
Speech production intelligibility,
Sign language (Signed English and American Sign Language-ASL),
Lipreading,
Reading: vocabulary, sentence and text level,
Written language tests.

Three factors: sign language, socio-economic status, and mainstreaming, do not contribute significantly to literacy. This result suggests that *the most important predictor of literacy in these hearing-impaired adolescents is oral English competence.*

Conclusion: Their mean grade level for reading comprehension on the SAT was 8th grade. Thirty percent were at or above the 10th grade level. Fifteen percent lie below the 3rd grade level which is the mean level for the general 16- and 17-year-old according to demographic studies.

Even though the students in this study had a mean dB loss of 100,
They have well-developed speech perception skills,
Well-developed spoken language skills.

However, this group had minimal sign language skills—only 9 percent had sign language proficiency.

Background:
Acquired language exclusively through oral methods,
Above average non-verbal intellectual ability as compared with normal
hearing adolescents,
Parents well educated and in professional and business careers,
(note 1)
Early amplification,
Special education at early age,
Most spent junior and high school in mainstream educational settings.

In spite of these positive characteristics and advantages, the majority of the subjects still did not achieve reading levels commensurate with normal-hearing adolescents at the end of high school. It is likely that vocabulary development was a contributing factor.

Results:
24 percent to 34 percent can obtain reading skills equal to hearing
students.
Can, on the average, obtain 7th and 8th grade reading levels.

Factors that are associated with literacy are:
1. Good use of residual hearing
2. Early amplification
3. Educational management
4. Oral English language including vocabulary, syntax, and discourse skills.

Dr. Ann Geers is Director of Clinical Services and Ms Jean Moog is

Principal at Central Institute for the Deaf in St. Louis, Mo. *The Volta Review,* February/March 1989 pages 69-86.

Note 1—Comment

I found that neither the level of parents' education nor the occupations were critical factors. An understanding of the special needs of the child, the encouragement and acceptance of the child, and the cooperation of parent and school were the deciding factors. —*M. Ferris*

. . . . .

Factors Predictive of School Achievement

Donald F. Moores, Catherine Sweet

Preparation of this chapter was supported by the National Institute of Neurology and Communicative Disorders and Stroke. It appears on pages 154-201 in *Educational and Developmental Aspects of Deafness* by Donald F. Moores and Kathryn P. Meadow-Orlans

This is a review of Chapter 7.

Deaf Adolescents with Hearing Parents

These 65 severely and profoundly hearing impaired 16- and 17-year old residential students had been in total communication programs from preschool years. These students had hearing parents.

They exhibited a wide range of literacy skills, as well as achievement in related areas. Communication skills also showed variability, with the exception in English-based sign and ASL conditions, where all had some level of fluency. There was ease of communication at home. All participated in school activities.

The individual tests for these deaf students with hearing parents correlated most highly with reading outcomes consisting of four subtests of the WAIS Verbal Scale, three tests of vocabulary and two tests of English grammar. Only three of the 31 independent measures correlated with writing outcomes.

Results suggested that literacy achievement in total communication subjects is closely tied to specific knowledge of English grammar and English vocabulary. Page 199.

Deaf Adolescents With Deaf Parents

Only 210 deaf children with deaf parents were identified from the slightly less than 7000 students in the United States of 16- to 17-years of age. The final selection was of 65 students of the 16- to 17-year-old group. Only 12 percent were minority status. Several had enrolled at Gallaudet University, but only two were from this level as the study wanted to show the general abilities of this age group.

The same battery of 31 tests were administered as had been used with the other two groups. Only four of the tests appeared to be predictive for reading scores:
Test of Syntactic Abilities
WAIS picture completion subtest
CAT vocabulary test
MAC Aided test

Predictive Factors for Writing for deaf children of deaf parents:
WAIS Vocabulary
Digital Symbol
MAC Vocabulary
English-based Sign

To quote a paragraph that sums up the study, page 184.
"The results suggest that knowledge of English grammar and vocabulary, along with the ability to utilize even minimum amounts of auditory input, are highly predictive of the reading skills of deaf adolescents whose deaf parents have signed to them from birth. The quality of the child's fluency in speech, English sign and/or ASL are not major related factors."

Both of these groups of deaf students attended residential schools which probably has increased their commonality.

At present it is unknown whether deaf adolescents in public schools total communication programs would evince the same characteristics. Page 200.

Author's Comment

When the *mainstreamed programs* that use sign interpreters have been available for a sufficient length of time, it will be interesting to do research to see how this group differs from the three hearing impaired groups in this study. Certainly, a residential school has a great influence on the academic programs. State residential schools use ASL in their socializing programs, dorms, and after school activities. The hearing impaired students in mainstreamed classes socialize, play on teams, and live in hearing neighborhoods.

Unlike the study of oral deaf adolescents, which gave the percentages at each reading level, this study, done at Gallaudet University, gave the grade range as 2.8 to 13.0 with the mean at grade 6.01.

These three recent studies indicate that the reading and writing levels are higher than previously indicated. With the knowledge of what fosters literacy, curriculums can be enriched.
· · · · ·

Oral Nursery
And On With An Oral Program

Today there are few all oral nursery programs for toddlers with hearing impairment. However, it is still possible and parents should have that choice. Here's how an all oral program will function. Right after identification—hopefully before six months of age, home visits will be started. Soon the parents will bring the nursery age child to a program.

"Talk, talk, talk" is the advice given to parents of hearing impaired children. However, there is something special about the way to talk to the infants and preschoolers.

Teachers: The teacher must be a trained teacher of deaf and hard of hearing children, knowledgeable in the ways to encourage speech and language, familiar with early childhood development. She must be able to stimulate and build the understanding and comprehension of spoken language. She sets the correct patterns, encourages natural, pleasant voices. By using the same phrases and simple sentences over and over the child comprehends meaning.

The teacher must check hearing aids daily. Keep a supply of batteries. Batteries can go dead at any minute.

For a class using assistive listening devices, which usually have rechargeable batteries, these too must be daily checked so that they function properly. The need for an Educational Audiologist is apparent.

The child will learn that spoken language gets him what he wants.

The talking the teacher does is "in situ"—is part of every activity. The teacher and aides must wash hands with the toddlers, be in the play area and play ground with the children, be in the hall when they take off their jackets or put on their boots. She has to take advantage of every wisp of experience and breathe life into it.

Parents: Parents need this same insight and guidance to know how to take advantage of every opportunity to introduce and re-inforce language. When the child is an infant a professional must visit the home regularly to show parents how to be effective in the child's development. And when the child is enrolled in the nursery program the parents must accompany the child. And if this cannot be arranged for each session, it should be as often as possible.

This does two things: It shows the parent how to work with the child. This may not be obvious, so a few minutes of explanation must be part of each visit. And secondly, it gives parents the opportunity to see what other toddlers are doing so that the parent realizes what is the norm. They see their child is regulation—some good days and some bad.

Speech: Speech is movement, a flowing thing, not static positions. Speech must arise from need, be the clothing of an idea, the manifest expression of thought. To drill "foo, foo, foo" or "ba, ba, ba" is a lifeless activity. It ignores the basic law of learning—meaningful experience is easier learned. The talking must emerge as a whole, no matter how imperfect. It is so with all hearing children. We do not censure the normal hearing child if the first words are not perfect. The important thing is that it is consistent. If the child says "wa" for water and uses it every time he wants a drink, that is welcomed and encouraged in the beginning. We repeat back the correct word just as all parents do and put it in a phrase or question: "You want a drink of water?" or "Here is your water."

Unlike the hearing child who lives in a sea of sound and talking, our child with a hearing loss—even a mild one—has a limited listening experience, regardless of how much help he gets through his hearing aids. So parents must be ever mindful of every opportunity to talk—talk about what he is doing.

Taction is helpful in saying words correctly. He can feel mother's face for vibration for voiced sounds. Or a puff of air on his hand if need be: the breath on the hand as you say the word "candy". One parent asked me what to name the pet dog so it would be visible and easy to say. "Bimbo" was such a name. Read Dr. Kile's article about vibrotactile aids (p. 102) which children with profound hearing losses can wear.

But again, your child must wear his hearing aid at all times. It should be the first thing put on in the morning and the last thing taken off at night. I know that parents often think that the aid is so expensive it might get broken in play. If your child had to wear a leg brace, would you let him take it off when he came home from school and then crawl around the rest of the day? Of course not. *Play is what children do.* This is when they need to wear their hearing aids. When a child goes out to play does he not need to hear a car horn? Yes, a hearing aid works best in a room with a rug and upholstered furniture to absorb much of the normal reverberations. It goes without saying that a classroom should also be carpeted.

Language: The development of language is the main goal of education so that the child may learn the many facts, theories, and tasks. Spoken English is the goal of Oral Education. No philosophy of Deaf Education has raised such furor as the controversy over the methods of educating hearing impaired children. In as much as 90 percent of our hearing impaired children have residual hearing and come from hearing families—these parents can request an oral method. Or at the very least, an emphasis on spoken language.

Social Development: Developing attention span, cooperation, learning to take turns, being considerate of others' feelings—all are part of the nursery program. Large muscle development requires space and toys to allow for this. A safe play ground area is required. Small children cannot safely share a play area with older children.

Self help skills are taught at both home and school. One year our nursery children brought their jackets and snow pants and boots and threw them on the floor expecting the aide and me to dress them. Guess what we discussed at the next parent meeting! These children had no physical handicaps. They could learn self help skills that all children must learn. Don't buy snow pants with confusing straps. In fact, do not leave the store until you see your child can work the zippers and struggle into the clothes himself.

After home visits oral nursery programs may be developed for toddlers under the age of three. They may be held in clinics or in universities. However, parking is such a problem around educational settings, that it would be best if an off campus location could be found. This should resemble a home with similar furnishings so that teachers can guide the parents in taking advantage of simple activities. A kitchen for baking cookies or preparing lunch—the names of the utensils and the activities of making a meal and cleaning up. A living room, bedroom, and bathroom—the locations where our toddlers live and play. All this seems over simplified, but how many parents make a point of actually including the toddlers in house-keeping tasks and talking about the activity as they do it? Most need guidance as to how and why it is necessary.

Again, speech and language are learned as one participates in the every day, normal activities.

Now we come to the educational program for three-year-olds when they are admitted into the public school. The same requirements hold for the teaching staff. Today speech therapists often take over the speech development. Gone are the days when the trained teacher encouraged and guided speech throughout the day in all activities. However, mainstreaming requires these speech lessons be relegated to a specialist.

We are still talking about an oral program. In addition to speech lessons, our hearing impaired student may benefit from added help in language and concept development from a teacher of the hearing impaired.

Consideration of the Needs
for the Oral Program for Hearing Impaired Students

Teachers: It goes without saying that there must be trained teachers for day classes and resource rooms.

Director: No discussion of the philosophy of all classes for the hearing impaired is complete without a word about the role of the director of the program.

The first ten years that I taught in Oshkosh the two men who directed the program were trained teachers of the deaf and also had masters degrees in audiology. They tested the children, kept checking the equipment and we teachers could ask for guidance. We all went to conventions and meetings. Our department library contained professional journals.

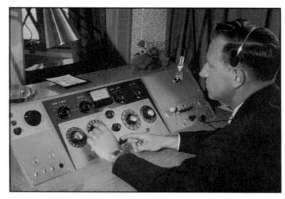

Leonard Becker.
Principal, teacher, and
audiologist for the day
class for the hearing
impaired in 1965.

This testing is still used for
older children and adults.
(1994)

Photo by James Auer

Unfortunately the Exceptional Education Needs (EEN) Departments in all school systems grew so large and demanding, that directors were hired.

These persons, even with doctorate degrees in special education, were not on the scene. Their offices were removed, they did not take part in the day to day activities. Few had more than an introductory course in education of the hearing impaired. The principals in each school took over the day to day direction of the classes for the hearing impaired. They were only specialists in regular education.

I would like to suggest that whoever directs the program for the hearing impaired be first a trained teacher in that disipline. Whatever the designation is, be it department head, or head teacher, that makes no difference—but his/her education and background is important. If there are only two, or more than ten teachers for the hearing impaired in a system, one must be designated head of the department and be responsible for the program.

This person should hold regular staff meetings, read all the journals, and attend conventions and encourage the staff to attend. Often there are funds to cover much of the cost of professional meetings. The program's library must subscribe to professional journals. And it goes without saying that this department or class must have parent meetings.

M-Teams: This is a group of professionals *who are familiar with the needs of hearing impaired children, and the individual child.* Parents must be an integral part of this assessement and the recommendations. Older children should also be a part of their team.

An Individual Educational Plan (IEP) is drawn up and becomes a legally binding document. It is reviewed yearly. *Parents have the right to challenge this plan at any time.*

Oral Mainstream Classes: Today nearly half of all hearing impaired children are placed in regular classes. Here again, supportive staff is a necessity. Speech therapy needs to be continued throughout school years. The student may need extra help from the regular teachers or hopefully a teacher of the hearing impaired may make scheduled visits to the school.

Suggested supportive help: There may be oral interpreters. However, if the student has come up with using assistive listening devices that are coupled with his/her hearing aid, this should be continued.

Videos and movies used in the regular class should be captioned.

And for lecture classes, a typist working at a computer in the class can record all that is said. Turn the screen of the computer toward the hearing impaired student. The print can be enlarged on the screen for easier reading. And a disk can be made for review.

Note takers—students who make carbon copies of their notes. The hearing impaired student must be continually lipreading or reading the information on the computer screen which means the hearing impaired student has no time to take his own notes.

If it is a class of all oral hearing impaired students, a projection panel placed on the over-head projector connected to the computer will project all the information up on a screen for all class members.

Parents need to know the options and then work with the school and let their child know they are there to help in every way.

* * * * *

Commission on Education of the Deaf

1988

A federal commission studied the appropriate educational opportunities that should be available to deaf individuals. The Commission on the Education of the Deaf, 1988 (COED) became the most crucial aspect of the new law. Today we see progress on many fronts.

1. Choice of appropriate educational settings.
2. Parents rights.
3. Newborn hearing tests.
4. Early intervention.
5. Use of technology, individual and in school.
6. Trained educational interpreters.
7. Television captioning.
8. ADA services and employment.
9. Research on language acquisition.
10. Adapt postsecondary programs.
11. Attention to students with additional handicaps.
12. Medical research.
13. Cooperation of federal, state and county agencies.
14. Public awareness.
15. Development of information and referral databases.

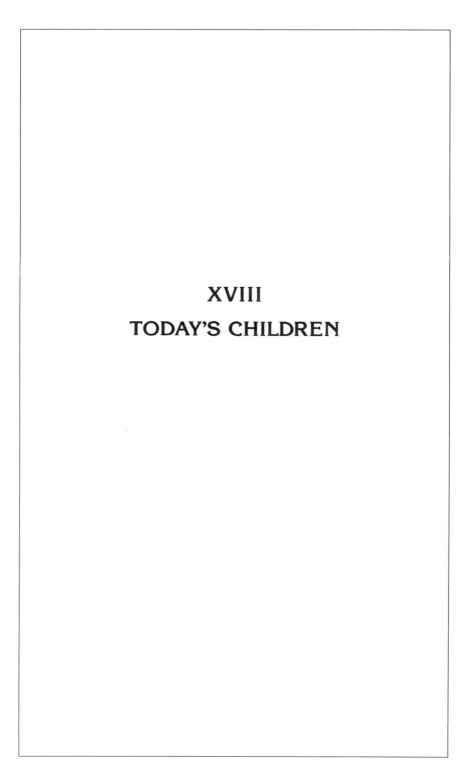

XVIII
TODAY'S CHILDREN

Today's Children

Parents today, more than ever, need to know the options for the education of their hearing impaired children. And the choices are many. The right choice requires that parents look down the path of years to come. How can they understand and know what the choice of an educational program will mean for their own child? Research is all well and good, but how can a parent with an infant wait for years to see what would be best? The only hope is that each family considers what is available, what has worked for children in the past, or by working with other parents and the school, develop a better program.

The upsurge of Deaf Culture is appropriate for Deaf parents. But not understandably for the 90 percent of parents who are hearing. It is unreasonable to think one method would fit all! There is not a business magazine nor a newspaper article about today's prospects for employment that does not cry out for better educated workers. And successful workers will be the ones who are educated and skilled in communication necessary for business today.

Regardless, parents must make the choice for their youngster. You have read the stories of many students who have moved through the various educational systems. What is available today? Let us study the options.

Early Intervention
All counties are now required to establish programs to help parents with handicapped infants. The counties contract for these programs and must hire professional people knowledgeable and experienced in early childhood hearing loss. These professionals visit the homes on a regular schedule. Contact with this service can be made through county agencies who then direct the parents and the professional.

Day Classes
These classes exist in public schools. A hearing handicap is one of low incidence—one child in a thousand children. Therefore many school districts combine this service. The classes may be self-contained and/or the students are mainstreamed as they are capable. In Wisconsin these classes have teachers who use Total Communication which means that they use English based sign. They may also speak as they sign. Children are taught speech, lipreading, and in some cases—Cued speech. Every attempt is made to accommodate the *needs of the child*. Some children, depending upon their hearing ability, and use of hearing aids and FM (frequency modulated) systems, are very oral. And they are mainstreamed into regular classes where they function in an optimum fashion. Often they are accompanied by educational interpreters. A dozen or so such programs exist in Wisconsin.

Mainstreamed Classes

Since the passage of federal law recommending that all handicapped children be educated in the least restricted fashion mainstreaming has proliferated. It is understandable that parents want their children to attend neighborhood schools, be in the scout troup, go to the YMCA with friends for swimming and activities. It is the best of all worlds. However, and this is a big however, are local school systems aware of the special needs the children require?

Does the system have the services of an audiologist who can check the FM systems and the child's hearing aid on a regular basis? Do the parents send a supply of batteries along with a battery tester to the teacher or the school nurse? Are all the children in the class educated as to the function of the hearing aid—that the hearing impaired student must be able to locate the student answering the questions. Does the teacher write out the assignments? Is the student of an age or the class such that a notetaker would help? To lipread or watch an interpreter the hearing impaired student cannot take notes himself.

Is there an interpreter? A teacher's aide? Are speech lessons provided by a speech pathologist? Is there an itinerant teacher of the hearing impaired to suppliment the regular class assignments?

Even today mainstreaming can mean that the child may have only half of his subjects in the regular class. A resource room may be the answer for part time mainstreaming. Less than half of the hearing impaired students are fully mainstreamed.

Is the child the only hearing impaired student in the building? What of the need for peer companionship?

Perhaps the *least restrictive environment* should read, the *most appropriate environment.*

Does the speech pathologist have adequate space—a room with good lighting, carpeting, and a supply of materials to set up a learning situation? The little room off the noisy gym or near the music room will not do. Nor a desk in the hallway. And she must collaborate with the classroom teacher to present the speech needed in the regular class.

What in-service training does the regular teacher have when she includes the various handicapped children? Can she give her regular students the attention they need if she does not have an aide? And she needs to know how to encourage the inclusion of the hearing impaired student in group activities. And she must encourage the hearing impaired student to speak for him/herself.

And now we come to the student him/herself. Is this student willing to wear the FM system? Can the teacher make the child comfortable? Teenagers are so very sensitive that they will forgo better hearing rather than wear the aid. Children must have a positive feeling and good self-esteem.

For the students using interpreters, teachers can overcome this sensitive behavior by including lessons for the whole class in sign language. It takes the strangeness out of the signing if the regular students can participate. And it encourages communication and friendships.

Residential Schools

At first bloom of mainstreaming it was thought that there would be no need for residential schools. Not so. This still is a real choice. Students who attend these schools have a real feeling of "belonging". They relax and enjoy themselves. The schools have all kinds of after school activities. For some years residential schools have arranged for the students to go home for weekends so they do not become estranged from their families and community. Great effort is placed upon family involvement. Families serve on committees, they are encouraged to learn sign language. Local technical schools give sign language courses. Videos are sent home to augment this skill.

Many Deaf parents want their children to attend a residential school. Many of the instructors and house parents are deaf so there are role models for the students. While there are speech therapists, still most of the interaction is carried on in sign language. Certainly ASL is the common language. They stress English and their students move on to work sites and to trade schools and Gallaudet University or other colleges. At age 14 the children become clients of the Division of Vocational Rehabilitation. This is true for all handicapped students in mainstreamed classes, and day classes as well.

These schools have outstanding libraries and teaching equipment. Their audio-visual departments are exceptional. They make videos to send home. They have computers and modems. They emphasis pre-vocational training.

Each dorm room has a strobe light should an emergency require the students to leave their rooms. Fire drills are not only during class time, but can be during the night.

There are a few private oral residential schools: Clarke School for the Deaf in Northampton, Massachusetts, and Central Institute for the Deaf and St. Josephs School for the Deaf, both in St. Louis, Missouri. And there are others.

The Multiple Handicapped Student

There are still 30 percent of the students who have additional problems: health, behavior now called Attention Deficit Disorder (ADD), celebral palsey (CP), learning disability (LD), and mental retardation. The schools call the programs for these children—Adaptive Education. Both residential schools and Day Classes have the largest enrollment in Adaptive Education classes.

General Considerations

The mainstreamed student is usually one with moderate to severe hearing loss. Although some children with profound losses have been able to function successfully in the mainstream setting.

Thus, each child must be evaluated where he/she may best develop academically and socially. Today equal stress must be put on the emotional and social needs of the student. So placement considers all these normal needs.

The Forgotten Child

Again one must be reminded that the child with a mild loss may have an educational problem. These children can be as many as one in 25, or one in every class. These children will need extra help with speech, vocabulary and concept development.

Today's Child

By being open to every possible way to educate our hearing impaired children, hopefully each child will receive the very best education. See how these three families selected the program which was best for their children.

* * * * *

Follow Your Instincts

By Charlene Becker
Appleton, Wisconsin
SHHH Journal March/April 1987

When I sit down to try and recall all of the events that took place since the realization that our first-born girl wasn't hearing us, it seems so long ago, so much has happened. I find it difficult to remember all of them.

One thing I do remember is the pain, the feelings of sorrow, the pity I felt for this baby who couldn't hear, and how helpless I felt because I didn't know anything about hearing loss or how to help her. I did know that I had to overcome all of those feelings before I could truly help our child.

It's funny, but the last thing I ever thought about during my pregnancy was whether my baby would hear or not. It never occurred to me that it was a possibility. I thought of every other problem or birth defect, but hearing loss never entered my mind. Lindsey seemed as normal as any baby at first, especially with no other children to compare her to. I look back and wonder why I didn't question her hearing loss sooner.

When Lindsey was about six months old, my husband, Greg, began questioning her ability to hear—almost daily. I would call our physician to have her checked, and he would make some noises, and she would always turn to look—mainly to see what he was up to, but he'd send me home feeling relieved that Lindsey could hear and foolish for taking up his time.

We repeated that scene several times until I felt we needed to see another doctor—one who specialized in ears. Not knowing who or what kind of doctor we needed, I talked with our family physician about our concerns and the need to be reassured that he was right and we were wrong. He agreed that he wanted to know for sure himself. He suggested a clinic in our town where there are three ear, nose and throat (ENT) specialists. We chose one based on the recommendation of a good friend who worked there.

During our initial visit with the ENT specialist, he found nothing missing and determined, following the visual check, that the mechanics of Lindsey's ears were working fine. I felt relieved and sure that we would be going home once again feeling we had made a mistake. However, before we left, the doctor suggested we should see his audiologist.

Because of Lindsey's age, about eight months, the test was not completely conclusive; however, the audiologist did feel her loss was severe. During that first session with the audiologist we tried desperately to understand the audiogram, but we returned home and realized we didn't know what that piece of paper meant at all. Even though we listened and nodded, we didn't understand anything except how severe he thought her loss was and that the evaluation was not necessarily conclusive. (We took that statement as a chance that he was wrong.) A few days later when I had time to sort out my thoughts, we wrote down questions we had, called the audiologist and tried to gain some knowledge about this new subject.

If I could change any part of the initial process of discovery, I'd take away the feeling foolish for needing additional information and for not under- standing when people would re-explain things to me. All this new information is not easy to understand and took time to learn.

Our audiologist referred us to a county agency called Early Intervention where speech-language pathology services are offered free of charge. We began working almost immediately with a speech clinician, Judith Gaines, after Lindsey was fitted for her first hearing aids, which, by the way, were taped to her bald little head because her ears were so soft and flexible.

Judith Gaines' initial visits were often made to try and help us determine if the hearing aids were set for the correct amplification. We were not able to ask Lindsey if they were helping or if they were too loud; how could she know! Later, the clinician came once a week and brought new noise-making toys and mirrors for us to use and play with. Several times every day we would do our "exercises" and I was told to talk, talk, talk to her. All of our activities were learning experiences, but we did spend as many hours a day as she would allow going from one game to another. Even listening to the toilet flush or for the telephone to ring was a big event at our house!

We also heard of a clinic for preschool children in California called the John Tracy Clinic. (John Tracy Clinic Correspondence Course for Parents of Preschool Deaf Children: 806 West Adams Blvd, Los Angeles, CA 90007.)

I wrote for information and they returned a correspondence course for parents. There were 12 lessons and we could move at our own pace. The lessons covered communication and its importance for growth and development in all aspects of a child's life. It helped us generate new ideas for teaching Lindsey speechreading skills, auditory training and for developing her sense of touch. With each lesson was a personal letter about Lindsey's progress and suggestions in response to my concerns from the previous lesson. I always felt a new burst of energy and excitement to continue working with Lindsey when I got a new lesson or when the speech clinician came. I don't remember any conflicts of interest between the correspondence course and the speech-language pathologist and I felt "the more help the better". I chose what I thought would work best with Lindsey and she knew exactly what she did and didn't like.

I gathered from the books I was reading on education, that our future decisions about her education were going to be difficult. By two and one-half years of age, Lindsey could communicate in two-word sentences and had begun to reject our therapy lessons at home. It was time for a school program.

Our city had no provisions for hearing impaired students and I had been battling with myself whether to sign or not to sign. The closest program for hearing impaired children was 25 miles away and since I had spent one and one-half years repeating ba ba ba ba, va va va va, etc., it was hard for me to jump at the only program available—a total communication program.

Many sleepless nights were spent wondering what choice we should make and hoping it would be right for our daughter. I observed many classrooms but wasn't sure what I was looking for despite all the books I had read. The school system assured me that they would test Lindsey and evaluate her before our M-Team (Multidisciplinary-Team) meeting so she would get the right placement in school. Our M-Team was made up of a panel which included people who had seen, tested and tried to evaluate Lindsey. We were accompanied by our speech-language pathologist (who had recommended Lindsey be placed in school) along with the director of special education, his assistant, the school psychologist, a teacher of hearing impaired children and the early childhood teacher.

I remember sitting around the table. It was a frightening feeling. I knew it would be hard not to cry while listening to the "experts" spill their feelings and reports on the table. I felt bombarded and alone since they all felt she was not going to "make it" in a regular classroom because her hearing loss was too severe (105 dB). I had thought before the meeting that my husband, our speech clinician, who knew Lindsey quite well, and I all felt she should try a speech and language early childhood class. The other members of the team disagreed, and soon Greg was on their side too. It was very difficult to listen to all the negatives about my child.

But, we "followed our instincts" and had Lindsey attend school in our town. She is now seven years old and is attending first grade in her neighborhood school. She has proven them all wrong and made us very proud of her accomplishments. We have tried to teach her sign language and realize she needs to learn more. She wears an FM unit at school and receives services from a teacher of hearing impaired children. She must also have teachers who understand and are willing to learn about her impairment and realize that she needs to "see" to hear. With help and support she compensates beautifully for her hearing loss.

She amazes the audiologists each time we have a check-up. Her speech and intonation are not perfect but she is very intelligible. She receives speech therapy daily and I can see progress.

Little did I know when I found out we had a daughter who could not hear the birds sing, chipmunks squeak or Rice Krispies pop, we would have one who could tell me the time of year or weather by the smell in the air. She is a real delight for both of us.

If you suspect a hearing loss in your child, here are a few suggestions:

1. See your doctor, talk to him or her and really explain what kinds of things are making you question your child's hearing.

2. Ask for a few referrals to an ear specialist to set your mind at ease, even if your doctor feels you are probably mistaken.

3. Find an audiologist who is experienced in testing children. This is important since many professionals delay because "the child is just too young". Children are never too young.

4. Ask where you can learn about community services, either through school or intervention programs. Red Cross referral agencies are good.

5. Talk to a few hearing aid dealers; find out about the brands they carry, cost, maintenance and their reputation in the community.

6. If you need help understanding the terms, ask and then ask again! Books are often available through local libraries, audiologists or hearing aid dealers. If not, The Alexander Graham Bell Association for the Deaf, Inc., and Gallaudet University Press sell books that are great. Self Help for Hard of Hearing People, Inc. (SHHH) can provide helpful information as well.

7. Become involved! You'll learn and your child will benefit. I have learned more about hearing loss since I've gotten introduced to other parents, to SHHH and through attending every seminar I can that concerns hearing loss. You can never know everything and what you do know is always changing.

Charlene Becker is a member of the SHHH Parent Involvement Committee.

• • • • •

Where Do We Find The Time?

By Charlene Becker

Appleton, Wisconsin
SHHH Journal November/December 1987

As children became older, parents begin to feel their child's independence taking hold. The breaking away and desire children have to be with their own friends or be involved in their own activities outside of the home is apparent.

The parent also gains some independence, but the newly acquired "time" is absorbed by car pools, basketball games, swimming lessons, etc. As our daughter has gotten older the actual caregiving time has lessened, but our lives seem busier each year. It gets harder to find the time to spend with each of our children on an individual basis.

My oldest daughter is hearing impaired. It is necessary to find time for her auditory and speech training. Without any other children then, there was more time for her, and we would spend as much time as she would allow working on auditory training. Since I could dictate much of that time and how it was spent, the change with her independence to choose her own activities is sometimes difficult to adjust to.

She always had input as to what she wants to wear, what books she wants to read, and what we'll work on or play, but these days her choices are not as eager for auditory and speech training activities.

I hear other parents asking each other and of myself, "How do you find time to keep up with all the individual time your child requires?" We by no means have the ideal solution when it comes to this, but I've learned to accept daily activities as learning opportunities. I feel that with a little boost in energy (a new article or idea), and a reminder that each time you speak to your child, it represents and opportunity to teach something new so we can see how much help we are really giving. A lesson in auditory training or speech doesn't have to be structured all the time. It can be a ten minute game of checkers, a card game, a look through a microscope, cleaning out a pet's cage, or picture bingo. A bedtime story on a new subject is a great time for language development. Introduce a new subject, animal or place, explain or show the meaning to one or two new words that to the child have no meaning as yet, and give a few examples of ways to use the new words. During dinner ask your child what was the favorite part of his or her day. Ask questions about it so you encourage sentence structure. "Did you meet a new friend today?" or "Who did you eat lunch with?" and "What did you have to eat?"

These "lessons" are the fun experiences to learn for them, and yet there's still the ever-dreaded "homework" that they get in the upper grades. Try to establish good study habits, but don't do so right after they come home from school. They need time to relax and do some of the things *they* want to do. If possible, during supper preparation or right after dinner is a good time to sit down and practice those math skills or sentence writing and story telling skills. Remember that what seems so simple and logical to us is a "foreign language" to them and it is complicated by their inability to hear exactly what has been said.

I've been told that it takes hearing impaired children ten times as many repetitions to learn something new as it does for children with normal hearing. After the hard work is finished, remember to thank the child for cooperating. Your child needs to know that his or her efforts are appreciated.

Here are some things to remember:
1. Speech training through natural, enjoyable interaction will seem easiest when fitted into today's busy life-styles.
2. When your child tells you something, casually repeat the sentence back to him or her, using correct English or a lengthened version of the statements. Ask your child to repeat occasionally.
3. Integrating speech and listening, language cognitive skills (listing, grouping, labeling), social and academic skills in the course of your child's day will give the child the ability to perform real life skills on his or her own as growth and development progresses.
4. If you're a person who needs organized play, set up a schedule for you and your child, even if it is one activity each day or every other day. Think of ways to incorporate the integrated training into that activity. They can be washing dishes, reading nursery rhymes, or changing doll clothes.
5. If it becomes boring to you, chances are it will also be boring for your child.
6. It is important not to get too focused on one deficit. Look at your child as a whole person. Consider what he or she needs as a whole person, but include the special needs to accommodate hearing loss so that your child can participate.
7. Include your hearing impaired child in the details of the family's schedule and activities. This will show your child that he or she is definitely a part of all the activity. It will also help build vocabulary.
8. The role of the parent as primary caregiver is a big responsibility for giving a good foundation for listening and verbalizing in a young hearing impared child. Remember to take time for yourself. You will feel better and be a better parent despite the busy schedule with work, school, lessons and housework if you feel good about yourself.

Author's Note

Charlene Becker is a member of the Fox Valley (WI) Chapter and a member of the National Parent Involvement Committee.

· · · · ·

271

Lindsey Becker

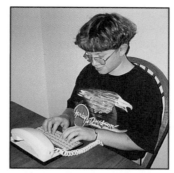

Lindsey Becker using the
TT, Telecommunication Text,
a portable telephone.

1993

Mrs. Becker writes about Lindsey and her school program today. "What you do know is always changing." And this is so as the Appleton parents have become actively involved.

Lindsey has grown up quite a bit since these first observations of her hearing impairment. Her maturity has taken her to a young lady who loves sports and hunting which confirms her attachment to her father and his love for the same.

She now attends Junior High and continues to be mainstreamed into regular education curriculum with support services to supplement her deficiencies due to her severe hearing loss.

She receives service from an educational interpreter daily in most of her classes. The interpreter reinforces her learning of sign language by individual lessons in sign language vocabulary two times a week besides what she picks up in context during classroom activity. In addition to that she meets with her speech and language specialist two times a week for 30 to 40 minutes per session and also meets with the teacher of the hearing impaired once per week to go over areas that need extra reinforcement from her regular class schedule. Lindsey also continues to use an auditory trainer in all of her classes.

Her first quarter of the new school year was very good for her and she was very excited to be on the honor roll. (Her parents were really happy about that too.)

The staff is learning to use sign language, and the English teacher is taking one day a week to have sign language be part of their English lesson. The students love the exposure and learning too.

This seems to be working quite well for the time being and most of Lindsey's educational needs are being met. The transition to Junior High went fairly well as there was much preparation for the staff before her arrival.

As her mother, I feel the social aspects will continue to be a struggle through High School even though she is active in sports in school and outside of school. There are some "normal" kinds of girl social situations that I am sure Lindsey is missing. How that will affect her remains to be seen.

She received a portable TT (Telecommunications Text) for Christmas and it is opening up her ability to communicate with family and friends. She uses the Telecommunications Relay System and can talk to her friends just as all teenagers do. This service is available 24 hours every day. Lindsey can now order a pizza or arrange to meet her friends and reach Mom and Dad at work if a need arises.

Yes, everything is changing and for the better!

John Tracy Clinic Works With Entire Family

By Kathy Walsh Nufer

Appleton Post-Crescent staff writer
Courtesy of the *Appleton Post-Crescent*

Parents of hearing impaired and deaf children are an isolated, and often desperate lot. Only about one tenth of one percent of the world population has a hearing impairment, and services in many countries are inadequate or difficult to find.

Thus, many families of young children who have been diagnosed with significant hearing losses look to the future feeling overwhelmed, confused, frustrated and rudderless.

Decisions on everything from hearing aids to schooling to the type of communication program, whether it be oral or sign language, or a combination of both, must be weighed carefully because all these factors will have a profound effect on the child's ability to take his or her place in a hearing society.

So it is no wonder that parents on the prowl for educational resources are thrilled when they discover John Tracy Clinic in Los Angeles.

John Tracy clinic was founded by Louise Treadwell Tracy, wife of actor Spencer Tracy. When the Tracys discovered that their son John was deaf at 10 months of age, they refused to be paralyzed by grief.

Rather than wait to do anything until John reached school age, as some advised, Mrs. Tracy halted her own acting career and turned her energies toward rounding up all the information and professional expertise she needed to help John.

Eventually, a parent study group she headed evolved into a clinic adjacent to the University of Southern California, which is designed specifically for families of young hearing impaired children.

Well aware that there is no time to waste in getting down to the formidable task of developing language and speech in children who cannot hear, Mrs. Tracy dreamed of offering parents not only the how-tos of building early communication skills, but the hope and encouragement they would need to persevere.

From the beginning, the clinic was self-supporting, taking no government funds. That policy continues today. Spencer Tracy provided the startup grant and several Hollywood celebrities, including Walt Disney, stepped forward to serve on the Board of Directors.

The Tracy's daughter Susie is a current member of the board. John Tracy, the clinic's namesake, seldom goes out in public today. He is in his late 60s and is losing his eyesight.

Since 1942, more than 70,000 families from 141 countries have enrolled in the JTC's correspondence and on-site programs during the school year and summer. The clinic's services are free.

Philip Strout, director of development, said the no-charge policy was established early on and has continued despite the high cost ($10,000 per family per year). "Parents are doing the work, so how can you charge them?" Strout said.

A key part of the clinic's outreach is its three-week summer sessions for families living outside the Los Angeles area. Each of the two sessions has up to 25 families from all over the world, selected on first-come, first-served basis.

Attending the July session this year were families from India, Mexico, Barbados, the Virgin Islands, the Philippines, Ireland, England, Greece and New Zealand as well as Colorado, Florida, Nevada, Texas, Michigan, Wisconsin and California.

The summer sessions are designed with the needs of three specific groups in mind—the parents, the hearing impaired preschoolers and their older siblings.

The hearing impaired children attend nursery school Monday through Friday and work individually with their speech tutors. Each undergoes audiological, language and developmental assessments.

Their older brothers and sisters, meanwhile, meet in another part of the clinic, combining fun and games with lessons on communication and serious talks about how it feels to have a sibling with special needs.

Parents immerse themselves in an intensive round of lectures on everything from language and speech development to behavior management, hearing aid maintenance and the special problems their children will face as they learn to read.

According to Maura Martindale, director of educational services, families coming to the clinic have a wide range of needs. Each family is at a different stage in its acceptance of the situation and knowledge of how to proceed, she said, "but all want some hope."

The program gives them hope, but also stresses the active role parents must play if their child is going to learn and use language. This is not a job they can simply turn over to the professionals.

Parents are encouraged to "talk, talk, talk" to their youngsters and practice every morning in the classroom under the watchful eye of teachers and speech tutors. As parent and child move around the room painting, playing with dough or sifting rice, mom or dad keeps an animated conversation going, even if it is one sided.

Eventually, parents are assured, with enough of the right stimulation, the child will give that language back.

Parents worry about oralism and whether their child will learn to talk, said Martindale. They are torn as to what communication program to pursue.

Although JTC is an oral program, staff members recognize that 70 percent of school programs use the "total communication" approach (signing, oral, speech reading, finger spelling) and take great pains not to be judgmental. Every child is different and parents have to decide what is best for their child, Martindale said.

Just as important as the lectures and the appointments with speech tutors and audiologists is the time parents spend with staff psychologists in support groups.

"Most people come here thinking they're going to learn how to teach their child, but we hope they get a broader perspective of their child as a child," said psychologist Pauline Corliss, who herself went through the JTC program as the mother of a hearing impaired daughter.

Corliss encourages parents not to see their hearing impaired child as "the family project" but as a full participating member of that family.

And she is relentless in pointing out that parents, in their eagerness to protect, often do not expect enough from the hearing impaired child.

The underpinning of the JTC program is the contacts parents of hearing impaired youngsters make with each other.

"When parents leave here they remember not so much the classes or the staff but each other and the help and support they received," Martindale said. "This is their time to grieve and cry and share their story with someone else who's been there."

As the July session drew to an emotional, tearful close, parents were full of praise for the John Tracy Clinic as they packed up to scatter across the globe.

Teresa and Harry Laird of Dublin, Ireland, enrolled in the correspondence program when their daughter Aoife, who has a profound hearing loss, was one-year old. They felt they had benefited greatly from the correspondence program and would learn even more by coming to the clinic.

"I thought I would learn better from live lecture situations than correspondence," said Harry Laird. Teresa Laird added that her experience at JTC was filled with such hope for what might be accomplished with Aoife that it confirmed her belief: "If you have a positive approach to life, you can achieve a lot."

The experience also renewed the couple's confidence in the quality of the services they receive for Aoife through the Irish government.

Unfortunately for many foreign families, the opposite is true. Jaime and Celia Lopez, whose four-year-old daughter Monica has a moderate to severe loss, moved from Mexico to Texas in order to give Monica a chance for better schooling and services. Carlos and Luz Alicia Madrazo did the same for their two-year-old daughter.

"We were desperate for a way to work with Monica," said Celia Lopez, who hopes to use what she has learned at John Tracy Clinic as the foundation of programming for the hearing impaired at home.

Four months ago Lee and Joy Farnum-Badley of Barbados saw the clinic advertised in a Peace Corp book on mainstreaming deaf children and wrote for literature.

With little or no services available in their country for their three-year-old son Wim—they waited four months to get a hearing aid repaired out of the country—the couple was desperate. "We tried to do everything ourselves but we were very frustrated because we didn't know if we were doing the right thing," said Joy Farnum-Badley, who hoped to pass on what she has learned to Wim's preschool teacher.

How To Contact The Clinic

Anyone with a pre-school child age six and under may take advantage of John Tracy Clinic services free of charge.

The correspondence courses—one geared to the parents of hearing impaired infants, another for ages three and older and a third for families of deaf-blind children—consist of 12 packets of lessons and activities and take about a year to complete. Parents report their progress to JTC staff members, who write back with ideas and suggestions to fit each child's needs.

Families who attend the summer sessions pay for their own travel expenses and meals. Housing in dorms on the University of Southern California campus is $14 per day per family.

For further information on the training programs, call JTC's toll free number 1-800-522-4582.

Training opportunities for professionals also are available at John Tracy Clinic.

· · · · ·

Unraveling The Mystery Of Lizzie

By Kathy Walsh Nufer
Appleton Post-Crescent staff writer

My husband and I were not sure what to expect when we signed up for a three-week summer session at John Tracy Clinic. We had heard of the clinic's fine international reputation and had enrolled in its correspondence course for hearing impaired preschoolers, but we did not know anyone who had actually gone to Los Angeles.

Any hesitation we had, however, was far outweighed by our need to find more clues that might help us solve the mystery of our daughter Elizabeth.

Lizzie, who turned five in Los Angeles, has a moderate sensory-neural hearing loss that frequently dips into the severe range because of chronic ear infections.

Her condition has been further complicated by a cholesteatoma that required a mastoidectomy last fall to clear out infection and debris that had destroyed two of three conductive hearing bones in her right ear.

She also has, among other things, low muscle tone and accompanying motor difficulties, which have slowed her production of speech greatly.

Needless to say, we could fill a dance hall with all the medical specialists, assorted speech, physical and occupational therapists, audiologists and special education teachers with whom we have come into contact during the last few years.

We did not get all the answers we craved at John Tracy Clinic, but we did come home with a truckload of useful information, and perhaps most important, the reassurance that we are headed in the right direction in trying to help our daughter become all she can be.

To us, that kind of reassurance was no small gift.

The opportunity for close association with other parents of hearing impaired children cannot be underestimated, either.

As cliche ridden as the words may sound, there is nothing more therapeutic than trading worries, doubts and fears with moms and dads who have bumped up against similar challenges and know precisely how it feels.

During three emotionally exhausting but highly motivating weeks in July, we and other parents had a chance to speak to each other from our hearts. We shared both the sadness of what we had lost when we learned that our children cannot hear like "normal" kids and the unexpected joys we had discovered in loving them anyway.

As one mom confided, as we sat on the lawn of our dorm one evening and watched youngsters with moderate, severe and profound hearing losses from all over the world play together with their hearing brothers and sisters, "Being here has helped me get over my grief. Now I see children, not just hearing impaired children, but children."

We talked and talked some more—during coffee breaks between lectures, while carting kids by caravan to the University of Southern California swimming pool, while hiking in cautious pairs to the market for such necessities as peanut butter, macaroni and Oreos, and while sitting in the dorm rec room waiting our turn to use the one and only available telephone.

Our togetherness in the classroom spilled over into birthday celebrations, and trips to Disneyland and to the beach.

As families drew closer it became easy to root for the success of one another's kids in their efforts to succeed in the classroom.

Everyone shared in the excitement of seeing Shanelle from the Virgin Islands try out, and love her new hearing aids, the delight of watching Catherine from New Zealand come out with a stream of intelligible phrases, and the pride of hearing Jennifer from Colorado complete one of the more difficult auditory listening tasks.

If Jennifer can do that, we all thought, maybe someday our kids can, too.

A huge bonus for us and other families was the sibling program that recognizes that older brothers and sisters have to make some major adjustments in their lives to accommodate a little one who requires extra time and attention.

As Margaret, our nine-year-old informed us, having a hearing impaired sister isn't much fun sometimes. At John Tracy Clinic she got to commiserate with brothers and sisters from all over the globe who get as exasperated as she does when their hearing impaired siblings monopolize Mom and Dad and "get away with stuff" they never could.

It's not exactly a vacation "camping out" in a drab dorm apartment with two children and no T.V. for three weeks, and breathing L.A. smog is a definite downer. But any hardships we put up with pale against the richness of the overall John Tracy experience.

From the professionals who were so tuned in to our need for both information and support, to the families who shared with us their deepest selves, we couldn't have dreamed up a better resource than this.

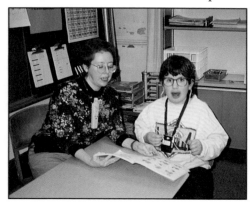

For us, July of 1989 will always be looked back upon as a turning point, and a memory our family can long cherish.

Lizzie Nufer with her teacher Susan Mitchler in school in Oshkosh Department for the Hearing Impaired. She is wearing the FM system, the teacher wears the microphone. (1994)

A Father's Experience

Bruce Nufer

At a Fox Valley Chapter-SHHH meeting Bruce Nufer filled in some added events.

We had an appointment to take Lizzie to the House Ear Institute. The doctor used a powder, an anti-bacterial powder that is puffed into Lizzie's ear. Her infections have been less and not as serious. What is probably a good development is that the doctor at the Children's Hospital in Milwaukee, and our doctors here have inquired about this medication and are prescribing it.

Lizzie has motor problems and did not walk until she was three years old. This probably accounts for her slow development of talking. She does seem to understand what is said to her. We have learned some sign language, but do not feel we need it all the time.

When we played with Lizzie at the clinic from 9:00 to 9:45 each morning, the teachers and therapists watched through one way windows. They wanted to see if we talked at eye level, talked naturally, expanded vocabulary, got eye contact and waited for the child to attend. After this session the parents went to lectures four hours a day. One very interesting session was having hearing impaired adults and teenagers speak to us of their experiences. Another lecture showed us the new technology and what the future promises.

Our goal as parents is to provide an enriched language environment.

We had sessions with the psychologist. Fathers met separately and for the first time we could express our fears and frustrations, and to actually cry. It is a strain on marriages to raise a handicapped youngster.

We learned to have high expectations and not be over protective. Also we learned that we are not to ignore our other children and to take time out for ourselves.

It was extremely reassuring to be with the 25 families that have the same problems.

Lizzie is going to Read School in Oshkosh and her teacher Donna Glasheen is excellent. Transportation was a problem in the beginning. It took an hour and a half to get to school and to get home after school. We parents went to the school board and the time was cut to half that time. Fortunately I work in Oshkosh so I drive Lizzie to school mornings which means we do not need to get up so early. And we enjoy this time together. Two mornings a week Lizzie has physical therapy in another school. One day the therapist asked why we were always late—guess I have to learn the routine of each school.

We are inquiring about a program in Louisville that may give us some help concerning Lizzie's motor problems as they infringe upon her speech ability. We are always searching for ways to improve Lizzie's education.

We are fortunate to live here where there is a school so near.

· · · · ·

A Least Restrictive Environment
Dream Come True

By Susan K. Perrault

Christmas 1993/January 1994
Diocese of Green Bay
The Bulletin for the Deaf Community, Family and Friends

Allow me to describe the placement offer every parent dreams of . . . a least restrictive environment (LRE) where my child will learn on grade level in a roomful of age-appropriate peers with a minimum of extra support services. An opportunity to earn a place on the honor roll without that damned asterisk which indicates "special educational programming". Free and easy communication will flow between my child, his teachers and his peers. Friendships and relationships will develop naturally (no one is receiving "extra credit" to become my child's pal). Extracurricular activities are wide open to my child! Imagine a chance to *earn* a position on the athletic team of his choice (no longer necessary to mandate this on the IEP). Theater Club? No problem. Debate team? Ditto! Student Council? Start your campaign! Homecoming Court, school dances, field trips, the prom, my child will have the same opportunity to participate in whatever he should so desire on a moment's notice. No advance requests necessary, no hurried meetings to adapt an IEP, no more frantic phone calls to PEP for advice and support! My child will have the opportunity to go out on a date—I can't wait to experience those "normal" headaches that *come with parenting teenagers!*

Nice dream you say. (Dream on! you smirk). But every word is true, every opportunity described is real and very soon all of it will be a reality for my child. Would you believe me if I told you I fought this placement offer, that I refused this very placement offer for years? This very "normal" educational experience is available for my son *only* at the state school for the deaf, a residential school where all the students are deaf or hard of hearing, located over 200 miles from our home. Certainly not our neighborhood school!

For too many years I put all my child's eggs in one basket, the least restrictive environment basket (read: neighborhood school). I chose to ignore the part of the law that requires "continuum of placement options". As far as I was concerned, there was no option, he was to go to school here. Period. End of discussion. He had to learn to live in our "hearing world"! Academic plans were modified and sometimes sacrificed. Friendships were limited and a social life really didn't exist.

Then I began to meet adults who were deaf. I began to listen to their conversations, their stories, their experiences about learning to live in our "hearing world". Slowly, oh-sooo veerry s-l-o-w-l-y, something began to nag me. A light bulb went on in my head and steadily burned brighter and brighter. As much as we love our son, as much as we are willing to advocate

280

for every right he is entitled to, my husband and I are still "hearing" people. We can never, ever possibly teach our son, who is deaf, how to live in a "hearing world". He can only learn that from the very people who have done just that since the beginning of time . . . other people who are deaf.

So, please, I am asking all of you who advocate LRE, integration *and* inclusion, to please tread lightly. What might be right for your child will not be right for mine. Don't overlook the guarantee of a "continuum of placement options". You may need that guarantee some day.

As for me, I gotta get to the store. I need a new outfit for the Homecoming Game. It's Parents Day and I wouldn't miss it for the world!

· · · · ·

Suggested Readings for Parents

Davis, J. ed. 1990. *Our Forgotten Children: Hard-of-Hearing Pupils in the Schools.* Washington, DC: Self Help For Hard of Hearing People, Inc., Revised.

Ferris, C. 1980. *A Hug Just Isn't Enough.* Washington, DC.: Gallaudet College Press.

Kisor, H. 1990. *What's That Pig Outdoors.* New York: Hill and Wang, a Division of Farrar, Straus & Giroux.

Ling, D. 1988. *Foundations of Spoken Language for Hearing-Impaired Children.* Washington, DC.: Alexander Graham Bell Association for the Deaf, Inc.

Moores, D.F. and K.P. Meadows-Orlans. 1990. *Educational and Developmental Aspects of Deafness.* Washington, DC: Gallaudet University Press.

Padden, C. and T. Humphries. 1988. *Deaf in America: Voices from a Culture.* Cambridge, MA: Harvard University Press.

Riekehof, L.L. (1978) *The Joy of Signing.* Springfield, MO: Gospel Publishing House.

Ross, M., Brackett, D., Maxon, A., (1991) *Assessment and Management of Mainstreaming Hearing Impaired Children — Principles and Practices.* Austin, TX Pro-ed.

Simmons, Daniel, *"In-Service Training — Luxury or Necessity?" SHHH Journal,* September/October 1992.

Simmons-Martin, A.A. and K.G. Rossi. 1990. *Parents and Teachers: Partners in Language Development.* Washington, DC: Alexander Graham Bell Association for the Deaf, Inc.

· · · · ·

This Year and Years Following

Attn: Physicians,
Health Care Agencies,
City and County Nurses:

All newborns should have audiometric screening.

Any infant may develop a hearing loss due to infections or injury.

Respect a mother's concerns about her baby's hearing.

Arrange audiometic testing immediately.

Recommend agencies which can give intervention and support.

Early intervention is essential for the most successful education and social development.

Act Immediately.

Sincerely,

Parents of Hearing Impaired Children
Birth to Three—Early Intervention
Educators of Hearing Impaired Children
Division of Vocational Rehabilitation

This page may be reproduced without permission of author.

Alexander Graham Bell Tour to Russia
September 1993

Comments from an article in *Newsounds* by Patrick Stone, President,
Alexander Graham Bell Association for the Deaf, November 1993

Some high lights from the two week tour to Moscow, St. Petersberg and Stavropol. A delegation of 54 educators, audiologists, psychologists, counselors, hearing instrument specialists, and adult hearing impaired members went on the tour sponsored by the Citizen Ambassador Program of People to People. The tour visited schools for the deaf. In every city we saw teachers and children who looked similar to the children and teachers at home. Oral methods were used. Emphasis on the arts. We were impressed with the music and dance activities.

It was frustrating to see the lack of amplification. Hearing aids are not manufactured in Russia. Amplification furnished by the schools was manufactured in Estonia. There are two school systems—one for hard of hearing children which are oral, and the schools for the deaf where fingerspelling is used to augment the oral education.

Kindergartens start at age 2 to 7. There was an abundance of toys and equipment to stimulate conversation. The older children attend schools age 8 to 18.

Mainstreaming is not practiced. The administrators feel they can educate children more effectively in separate schools.

The large cities have trained teachers, but generally only 17 percent are trained.

Four days before we left Russia, Boris Yeltsin dissolved the Parliament. However, there was much hope and dreams for the future not only for the hearing impaired students, but for their country.

Following articles of the tour will appear in *Volta Voices,* a magazine to replace both *Newsounds* and *Our Kids* magazines.

* * * * *

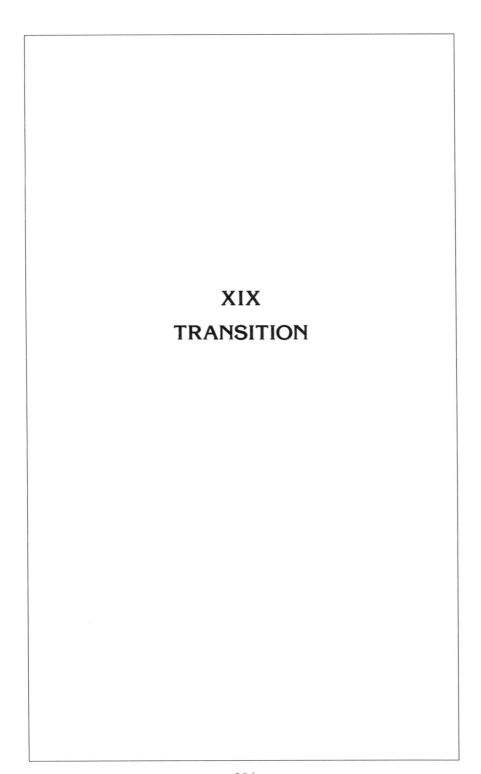

XIX

TRANSITION

Transition
1990's

The most successful hearing impaired students are those who have had early intervention, parents have been helped, and the children were able to progress in communication and social development.

The Birth to Three program is a national mandate that requires all counties to have such a program in place by 1992. This program is under the direction of the Department of Health and Social Services—not the schools who accept handicapped children at age three. The counties contract agencies to carry out this mandate. Trained teachers of the hearing impaired and speech therapists along with teachers of early childhood development work together. One member of this staff visits a home with a handicapped infant on a weekly basis to guide the parents. An Individualized Family Service Plan—IFSP—is developed with the parents. It draws on the family strengths and knowledge about their own child.

At age three the hearing impaired child may enter the public school system in a class for hearing impaired children or in a class of Early Childhood Development. This transition requires preparation that must be outlined in the IFSP. All the child's milestones are recorded and made available to the new setting. Usually transportation must be worked out. In-service training may be necessary if the class is one of Early Intervention that has not worked with a hearing impaired child. Usually speech therapy and possibly physical therapy are in place, but sign language needs may be new. Also special equipment such as an FM system must be obtained. It is also obvious that the services of an audiologist must be available on a regular schedule to check the equipment and periodically examine the youngster.

Transition within the school programs must be prepared for and stated in the IEP—the child's Individual Education Plan. The changes necessary for a child to move from the elementary to the junior high school must be anticipated. Read the ease with which Lindsey Becker moved into the junior high program. There were in-service sessions for the new teachers and her same speech and language therapists moved along as did the teacher of the hearing impaired. When this program started eight or so years ago, the school system did not have such an exemplary program. Here the parents played such a crucial role in the development of the services for their children.

The program at the Oshkosh Day classes grew and changed over the better than a hundred years of its existence. In 1959 when I was hired, the principal of the department had held a summer session for parents of young children. Several years later when I had a new class of young children I realized the need for better parent sessions than infrequent visits to the classroom and monthly parent meetings at school. It was then that I spent a summer visiting families of young children throughout the ten counties that sent children to our Oshkosh classes. Shortly after that the school instituted the program of having the mothers attend class with the children. As we had worked with the parents of the very young children and enrolled them in school much before the age of three—there was no transitional problem.

Today the same staff works in the home and then at school. There are some communities that must make the transition, but generally the children enter the Oshkosh system at a very young age.

. . . . .

IDEA —
Individuals with Disabilities Education Act

The 1990 Amendments of the Education for All Handicapped Children Act, retitled the Individuals with Disabilities Education Act (IDEA)[1], requires that all secondary students with disabilities have a transition service component included in their Individualized Education Program (IEP). This is to ensure that planning is provided to prepare students for adult life including such areas as: postsecondary education, vocational training, employment and/or adult services. This is to see that each student with a disability is linked to appropriate services in the adult system.

This means there must be a coordinated set of activities within an outcome-oriented process which promotes movement from school to post-school activities.

The IDEA requires that such services are stated in the IEP. This must be started no later than age 14. A statement of interagency responsibilities or linkages before the student leaves school.

In case agencies do not respond, the educational agency shall reconvene the IEP team to identify alternative strategies.

To assure that the student's needs are addressed:
1. Students must be included in the planning.
2. Students must be told of the options.
3. Students must have experience in work situations and community activities.

The students, parents, adult services agencies, and Committee on Special Education must jointly consider the total life needs of the student and identify transition services which both support the individual needs of the student in school and after the student leaves school.

1. Review of article in *NEWS 'N' NOTES*, Summer Issue of *The Convention of American Instructors of the Deaf*. Editor: Judy Egelston-Dodd, Vol. V, Number 4.

XX

TOMORROW

Tomorrow

The remarkable advances in technology and the new insights in education, not only for our hearing impaired children, but for all children, make the future look bright.

When I began teaching I wondered why the children's head sets had to be attached by short cords to a stand or their desks. Today new technology has solved the problem. No cords. Then I had to clip pictures from magazines and catalogues. I hoped for standardized picture cards, both large for charts and individual ones for the children to handle. Peabody Picture Kit started the process. Schools are inundated with catalogues offering not only pictures, but also readers, math, science series, and videos. The beginning text books incorporate the language development so we no longer need to rewrite the text books. Videos with captions are available for school. Parents, even those living far from the schools or who cannot avail themselves of signing classes, can borrow videos to learn sign language of the various topics covered in school. The ADA now requires all new televison sets of 13 inches and larger to have captioning capabilitiy.

Now computers are everyday teaching tools with programs and printers. To make copies of seatwork papers in the past there was a ditto machine. Today copy machines are in every school.

Medically we thought nothing could be done for the child with a profound hearing loss. Today cochlear implants are changing that prediction.

It seems strange that the advocates of Deaf Culture are taking such a pessimistic stand. They worked so hard and long to bring the Americans with Disabilities Act—ADA—into being. Alexander Graham Bell invented the telephone in 1876, and it took 117 years to make the telephone completely accessible for the deaf and hard of hearing population via the Telecommunications Text—TT. The ADA requires all states to have 24 hour, every day, relay service which gives the hearing impaired the ability to contact hearing people. It took an act of Congress so the hearing impaired can order a pizza!

And the legislation to secure volume controlled phones help the hard of hearing. Now interpreters for medical appointments, court sessions, agencies and businesses are becoming routinely expected. Hotels have equipment for the use and safety of hearing impaired people.

And employers must make "reasonable" accommodations for *qualified hearing impaired workers*. Here the operative word is *QUALIFIED. The responsibility falls on the shoulders of the educators, the students themselves, and their parents.* Also, no public place is required to make meetings accessible unless asked, so the deaf and hard of hearing people must request these services in advance to allow for compliance.

The ADA of 1990 is probably the most important social legislation of our time.

Deaf Empowerment, born of the Gallaudet demand for a Deaf President for the University, is to be applauded. It is time that the Deaf do move into more positions in business, industry, the professions, and social areas.

Education is the key. The deaf and the hard of hearing students, their parents, and the teachers are challenged to do a better job. The work places presently demand skilled workers. Most jobs today require technical training above the high school level.

It is unconscionable to delay the teaching of standard English to both deaf and hard of hearing young children. Young children under three years of age are at the ready. Hearing aids need to be introduced at the time of diagnosis. Hopefully this will occur within the first year. Parents and caregivers need guidance in following normal development of speech and language. Signed English can be an added pathway. Naturally Deaf parents will use sign language, but standard English should be taught in school from age three. English is the accepted language of the land. Command of English will open doors for our children.

The natural approach to encouraging speech has long been followed in many programs. It is the face-to-face, repetitive simple language all parents use to bring meaning and shape the speech. Isolated drill for the preschool child has very little carry-over. The speech has to be developed "in situ", as the situation unfolds. In those first formative years it is the family that is most important. They need guidance. Hopefully the Early Intervention personnel understand this approach to speech and language.

A Picture Can Elicit A Thousand Words

It is recommended that parents use two cameras. A regular camera to take the many activities throughout the day. And a Polaroid camera for quick reproduction of an activity. These pictures need to show the normal activities such as putting on the child's shoes, eating breakfast, or an ice cream cone. Dad reading the paper, washing the car, mowing the grass, shoveling the snow. Brother Dan putting on his jacket, looking in the refrigerator, eating a hamburger, drinking pop. Sis combing her hair, helping wash the dishes, telephoning her friends. Mom at the store, doing the washing, making the beds, sweeping the kitchen floor. The baby crying, being bathed, eating prunes—what a mess!

And talk about these activities over and over.

Be sure to have pictures of all relatives, friends and playmates and special get-to-gethers as holidays and birthdays. Take pictures of furniture, the child's bed, tricycle, brother's bike, a favorite stuffed toy. You get the idea.

In the beginning all children are interested in the immediate present. But language must be able to convey ideas and events that are either past or will happen or are in another location. With the pictures we can talk about what happened last week when Betty fell down or Jim got a hair cut.

When parents leave the house, the child should know where they are going—to work, to the store, to get gas in the car, to get the car fixed, to the hardware store or the drug store.

These many pictures need to be in albums and organized—places, people, activities around the house, and toys, and things to eat. Catch the child crying, busy playing, fighting, loving the pet, bathing, and sleeping.

I took many pictures in school and on our many trips in the community. When the former students visit, they want to look at those albums and talk about what we did. Your children will enjoy them through the years.

While movie cameras are good for special activities, the pictures are not available for daily review. Plus they are expensive.

It is hoped that the many stories recorded in this book show that there are many paths to adulthood.

· · · · ·

XXI
DEDICATION OF ALL OUR CHILDREN

Educators and therapists stress the need to accept the hearing impaired child first as a child. Your child needs what every child needs—lots of love and guidance.

I close with the dedication by Dr. William and Lynn Carlson of their three daughters. Dr. Carlson is a family physician and his wife, Lynn Carlson was an elementary teacher.

Give Yourself To Life

By Dr. William & Lynn Carlson
The Dedication Of Our Three Daughters

Seek sunsets, fishing moons, northern lights and falling stars.

Enjoy the good health you were blessed with.

If a mountain meadow is named "Oh, Be Joyful", hike to it.

Visit libraries.

Think YES, yet say no when necessary.

Be playful . . . play throw the mat, pile driver and airplane.

Play SPOONS at the cottage, bake gingerbread houses, make home made valentines, read *A Very Special House* and *Cloudy With a Chance of Meatballs*.

Protect the things that you need and risk them as little as possible.

You are in charge of celebrations . . . Don't let them pass you by.

Learn from your mistakes.

When you appreciate someone, tell them.

It is good to go hungry once in awhile.

Make friends with uncertainty.

Enjoy the good planet that you were blessed with.

Have wild imaginings and feel electrified, as well as perfect calm and inner peace.

Be responsible for the ways that you make yourself feel.

Plant flowers in your yard, feed the birds, hug a tree and be at eye-level with ladybugs.

Take good care of the relationships that have meaning for you.

Be honest with yourself and with other people.

Acknowledge the potential for the Dr. Jekyll and Mr. Hyde within you and be responsible for it.

Over root beer floats, listen and learn from your Grandparents and Great-Grandparents and join hands around the Granny Laura tree (planted in her memory).

· · · · ·

The challenge is for each of us to write our own personal family dedication. To enjoy a full and healthy family life we need to be cognizant of the good and real experiences that make our lives whole.